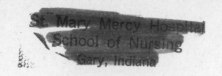

D1482876

PRINCIPLES AND
METHODS OF
STERILIZATION

Principles and

Second Printing

Methods of

Sterilization

By

JOHN J. PERKINS, M.S.

Director of Research
American Sterilizer Company
Erie, Pennsylvania

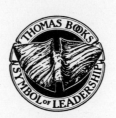

CHARLES C THOMAS · PUBLISHER

Springfield · *Illinois* · *U.S.A.*

CHARLES C THOMAS • PUBLISHER
BANNERSTONE HOUSE
301-327 East Lawrence Avenue, Springfield, Illinois, U.S.A.

Published simultaneously in the British Commonwealth of Nations by
BLACKWELL SCIENTIFIC PUBLICATIONS, LTD., OXFORD, ENGLAND

Published simultaneously in Canada by
THE RYERSON PRESS, TORONTO

Library of Congress Catalog Card Number: 56-6401

First Printing, 1956
Second Printing, 1960

Printed in the United States of America

EXCERPT:—

The mode of life of modern men is profoundly influenced by hygiene and medicine and the principles resulting from the discoveries of Pasteur. The promulgation of the Pasteurian doctrines has been an event of the highest importance to humanity. Their application rapidly led to the suppression of the great infectious diseases which periodically ravaged the civilized world, and of those endemic in each country.

—ALEXIS CARREL: *Man The Unknown*

Preface

THIS BOOK is an attempt to integrate basic principles upon which conventional sterilizing processes depend with practical methods for the preparation and sterilization of materials and supplies. It was written primarily to serve as a reference guide for sterilization practices in hospitals, clinics, laboratories, allied institutions and services. It is in this institutional environment that we find a host of professional and non-professional workers daily depending upon the science of sterilization and surgical asepsis as the chief means of protecting the patient against the ravages of infectious disease. The need for helpful information on the subject is acute, particularly among operating room supervisors and central service supervisors—the key persons largely responsible for sterilization techniques in hospitals.

The goal of the author has been to systematize the study, giving all of the important principles and methods of which he is aware, at the same time keeping the work within the limits of a textbook rather than an extensive reference volume. Many important references on the subjects of sterilization and disinfection have been freely consulted. Without the long list of reference material this book should not have been written. Any subject as extensive as that of sterilization which, conservatively, covers the past seventy-five years, is not the work of a few, but many people. Scientific minds pave the way and open the door to progress, but actual advancement does not take form until industry through the designing engineer is able to build the necessary equipment. Even then, the maximum benefits of progress in sterilization are not realized by the patient until hospital personnel are thoroughly trained to apply the principles and to intelligently operate the equipment.

The question may logically arise as to whether nurses or nursing students, as a group, are sufficiently prepared to profit by the study of scientific journals and technical publications. It is the author's opinion that if nurses are to be charged with the responsibility for sterilization in hospitals they must be encouraged to read and search for pertinent reference material. Certainly it is desirable to stimulate an open-minded questionable attitude on the part of all nurses for the subject of sterilization. The operating room supervisor and the central service supervisor particularly should realize that sterilization is an expanding subject with the constant addition of new knowledge, the discarding of old theories or their reinterpretation in the light of new experimental evidence.

For any errors, omissions or misstatements found in this book, the author must assume full responsibility. The long hours spent in the preparation of the manuscript have been a work of love rather than labor. It is hoped that it will be found useful in some measurable degree by those for whom it is intended.

JOHN J. PERKINS

Written at Lake Placid, N.Y.

Acknowledgments

THE AUTHOR wishes to acknowledge his indebtedness to the American Sterilizer Company, for the generous grant of time expended in preparing the manuscript, and for permission to use the large number of photographs and diagrams from which many of the illustrations have been made. An expression of gratitude is also due the American Sterilizer Company for permission to use certain copyrighted material from the Textbook on Sterilization by the late W. B. Underwood.

Sincere thanks and appreciation are extended to the friends and colleagues of the author who have rendered valuable assistance, in particular: to Miss Edna Prickett, of the National League of Nursing, for review and criticism of the sections dealing with surgical sterilization; to Miss Marian Fox, of the American Hospital Association, and Miss Margaret Giffin, of the National League of Nursing, for the opportunity to observe the everyday problems of the operating room supervisor and the central service supervisor through the medium of Institutes; to the Research Staff of the American Sterilizer Company for skillful assistance in the accumulation of material and the reading of proof.

Grateful acknowledgment is also made to the many authors whose works have been quoted in this book. Finally, thanks are extended to the various publishers who have generously granted permission for the reproduction of illustrations and quotations from their publications. In these cases, specific acknowledgment has been made in the appropriate places throughout the text.

J. J. P.

Contents

PRINCIPLES AND
METHODS OF
STERILIZATION

CHAPTER I

Historical Introduction

IT HAS OFTEN been said that "nothing is more difficult than the beginning." This remark seems particularly appropriate as the opening phrase to the Historical Introduction on the subject of sterilization. To be sure, one cannot claim that related material is lacking as a preparatory measure, because the literature contains a wealth of information dealing either directly or indirectly with the subject. However, any attempt to trace the origin of various practices which form the basis of our modern concept of sterilization leads eventually to the conclusion that gradual development of the art has been so closely allied with the development of bacteriology that it is difficult to discuss the former without bringing into the picture more than the desirable amount of the latter. Just as the science of bacteriology is said to have originated from the various attempts to solve the origin of life and the origin of death, so has the advancement of our knowledge of sterilization kept pace with each important contribution to these age-old problems of nature. To the historian, it is also evident that the many investigations and researches which have led us to our present state of knowledge on this subject, as well as that of bacteriology, were actually stimulated by certain controversies and ideas originating hundreds of years before the beginning of the Christian era.

OUR ANCIENT HERITAGE

From the dawn of recorded history man appears to have practiced in one form or another the process of purification or disinfection, the latter a precursor of sterilization. The use of antiseptics, such as pitch or tar, resins and aromatics, was widely employed by the Egyptians in embalming bodies even before they had a written language. From the work of Herodotus[1] (484-424 B.C.), there are indications that the Egyptians were acquainted with the antiseptic value of dryness resulting from the use of certain chemicals such as niter and common salt. The fumes of burning chemicals were also used by the ancients for deodorizing and disinfecting purposes. Of early importance was sulfur, apparently the first of the useful chemicals to be mentioned. In the Odyssey[2] the following passage may be found:

> *To the nurse Eurycleia then said he:*
> *"Bring cleansing sulfur, aged dame, to me*
> *And fire, that I may purify the hall."*

The purification of premises and the destruction of noxious and infectious material by fire also seem to have originated among the Egyptians. The cremation of bodies of animals, and of persons, especially in the case of war, was often resorted to by the ancients as a means of their disposal, as well as to destroy putrefactive odors.

Moses was the first to prescribe a system of purification by fire, and we learn from the books of Leviticus and Deuteronomy that he also developed the first system for the purification of infected premises. The stern mandates given by Moses (about 1450 B.C.) on the disposal of wastes, camp sanitation, treatment and prevention of leprosy, the touching of unclean objects or eating of unclean foods, formed the basis of the first sanitary code as established by the ancient Hebrews. From the precepts as laid down in the Mosaic law are based the various systems of purification of the succeeding ages.

History has recorded that the thinkers of antiquity never seem to have doubted that under favorable conditions life, both animal and vegetable, might arise spontaneously. Certain of the early Greek philosophers held the theory that animals were formed from moisture. Empedocles (450 B.C.), an early advocate of fumigation as a means of combatting epidemics, attributed to spontaneous generation all of the living beings which he found inhabiting the earth. Aristotle (384 B.C.) also asserted that "sometimes animals are formed in putrefying soil, sometimes in plants, and sometimes in the fluids of other animals." He also formulated a principle that "every dry substance which becomes moist, and every moist body which becomes dried, produces living creatures, provided it is fit to nourish them." During this era it is worthy of note that Hippocrates (460-370 B.C.), the greatest of all physicians, and who was responsible for the dissociation of philosophy from medicine, recognized the importance of boiled water for irrigating wounds, the cleansing of the hands and nails of the operator, and the use of medicated dressings for wounds.

THE MIDDLE AGES

In the period from 900 to 1500 A.D. progress from the standpoint of noteworthy contributions having a direct bearing on the development of the art of sterilization was virtually at a standstill. For medicine this period is also regarded as an age of decadence and stagnation. Filth, pestilence and plague ravaged all Europe in the Middle Ages. Attempts were made to combat the pestilence in hospitals, lazarettos and infected houses by means of cleansing solutions, aeration, the smoke of burning straw, fumes of vinegar, and, not the least, by the fumes of sulfur, antimony and arsenic.

THE DISCOVERY OF BACTERIA

The existence of bacteria was considered possible by many people long before their discovery. However, actual proof of their existence had to await the development and construction of a compound microscope suitable for the observation and study of forms of microbial life. For this achievement, credit must be given to Anthony van Leeuwenhoek, a Dutch linen draper, for marked perfection of lenses of short focal distance with

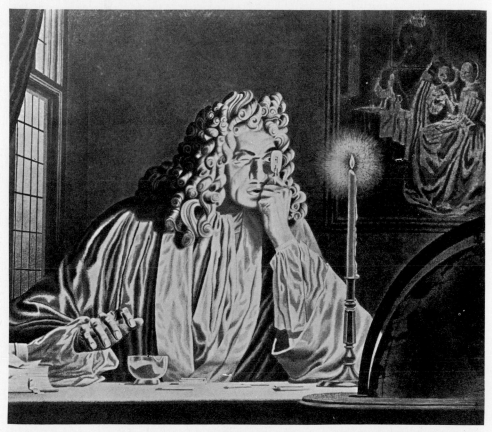

Courtesy Lambert Pharmacal Co.

Fig. 1. Antonj van Leeuwenhoek.

which he was able to see for the first time some of the larger forms of bacteria. In 1683, he observed and described a great variety of microbial forms in various body fluids, intestinal discharges from animals, water and beer with a high degree of accuracy and painstaking detail. He also made important contributions to microscopic anatomy and is regarded by certain authorities as the real discoverer of the blood corpuscles.[3] Leeuwenhoek's observations and development of the microscope provided the foundation of bacteriology and reopened the question concerning the causation of fermentation and disease.

THE DOCTRINE OF SPONTANEOUS GENERATION

Following the discovery of bacteria, the age-old question of spontaneous generation of living things again became a subject for discussion. Some few individuals did combat the theory, but the belief was general that bacteria did originate spontaneously and this belief persisted until Louis Pasteur finally settled the question with convincing experimental data in 1862. One of the early opponents of the theory was L. Spallanzani,[4, 5] who in 1765 demonstrated that boiling an infusion of decomposable matter for two minutes did not suffice to destroy all the microbes, but when the infusion was placed in a hermetically sealed flask and boiled for an hour no generation of microbes or fermentation occurred, so long as the flask remained sealed. Although Spallanzani proved to his own satisfaction that vegetative power does not exist in inanimate material, it was still maintained by some, notably John Needham (1713-1781) and George Buffon (1707-1788), that the boiling process had weakened or destroyed the "vegetative force," thereby preventing spontaneous generation from taking place.

The attack on spontaneous generation was continued by Franz Schulze,[6] in 1836, who failed to find evidence of living organisms in boiled infusions to which air had been admitted only after passage through sulfuric acid. Similar experiments were conducted by Theodor Schwann,[7] in 1837, except that the air admitted to the infusions was first heated to a high temperature, but the results were the same—no evidence of fermentation or bacterial growth. In connection with the work of Schwann, it is interesting to note that he considered the process of fermentation could be arrested or inhibited by an agent capable of destroying fungi, such as heat, potassium arsenate, etc. Because of this belief, Schwann is regarded by certain authorities as the founder of the science of disinfection.[8]

In 1854, H. Schroeder and T. von Dusch[9] made additional contributions in favor of the opposing forces to the theory of spontaneous generation. These workers employed a new technique of admitting air into flasks of boiled infusions by filtering the air through a layer or plug of cotton wool. This was done to combat the argument against any possible change in the properties of the air which could have occurred in the experiments of Schulze and Schwann, and which might give rise to a condition unfavorable to the support of life. Although the results showed that sterile solutions were obtained by this method, it was later demonstrated that the same procedure was unsuccessful in preventing fermentation of milk, meat or egg yolk unless these materials were subjected to prolonged boiling at 100°C., heated in an oil bath to 130°C. or heated in Papin's "digester" under a pressure of 15 to 75 pounds (see Fig. 2).

By the year 1859 the problem of spontaneous generation was still in a state of uncertainty. The primary issue at stake was decisive proof of the presence of microbes in the atmosphere. The controversy was further aggravated by the appearance of a publication entitled *Heterogenie*, by F. A. Pouchet.[10] Apparently the author had repeated the experiments of Schulze and Schwann and his results were diametrically opposed to the

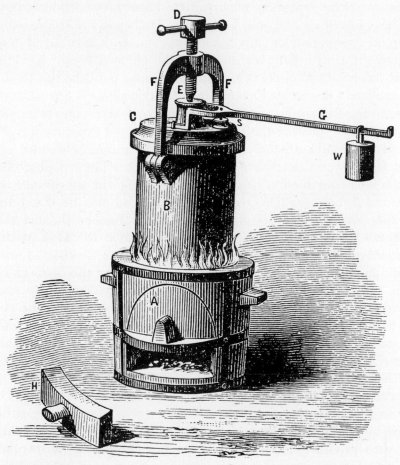

Fig. 2. Papin's "Digester." Invented by Denys Papin in 1680—a collaborator of Robert Boyle in the study of pneumatics. The "digester" consisted of a vessel, B, capable of being tightly closed by a screw, D, and a lid, C, in which food could be cooked in water raised by a furnace, A, to the temperature of any desired safe pressure of steam. The pressure was determined and limited by a weight, W, on the safety valve lever, G. Papin is given credit of having first made use of the safety valve to control the pressure of steam.

findings of the earlier investigators. Pouchet also ridiculed the assumption of organisms being present in the atmosphere—a view in direct conflict with the current reasoning of Pasteur that micro-organisms responsible for fermentation came from outside the fermenting material.

LOUIS PASTEUR

For an account of Pasteur's contributions to the development of the art of sterilization, it is necessary to begin with the year of 1860. Here we find Pasteur, having previously completed his brilliant researches on the microbic cause of fermentation, now ready to begin his epoch-making studies on the problem of spontaneous generation. He began his attack with a microscopic investigation of atmospheric air and with the aid of the most ingenious devices he demonstrated that the air in different localities differed in its content of micro-organisms. His paper published in 1862,[11] "On the Organized Corpuscles Existing in the Atmosphere," was destined, according to some scientific minds of that day, to remain forever as a classic. With a severity typical of the thoroughly-disciplined experimenter, Pasteur repeated and confirmed the experiments of Schwann, Schroeder and von Dusch. He showed that after passing air through a filter or plug of cotton wool the filter contained organized particles similar in appearance to mold spores, and if these particles were then introduced into sterilized nutritive fluids they would induce fermentation. Finally Pasteur showed that fermentation in boiled infusions could be prevented if the neck of the flask was drawn out and bent in a simulated U-tube form, so that micro-organisms and dust particles present in the air could enter the open end of the U-tube, but then due to the absence of air currents the micro-organisms were unable to ascend the other arm of the tube to reach the contents of the flask. With this type of flask, he also showed that fermentation could be immediately induced by tilting the apparatus so as to permit the infusion to contact the organisms deposited in the bent arm of the U-tube. In brief, this experiment constituted the greatest blow yet delivered against the doctrine of spontaneous generation.

The importance attached to this phase of Pasteur's work can best be summarized by saying that, where previous investigators had concerned themselves with experiments to demonstrate the absence of fermentation in sterilized infusions in contact with germ-free air, he not only did this, but also proved that the micro-organisms present in the air were unquestionably responsible for the changes which occurred in his sterilized infusions. In the words of W. W. Ford:[12]

> The great practical result of this phase of Pasteur's work is not so much that he finally settled the controversy regarding spontaneous generation, but that his observations on the pollution of the atmosphere by bacteria paved the way for Lister's antiseptic surgery which has revolutionized surgical practice throughout the world.

One of the last defenders of spontaneous generation was the English physician Bastian. In 1876, he attacked the previous work of Pasteur in which it had been stated that urine, sterilized by boiling, did not undergo fermentation or show evidence of bacterial growth upon incubation. Bastian claimed that such sterility was attainable only under certain conditions, and if the urine were made alkaline in the beginning bacterial growth would frequently take place. This led Pasteur to reconsider certain phases of his past work, and together with his collaborators, Joubert and Chamberland, he repeated and confirmed Bastian's experiments. As the result, it was demonstrated that liquids with an acid reaction could be rendered *apparently sterile* by boiling, because certain organisms not destroyed by the process were unable later to develop in the notably acid media, but if the liquids were made slightly alkaline beforehand the surviving bacteria would grow and multiply freely.

This controversy with Bastian finally led to the establishment of the fact that certain microbes exist in nature which are capable of resisting prolonged boiling at 100°C.; for example, the spores of *B. subtilis* discovered by Cohn in 1876.[13] Where formerly Pasteur had been content to boil his liquids, he was now forced to heat them to a temperature of from 108° to 120°C. in order to insure sterility.

> The custom of raising liquids to a temperature of 120°C. in order to sterilize them dates from that conflict with Bastian.[14]

In addition, other articles common to sterile technique, such as glassware, vessels, tubes, etc., were required to be put through a flame at a temperature of from 150° to 200°C. Vallery-Radot[15] has given Pasteur's definition of what he meant by putting glass receptacles, tubes, cotton, etc., through a flame:

> In order to get rid of the microscopic germs which the dusts of air and of the water used for the washing of vessels deposit on every object, the best means is to place the vessels (their openings closed with pads of cotton wool) during half an hour in a gas stove, heating the air in which the articles stand to a temperature of about 150° to 200°C. The vessels, tubes, etc., are then ready for use. The cotton wool is enclosed in tubes or in blotting paper.

To meet the requirement of more effective methods of sterilization at temperatures higher than boiling demanded of Pasteur the invention of new apparatus. During this period (1876-1880) of marked advances in bacteriological technique, Pasteur's pupil and collaborator, Charles Chamberland,[16] developed the first pressure steam sterilizer or autoclave with which it was possible to attain temperatures of 120°C. and higher (Fig. 3). This sterilizer was patterned after the steam "digester," invented by the French physicist, Denys Papin, in 1680 (Fig. 2). It resembled the modern pressure cooker, with the cover held in place by means of toggle bolts. It was equipped with a safety valve and a small petcock in the cover which could be opened for expulsion of air as pressure developed from heating. It contained a small quantity of water and the materials to be sterilized were suspended above on a rack. Although this sterilizer which became known as "Chamberland's Autoclave," an indispensable apparatus for hospitals and laboratories, was criticized later by the German school and other investigators because the higher and more uncertain temperatures developed were harmful to heat-sensitive forms of media, it did, nevertheless, usually sterilize in one performance, and it must be considered as the father of our modern precision sterilizers.

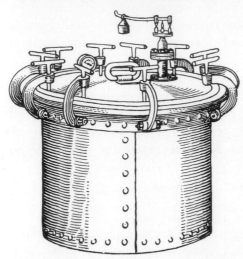

Fig. 3. "Chamberland's Autoclave." The first pressure steam sterilizer (autoclave) was built in 1880 by Charles Chamberland, a pupil and collaborator of Louis Pasteur. It was patterned after Papin's steam "digester" and resembled the modern pressure cooker.

Pasteur's researches were not restricted to fermentation nor to the settlement of the spontaneous generation theory. Of even greater importance were his accomplishments culminating in the establishment and laboratory verification of the true germ theory of disease. This, however, is a story so well known and so competently recorded in the literature that it would be an injustice to attempt to recount the events in the limited space available. Perhaps it will suffice to say that, in the author's opinion, the literature records no greater contribution to the development of applied sterilization than the statement made by Louis Pasteur in his celebrated lecture on the germ theory, delivered on April 30, 1878 before the Académie de Médecine:[17]

If I had the honour of being a surgeon, convinced as I am of the dangers caused by the germs of microbes scattered on the surface of every object, particularly in the hospitals, not only would I use absolutely clean instruments, but, after cleansing my hands with the greatest care and putting them quickly through a flame (an easy thing to do with a little practice), I would only make use of charpie, bandages, and sponges which had previously been raised to a heat of 130°C. to 150°C.; I would only employ water which had been heated to a temperature of 110°C. to 120°C. All that is easy in practice, and, in that way, I should still have to fear the germs suspended in the atmosphere surrounding the bed of the patient; but observation shows us every day that the number of those germs is almost insignificant compared to that of those which lie scattered on the surface of objects, or in the clearest ordinary water.

THE DISCOVERY OF THE HEAT RESISTANCE OF BACTERIA

Any history of sterilization would be considered incomplete unless something more than passing recognition were given to the discovery of the heat resistant phases of bacteria. For this enduring contribution we are indebted to the English physicist, John Tyndall. In 1876,[18] he made his entry into this field with a series of researches devoted to the phenomena of fermentation and putrefaction. Prior to this time, Tyndall had concerned himself with the problem of atmospheric germs and dust, and by means of a concentrated beam of light he developed a most searching test for suspended matter both in air and in water. He firmly believed that microorganisms present in the air were associated with dust particles. With the aid of an ingenious wooden chamber fitted with a glass front and side windows through which was passed a beam of light, he demonstrated that dust-free air which did not scatter the beam of light would not initiate growth in tubes of boiled infusions exposed to it.

Further studies made by Tyndall revealed that infusions prepared from old dried hay were far more difficult to sterilize by boiling than those prepared from fresh hay.[19] This observation led him to investigate extensively the heat resistance of bacteria. From numerous exacting experiments, he finally concluded that at certain times in the life history of organisms they developed heat resistant phases in which they were most difficult to kill even by prolonged boiling. This heat resistant (spore) stage of bacteria was also recognized by Pasteur and independently discovered by the German botanist, Ferdinand Cohn, in 1876.[13] Typical of Tyndall's conclusions on this subject is the following quotation taken from one of his detached essays:[20]

> As regards their power of resisting heat, the infusorial germs of our atmosphere might be classified under the following and intermediate heads:— Killed in five minutes; not killed in five minutes but killed in fifteen; not killed in fifteen minutes but killed in thirty; not killed in thirty minutes but killed in an hour; not killed in an hour but killed in two hours; not killed in two but killed in three hours; not killed in three but killed in four hours. I have had several cases of survival after four and five hours' boiling, some survival after six, and one after eight hours' boiling. Thus far has experiment actually reached; but there is no valid warrant for fixing upon even eight hours as the extreme limit of vital resistance. Probably more extended researches (though mine have been very extensive) would reveal germs more obstinate still. It is also certain that we might begin earlier and find germs which are destroyed by a temperature far below that of boiling water. In the presence of such facts, to speak of *a* death-point of bacteria and their germs would be unmeaning—but of this more anon.

It is also apparent from Tyndall's publications that he was quite aware of the role played by moisture in the growth and destruction of bacteria.

His early analysis of the importance of prompt interchange of moisture (wetting action) from the surrounding liquid to the bacterial cell for destruction is strikingly similar to present day theory advanced in explanation of bacterial destruction by means of moist heat. In one of his papers published in 1877[21] there appears the following remark:

> It is not difficult to see that the surface of a seed or germ may be so affected by desiccation and other causes as practically to prevent contact between it and the surrounding liquid. The body of a germ, moreover, may be so indurated by time and dryness as to resist powerfully the insinuation of water between its constituent molecules. It would be difficult to cause such a germ to imbibe the moisture necessary to produce the swelling and softening which precede its destruction in a liquid of high temperature.

Tyndall is probably best known and generally recognized as the originator of the method of *fractional sterilization* by discontinuous (intermittent) heating. This method was originally developed as a practical means of sterilizing infusions containing heat resistant forms of bacteria The process involved heating the infusions to the boiling-point on 5 consecutive occasions with appropriate intervals of holding at room temperature (10, 12 or 24 hours) in between each period of heating. The purpose of the intervals of holding between the heating periods was to allow sufficient time for the resistant bacterial spores to change or germinate into the more susceptible vegetative stage. Tyndall[22] has described the process as follows:

> An infusion infected with the most powerfully resistant germs, but otherwise protected against the floating matters of the air, is gradually raised to its boiling-point. Such germs as have reached the soft and plastic state immediately preceding their development into bacteria are thus destroyed. The infusion is then put aside in a warm room for ten or twelve hours. If for twenty-four, we might have the liquid charged with well-developed bacteria. To anticipate this, at the end of ten or twelve hours we raise the infusion a second time to the boiling temperature, which, as before, destroys all germs then approaching their point of final development. The infusion is again put aside for ten or twelve hours, and the process of heating is repeated. We thus kill the germs *in the order of their resistance*, and finally kill the last of them. No infusion can withstand this process if it be repeated a sufficient number of times.

Fractional sterilization, which later became known as Tyndallization, was actually the forerunner of developments leading up to the non-pressure steamer type sterilizer (Fig. 5) devised by Robert Koch and his associates in 1880-1881. The process of Tyndallization constituted an important advance in the development of practical sterilizing methods. Its usefulness and popularity can best be judged by the fact that to this day the procedure is followed in many laboratories for the sterilization of heat-sensitive media by steaming for thirty minutes on three consecutive days.

JOSEPH LISTER AND ANTISEPTIC SURGERY

Lord Joseph Lister has been recognized the world over as the "Father of Antiseptic Surgery." His work is too well known to justify any extensive presentation of his achievements here. Without doubt he was the first

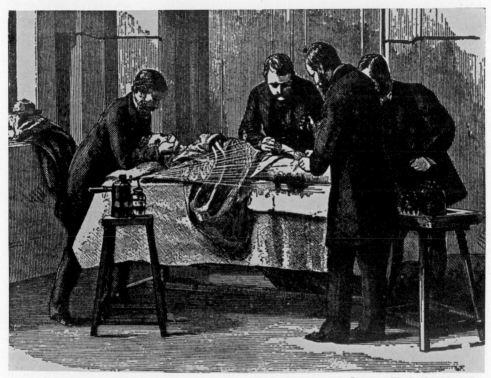

Courtesy W. B. Saunders Co.

Fig. 4. Lister operating with carbolic spray.

surgeon to employ a chemical disinfectant for the maintenance of an antiseptic atmosphere designed to prevent the entrance of bacteria into surgical wounds. Lister's antiseptic system was prescribed long before the germ theory had been accepted. In fact, it was toward the end of 1864 that he first became interested in Pasteur's work on the causes of fermentation and putrefaction. After carefully repeating and confirming many of Pasteur's experiments, Lister conceived the theory that air-borne bacteria are responsible for suppuration and putrefaction in operative wounds. This led him to the formulation of certain principles which ultimately comprised the basis of the antiseptic system:[23, 24]

1) Germs must be prevented from entering the wound during or after operation.

2) If germs are present in the wound they must be prevented from spreading after operation.

3) Germs on the outside or surrounding the wound should be destroyed.

4) All instruments, dressings and everything else in contact with the operation, including the hands of surgeon and assistants, should be rendered antiseptic.

In order to carry out the principles of the antiseptic system, Lister was obliged to develop suitable methods and materials. In his search of chemical compounds as a possible means of destroying bacteria, his attention was directed to a newspaper account describing the use of carbolic acid for the destruction of sewage in the town of Carlisle, near Glasgow. He immediately recognized this antiseptic as peculiarly adapted to his experiments. His first application of the antiseptic principles occurred in March 1865, Glasgow Royal Infirmary, in a case of compound fracture. The air about the wound was subjected to a fine spray of carbolic acid solution. Also, the hands, instruments and ligatures were washed and soaked in the same solution. Although this first test of the antiseptic system proved unsuccessful, Lister attributed it to improper management. Then followed a long series of experiments with repeated attempts at improvement of dressings and techniques that would permit more effective application of the antiseptic principles. Finally, in 1867 his first papers "On the Antiseptic Principle in the Practice of Surgery" appeared in the *Lancet*.[23, 25] Here it was recorded that with the application of the antiseptic treatment his mortality in cases of compound fracture was reduced from 45 per cent to 9 per cent—a remarkable stride toward the elimination of postoperative sepsis.

It is to Lister that full credit must be given for an organized system of antiseptic surgery—the basis upon which our modern aseptic surgery has been founded. He is responsible for introducing the sterilization of instruments, dressings, glassware and other supplies used in the operating room. Although equipment and methods employed in modern surgery differ greatly from those used by Lister, it should not be forgotten that the original Listerian principles remain as inviolable today as when they were first proclaimed. To emphasize the necessity of becoming bacteriology-minded, Lister offered the following advice:[26]

> In order, gentlemen, that you may get satisfactory results from this sort of treatment, you must be able to see with your mental eye the septic ferments as distinctly as we see flies or other insects with the corporeal eye. If you can really see them in this distinct way with your intellectual eye, you can be properly on your guard against them; if you do not see them you will be constantly liable to relax in your precautions.

It is of interest to note that Lister did not introduce the term antiseptic. Robinson[27] has stated that "perhaps the first who used it was the wholly unknown Place, who wrote in his *Hypothetical Notion of the Plague* (1712): 'As this phenomenon shows the motion of the pestilential poison to be putrefactive, it makes the use of (antiseptics) a reasonable way to oppose it, and whatever resists and is preservative against putrefaction, admits not of the generation of insects.' In the next generation, Sir John Pringle, father of military sanitation, published his important *Experiments upon Aseptic and Antiseptic Substances* (1750). By this time the word was evidently familiar to the public, for it occurs in the *Gentlemen's Magazine* (1751): 'Myrrh in a watery solution is twelve times more antiseptic than sea salt.' Yet over a hundred years later, Lister had to begin at the beginning."

It is a rather remarkable fact that Lister's extensively practical results were secured, in the destruction of bacteria in his surgical work, with no definite knowledge of pathogenic bacteria. To be sure, Pasteur and others had suggested the relationship between bacteria and infection but no one had proved that relationship. A great part of Lister's presentation occurred in the eighteen-sixties while it was not until 1876 that Robert Koch was able for the first time to cultivate artificially, outside the body, a pathogenic organism (anthrax) and to produce the disease in animals with his cultures. Shortly thereafter Pasteur was able to confirm all of Koch's observations and in 1878, in association with Joubert and Chamberland, he threw his great influence in favor of

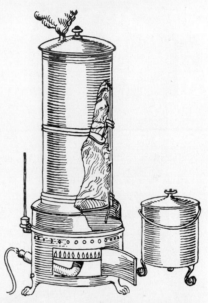

Fig. 5. This shows the non-pressure steamer type sterilizer devised by Robert Koch and his associates in 1880-1881. It was utilized broadly by the Germans for the intermittent or fractional sterilization of media.

the thesis that all infectious disease is caused by the growth of micro-organisms within the body.

CONTRIBUTIONS FROM THE GERMAN SCHOOL

The researches of Koch and his associates in 1881 on the disinfecting properties of steam and hot air mark the beginning of the science of disinfection and sterilization. In collaboration with Wolffhügel,[28] Koch demonstrated that there was a marked difference in the effect of dry heat on bacteria as contrasted with that of moist heat. These investigators determined that dry heat at a temperature of 100°C. would destroy vegetative bacteria in 1½ hours, but the more resistant spores (anthrax) required a temperature of 140°C. for 3 hours in order to insure their destruction. In

conjunction with Gaffky and Loeffler,[29] Koch also investigated the germicidal action of moist heat. This study showed that the spores of anthrax
were destroyed in boiling water at 100°C. in from one to twelve minutes.
It is certain that Koch was not impressed with dry heat as an efficient
method of sterilization because in one of his experiments he demonstrated

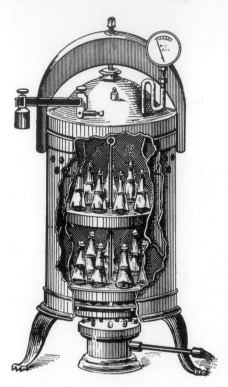

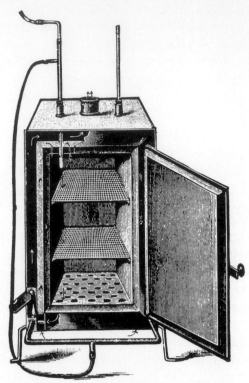

Fig. 6. An early modification of the Pasteur-Chamberland type of laboratory autoclave, probably of German make. It had
an improved type of cover lock and was
equipped with a pressure gauge but no
thermometer. There was no apparent
means for expelling air from the chamber.
Steam was generated from water contained in the bottom of the chamber and
heated by a gas flame.

Fig. 7. One of the early types of hot air
sterilizers used in bacteriological laboratories in the 1890's. It was patterned after
the design developed by the German
school, double walled, gas heated, in
which an attempt was made to circulate
the heated air by gravity convection. Relatively it served its purpose to much greater
advantage than the steam sterilizers of
that day because the actual temperature
of the heated air was measured by a thermometer.

clearly the greater powers of penetration of moist heat. This particular
experiment has been summarized by Zinsser[30] as follows:

> Small packages of garden soil were surrounded by varying thicknesses of
> linen with thermometers so placed that the temperature under a definite
> number of layers could be determined. Exposure to hot air and to steam
> were then made for comparison, and the results were as tabulated:

Temperature	Time of Application	Temperatures Reached Within Thicknesses of Linen			Results
		20 Thickness	*40 Thickness*	*100 Thickness*	
Hot Air 130°-140°C.	4 hours	86°C.	72°C.	Below 70°C.	Incomplete Sterilization
Steam 90°-105.3°C.	3 hours	101°C.	101°C.	101.5°C.	Complete Sterilization

The German school seems to have preferred the non-pressure steamer type sterilizer for the sterilization of media by the fractional or intermittent process. This may have been due, in part, to the difficulties experienced with the early models of autoclaves of the Chamberland type developed by Pasteur and his group. In any event, it is known that Koch and his associates devised the first non-pressure flowing steam sterilizer in 1881, and studied its bactericidal value (Fig. 5). In brief, it consisted of a metal cylinder in which water was heated through the bottom by a gas flame, the resulting steam enveloping shelves above the water on which materials were placed. It should not be construed, however, that interest on the part of the German

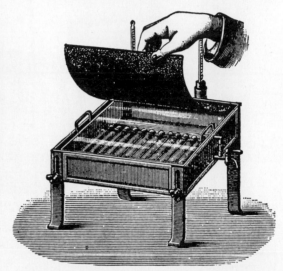

Fig. 8. Koch's Inspissator. A water bath type of apparatus developed for the coagulation and sterilization of blood serum media. The temperature was maintained at 60°C. (140°F.) or higher for one hour on each of five or six consecutive days.

school was confined solely to the development and usage of the non-pressure sterilizer. On the contrary, Koch and other workers showed that steam under pressure is a more efficient sterilizing agent than steam at atmospheric pressure. Also, one may gather from the literature of the first sterilizer manufacturers that the original autoclave of the Pasteur-Chamberland type underwent early modification at the hands of the Germans, and later became known as the Koch (Upright) Autoclave (Fig. 6).

Koch also developed methods and equipment for the disinfection of clothing. In this application he likewise found moist heat to be superior to dry heat because of its greater penetrating power. His studies revealed that upon exposing a roll of flannel contaminated with spores to dry heat at

140-150°C. for 4 hours, the temperature inside the roll was only 83°C., and the contained spores germinated freely. When the flannel was exposed to moist heat at 120°C. for 1½ hours, the temperature inside the roll was 117°C., and all the spores were destroyed. The apparatus shown in Figure 9 is typical of a flowing steam disinfector for clothing constructed according to Koch's specifications by the firm of W. Budenberg, Dortmund, for the King's Government at Arnsberg in 1888.

Although Ernst von Bergmann (1836-1907) is sometimes credited with

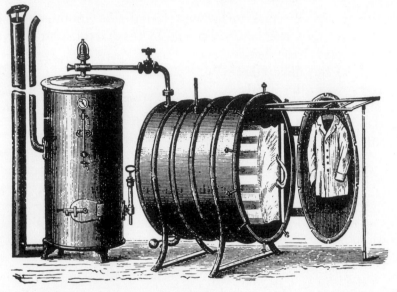

Fig. 9. The Budenberg Steam Disinfector. This apparatus was built in 1888 by W. Budenberg, Dortmund, Germany, according to the specifications of Koch and his associates. The assembly consisted of a small boiler for the generation of low pressure steam which was connected to an oval-shaped disinfecting chamber. It was used for the disinfection of clothing, mattresses, etc., by means of flowing steam.

having introduced steam sterilization into surgery, it has been pointed out by Walter,[31] in his discussion on the development of the concept of asepsis, that Schimmelbusch, one of von Bergmann's assistants, first used the steam sterilizer for the sterilization of surgical dressings in 1885. Apparently Schimmelbusch devoted much of his time and efforts to the establishment of a highly formalized pattern of operating room asepsis. He also recommended the addition of alkali, 1% sodium carbonate, to boiling water for the sterilization of instruments in order to prevent corrosion and to increase its bactericidal value. On this same subject, it is interesting to note that Hugo Davidsohn, another of Koch's assistants, first demonstrated in 1888[32] the practicality of boiling water as a means of sterilizing surgical instruments.

Following the discoveries and advances made by Robert Koch in the etiology of wound infections and in bacteriologic technic, other workers made significant contributions to the science of disinfection and sterilization. Von Esmarch,[33] for example, emphasized the great practical importance of using saturated steam containing the maximum amount of water vapor in all methods of steam sterilization. Max Rubner[34] also proved that the bactericidal effect of steam is diminished in proportion to the amount of air present in the sterilizer. From the literature it is evident that during the period of 1885 to 1900 the Germans made many notable contributions to the principles governing steam sterilization and chemical disinfection. Widespread application of these principles, including their adaptation to sterilizing equipment, did not, however, take place until some thirty years later with the introduction of the modern temperature-controlled sterilizer —a product of American manufacturers.

EARLY AMERICAN DEVELOPMENTS IN STERILIZATION

During the period of brilliant researches and discoveries in bacteriology in Europe, workers in this country were also engaged in furthering progress in the same field. By 1890, the new science of bacteriology had become well known in the United States. It is believed that Thomas J. Burrill (1839-1916) first introduced the study of bacteriology into this country at the University of Illinois sometime in the seventies.[35] Perhaps the earliest contributor to the subject of disinfection and sterilization was George M. Sternberg, who in 1878 conducted experiments on the evaluation of certain commercial disinfectants including chlorine. He also studied the thermal death point of pathogenic bacteria[36] and determined that non-spore bearing organisms were killed in ten minutes' exposure to a temperature of 62°-70°C. (143.6°-158°F.) and spore bearers were destroyed in five minutes' exposure to moist heat at 100°C. (212°F.).

Much of the bacteriological apparatus and sterilizing equipment used by the early American bacteriologists was brought to this country from Europe. Precise records of the early sterilizers produced in the United States seem not to exist, but certain it is that sometime prior to 1895 the industry of sterilizer manufacture had its origin. The best records available to the author have been taken from a publication entitled:

Pressure Sterilization
THE NECESSITY TO THE BEST RESULTS IN
ASEPTIC SURGERY

SPRAGUE-SCHUYLER COMPANY
Works: Rochester, N.Y., Main Office: 136 Liberty St., New York City
(Dated 1895)

Pertinent information may be gathered from the introduction to this brochure with respect to the first comprehensive installations of sterilizers in hospitals in this country:

The first complete plant for pressure sterilization of surgical appliances in the history of the art was installed in the Whitbeck Memorial Surgical Pavilion, connected with the Rochester City Hospital, Rochester, New York, in the year 1890, by A. V. M. Sprague, and is now in daily use, and appreciated as an invaluable auxiliary to their work. We illustrate the sterilizers for surgical dressings, for water, and the irrigation outfit employed. (See Figs. 10 and 11, *author.*) In the year 1892 we installed in the W. J. Syms Surgical Theatre, Roosevelt Hospital, New York City, an object lesson for

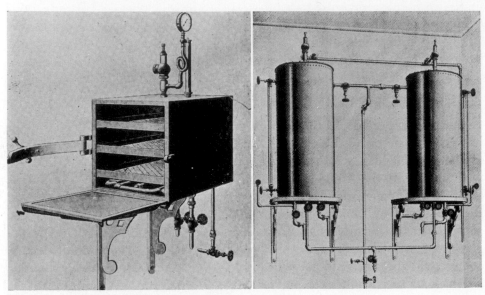

Fig. 10. This Rectangular Dressing Sterilizer was part of a group installed at City Hospital, Rochester, N. Y. in 1890. It was described by the producers, Sprague-Schuyler Co., as "The first complete plant for pressure sterilization of surgical appliances in the history of the art." The sterilizer was heated by direct steam from the institutions service lines. The chamber had dimensions of 15″ x 15″ x 20″ long and was made of cast bronze, highly polished. Fittings included a thermometer, pressure gauge and safety relief valve.

Fig. 11. Pair of steam heated pressure water sterilizers, 25 gallons capacity, part of the group mentioned in Figure 10, installed at City Hospital, Rochester, N. Y. in 1890. Water filters were not provided and there were no thermometers or pressure gauges. Evidently the control necessitated blowing of the safety valves to indicate adequate pressure. Certainly these were among the first pressure water sterilizers used in this country.

the world in the way of a perfect plant for sterilization under pressure. Embraced in this outfit are two tanks for the sterilization of water, each having a capacity of 100 gallons; six of our No. 3 horizontal dressing sterilizers; two special instrument sterilizers; beside the innumerable small items by aid of which the operations are carried on, and the articles processed safely and conveniently. (Refer to Figs. 12, 13 and 14.)

Historically, it is known that the major parts of the Sprague-Schuyler

Company sterilizers were built by the Shipman Engine Company of Rochester, hence the reference to "Works: Rochester, N. Y." This latter firm together with the Sprague sterilizer patents were taken over early in the 1900's by J. E. and G. F. Hall, the founders of the American Sterilizer Com-

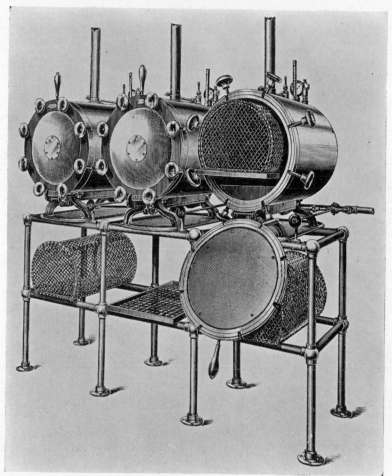

Fig. 12. Group of three dressing sterilizers installed in 1892 in the W. J. Syms Surgical Theatre, Roosevelt Hospital, New York City, produced by Sprague-Schuyler Co. They were heated by steam direct from the service lines and were equipped with pressure gauges and thermometers located in the extreme tops of the chambers.

pany, Erie, Pa. These men originally began their activities under the name of Hall Bros. in 1894. It is also known that the Sprague-Schuyler Company, together with another pioneer producer in this field, the Kny-Scheerer Company of New York (1888), were responsible for the introduction of the steam-tight radial locking arm door on pressure sterilizers—a door which could be opened or closed simply by the manipulation of a single hand-wheel. Figure 15 illustrates this feature.

Another early contributor to the sterilizer industry was the Wilmot Castle Company, who began operations in 1883[37] by producing the Arnold steam cooker which was later transformed into the Arnold (flowing steam) sterilizer (Fig. 16). This device and modifications thereof have continued throughout the years as a popular means of sterilization of heat-sensitive forms of media in laboratories. The Arnold sterilizer largely replaced the non-pressure steamer devised by Koch and his associates.

A significant advance in the development of sterilization in this country came about through the introduction of the Kinyoun-Francis steam and formaldehyde disinfecting chamber (Fig. 20). The fundamental principles and design of this equipment were conceived and developed by J. J. Kinyoun, Past Assistant Surgeon of the U. S. Public Health and Marine Hospital Service, working in conjunction with W. H. Francis, one of the founders of the Kensington Engine Works Co., Philadelphia. In 1888, on the recommendation of Kinyoun,[38] the Louisiana Quarantine Board constructed the first steam chamber in the United States for the application of steam under a pressure of 1 to 2 atmospheres, to be used for the disinfection of garments, mattresses, bedding, etc. Prior to this time the only bulk disinfecting apparatus available was of the Dumond or French model type, con-

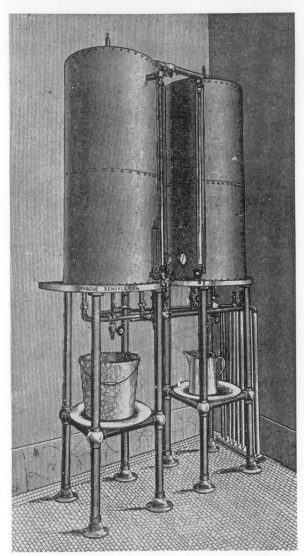

Fig. 13. These water sterilizers were also installed in the W. J. Syms Surgical Theatre, Roosevelt Hospital, New York City in 1892. Tanks were equipped with thermometers and pressure gauges but no water or air filters.

structed for operation at a maximum steam pressure of 7 pounds, equivalent to 111°C. The Dumond disinfector, as shown in Figure 19, consisted of a cylinder 4½ feet in diameter by 7 feet in length, equipped with a door

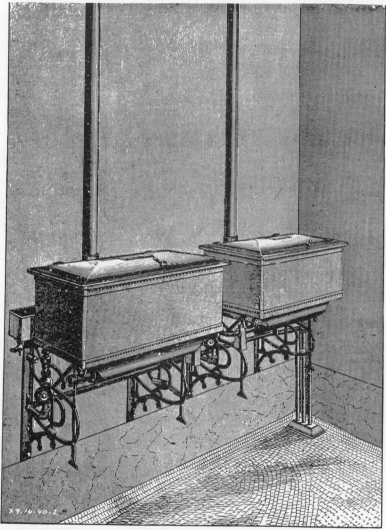

Fig. 14. Pair of instrument sterilizers (boilers) on wall brackets, heated by gas. Installed in Roosevelt Hospital, New York City in 1892 by Sprague-Schuyler Co. The covers were elevated by hand and the chambers were vented for disposal of excess steam.

at either end. It was also equipped with heating coils or radiators on top and bottom of chamber to maintain temperature of the desired degree without condensation of the steam in the chamber. Steam was admitted to the chamber by means of a perforated pipe extending the whole length of the cylinder.

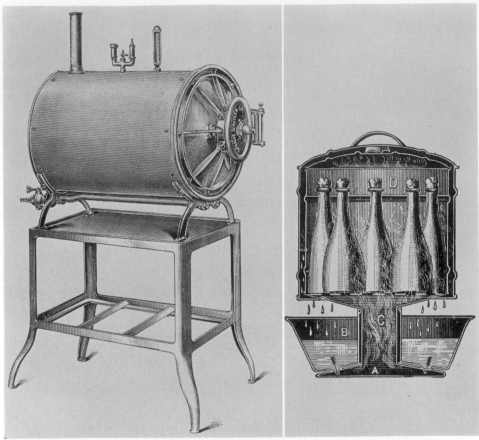

Fig. 15. An early type of horizontal pressure sterilizer, known as the Kny-Sprague Steam Sterilizer. This type was steam jacketed and the water from which the steam was generated was contained in the jacket to which heat was applied directly. There was no precise system of air elimination provided. A pressure gauge was furnished but no thermometer. The door was one of the first equipped with radial arms for locking.

Fig. 16. An early form of the Arnold flowing steam sterilizer, modified from the original steam cooker invented by W. E. Arnold in 1883. This constituted an improvement on Koch's non-pressure steamer. When water was placed in the reservoir B, it flowed into the shallow receptable A, formed by the double bottom. Upon applying a flame to the bottom, steam was generated in the area C, and then circulated through the main chamber D. Steam which escaped through the lid at the top of the chamber condensed under the outer hood and ran back into the reservoir.

Kinyoun devoted considerable time to remedying defects of the early steam disinfectors. The pattern which he eventually recommended consisted of an oblong cylinder, jacketed, with an outer and inner shell, instead of heating coils, and the entrance of steam at the top of the chamber rather than the bottom. By this system it was claimed that the currents of steam in the chamber could be easily controlled. A partial vacuum was also recommended for the rapid removal of air from the chamber prior to the introduction of steam.

In his experiments with formaldehyde as a disinfecting agent, Kinyoun[39] found that a greater penetration of formaldehyde could be obtained if the

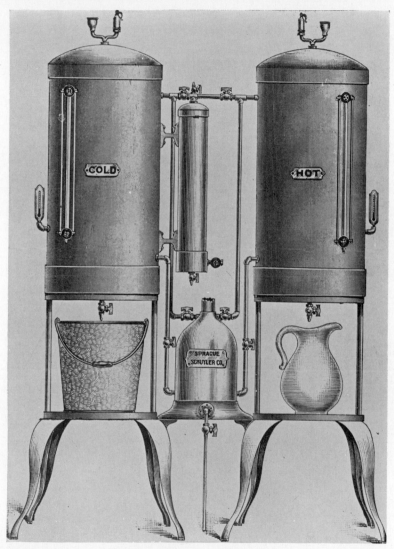

Fig. 17. Typical water sterilizers produced in 1895. Here for the first time we find evidence of an attempt to filter the air drawn in as water was drawn out. A small cup located on the top of each tank, fitted with a check valve, prevented the escape of steam under pressure and also opened to let air in as water was withdrawn. These cups were supposedly filled with fresh cotton daily for air filtration. Actually they were more hazardous than helpful. The tanks were equipped with thermometers, a water filter containing granulated quartz rock and animal charcoal as the filtering medium, and a combination gas heater. Sterilization was accomplished by maintaining the water at 240° F. (116° C.) for fifteen minutes.

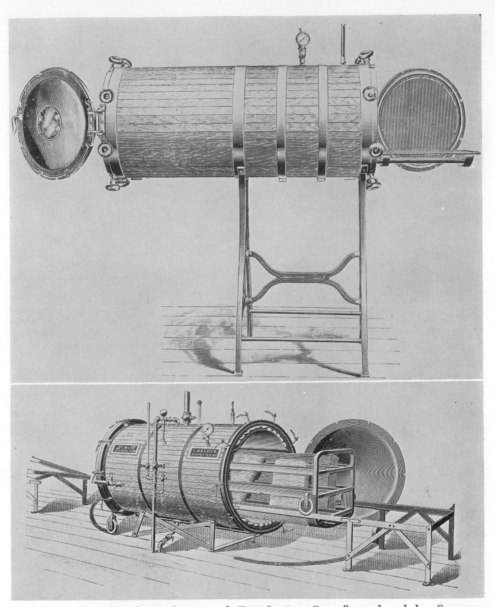

Fig. 18. A "Combined Sterilizing and Disinfecting Oven," produced by Sprague-Schuyler Co. in 1895. The apparatus was steam jacketed and the outer walls were insulated with hard wood strips. Doors were provided at each end of the oven, the design being to receive contaminated articles at one end and remove them, following disinfection, at the other end. It was arranged for building-in—a feature which apparently had its origin with the German school.

Fig. 19. The Dumond Disinfector—a development of the French school. This apparatus, widely used in Europe, was designed for the pressure steam disinfection of mattresses, pillows, fabrics, etc. It consisted of a cylinder 4½ feet in diameter by 7 feet long, with a door at either end. The radiators (heating coils) along the top and bottom of the chamber reduced condensation of the steam and permitted rapid drying of the goods following exposure to steam. The great advantage claimed for this apparatus was to the effect that one man could disinfect as many as one hundred mattresses in a day—a remarkable feat difficult to accomplish even with present day equipment.

process was conducted in a steam disinfector, provided with special apparatus, such as shown in Figure 20. The main feature of the process consisted of the partial displacement of the air in the chamber by means of a vacuum apparatus and then admitting formaldehyde gas into the chamber so as to replace the exhausted air. Steam was admitted to the jacket only of the disinfector in order to heat the articles and to maintain the chamber at a temperature of about 90°C. (194°F.).

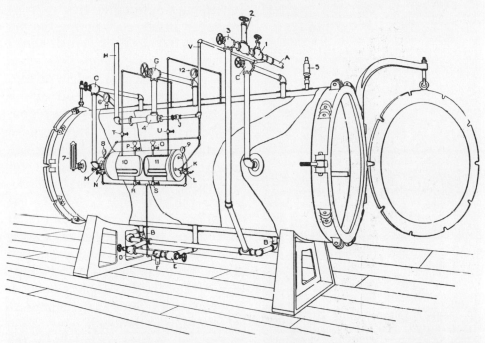

Fig. 20. The Kinyoun-Francis Steam and Formaldehyde Disinfecting Chamber. This apparatus constituted a marked improvement over earlier forms of pressure steam sterilizing equipment. It could be used for the application of steam under pressure at 1 to 2 atmospheres or for formaldehyde disinfection, combined with dry heat in a vacuum chamber. It was widely used for the disinfection of clothing, bedding, etc., in quarantine stations, municipal disinfecting plants and hospitals. The Kinyoun-Francis disinfectors ushered in the era of bulk (large cylindrical and rectangular) sterilizer design and application.

The efficiency of the formaldehyde disinfection process in a vacuum chamber was studied in detail by E. K. Sprague, Past Assistant Surgeon, U. S. Marine Hospital Service in 1899.[40] His report stated, in part:

The writer would be distinctly understood as not recommending formaldehyde, even when combined with a high degree of heat, as a disinfecting agent upon which reliance can always be placed for the treatment of articles requiring much penetration, especially when the exposure is limited to one-half hour. A critical examination of nearly all the published experiments with this agent will reveal instances in which organisms that there was every reason to expect would be killed have survived, and vice versa.

It is that occasional unaccountable uncertainty of action that calls forth the warning not to attempt disinfection with formaldehyde in a case in which there is any doubt as to the result.

The evolution and approach toward perfection of the pressure steam sterilizer has been, like all other apparatus of kindred nature, slow in development. Practically all of the pressure steam surgical dressing sterilizers employed in hospitals during the period from 1900 to 1915 were designed for operation by what was then known as the vacuum system of control. This system or method of operation, with few exceptions, consisted of the partial evacuation of air from the sterilizer chamber obtained by means of a steam ejector or vacuum attachment, and then subjecting the dressings or load in the chamber to steam at a pressure of 15 to 20 pounds for a period of from 20 to 30 minutes. The stated purpose of the initial vacuum (5 to 15 inches) was to aid in the displacement or removal of air from the chamber so as to insure a thorough penetration of the dressings or materials by the steam when it was next admitted to the chamber.

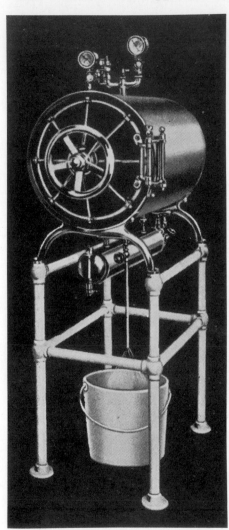

Fig. 21. Typical pressure steam sterilizer of 1915, utilizing the newly developed principle of gravity air discharge from the chamber—the first approach to the modern temperature-controlled sterilizer.

About the year 1915 there was introduced to hospitals in this country an entirely new conception of pressure steam sterilizer performance, in which the newly discovered gravity process of eliminating air from the chamber was substituted for the previously accepted standard of vacuum system of control. Much of the credit for the establishment of the gravity process of eliminating air from the chamber of the sterilizer, together with certain mechanical features of design, must be attributed to the efforts and accomplishments of the early investigator, W. B. Underwood and his co-workers, who were responsible for notable advances in this field.[41] Whereas the advantage of gravity air clearance from the pressure steam sterilizer was recognized by other workers[42] prior to this time, it is generally conceded that the first sterilizers for operation on this newly developed principle appeared about the year 1915, thus constituting the first approach to modern methods of steam sterilization.

A typical pressure steam sterilizer of early design and construction for gravity air discharge from the chamber is shown in Figure 21. The chamber was equipped with a drain outlet at the extreme bottom near the front end. This drain emptied into a pail on the floor, discharging into the open air so that the quality of the discharge could be observed by the operator. It was known, of course, that when steam is admitted to such a chamber with the bottom drain open, the lighter steam would literally float to the top of the chamber, and as the pressure was permitted to build up from the incoming steam it would force the air out at the bottom. The drain was left open until a full body of steam was observed to discharge into the pail, then the drain was closed in part so that only a slight discharge of steam occurred. When this process was followed with proper care, it left little to be desired from the standpoint of insuring the use of pure steam as the sterilizing medium.

Shortly after the introduction of the gravity system for air discharge as described above, a serious obstacle was encountered. The required performance of the sterilizer necessitated close attention on the part of the operator and in many cases, hospitals in particular, this close attention was not given. As the result frequent failures in sterilization occurred. Fortunately, certain sterilizer manufacturers were prone to recognize the need for a more effective system of air discharge that would eliminate the hazard of faulty operation. Consequently, there appeared several modifications to the non-vacuum system described above, each contributing its share to the development of the modern (automatically-controlled) pressure steam sterilizer. Because operators did not like the idea of the pail on the floor to catch the discharge from the chamber, the use of steam traps (thermostatic valves) to control the chamber discharge was introduced on sterilizers shortly after 1915. In 1919, Scanlan, Larson and Clark[43] showed the value of the automatic air and condensate ejector and its influence on the efficiency of steam sterilization in an autoclave. Following these advances, serious attention was given to the introduction of sanitary water and waste connections to sterilizers. These protective features were provided for the elimination of the so-called cross connections through which, under all possible conditions, the sterilizers were freed from contamination influences from water and waste connections, and which also guarded against pollution of the water supply system from the sterilizers. Slowly but surely progress had been made toward safer and more efficient sterilization.

IMPORTANT (PAST) CONTRIBUTORS TO THE DEVELOPMENT
OF THE ART OF STERILIZATION

1680 PAPIN, DENYS: French physicist (1647-1714). Invented steam digester (pressure cooker) to which was later added first safety valve on record. He also discovered that the boiling points of liquids vary with the pressure.

1765 SPALLANZANI, LAZZARO: Italian naturalist (1729-1799). A leading opponent of the theory of spontaneous generation. Studied the effectiveness of heat in the destruction of bacteria and the sterilization of liquids. Proved to his own satisfaction that there is no vegetative power in inanimate material.

1807 DALTON, JOHN: English chemist (1766-1844). Investigated the properties of gases and formulated the Law of Partial Pressures. His greatest work was the establishment of the Atomic Theory.

1810 APPERT, NICOLAS: Parisian confectioner (?-1841). Credited with discovery of process of food preservation by canning. Introduced the use of sealed containers followed by heating in boiling water. Published first treatise on canning.

1832 HENRY, WILLIAM: English chemist (1775-1836). Investigated the disinfecting powers of increased temperatures and demonstrated that infected clothing could be rendered harmless by heat. He devised a jacketed dry heat (hot air) sterilizer.

1847 SEMMELWEISS, IGNAZ: Hungarian physician (1818-1865). Recognized as the true pioneer of antisepsis in obstetrics. He proved the contact transmissibility of puerperal (childbed) fever from physician, midwife or nurse to the patient.

1861 PASTEUR, LOUIS: French chemist-bacteriologist (1822-1895). Generally recognized as the "Father of Bacteriology." Noted for his brilliant researches on fermentation and the prevention of anthrax and rabies. He disproved the doctrine of spontaneous generation and proved that putrefaction is a fermentation caused by the growth of microbes. He also originated the process of pasteurization; postulated the role of bacteria in disease, and contributed greatly to the foundations of modern surgical asepsis.

1867 LISTER, JOSEPH: English surgeon (1827-1912). Founder of antiseptic surgery. He applied Pasteur's principles of fermentation to surgical practice and postulated the theory that "infection was due to passage of minute bodies capable of self multiplication from infector to infected." Lister's contributions led directly to the establishment of sterile technic in the operating room.

1877 TYNDALL, JOHN: English physicist (1820-1893). Discovered the heat resistant phase (spore stage) of bacteria. He was the originator of the method known as fractional (intermittent) sterilization or Tyndallization.

1880 CHAMBERLAND, CHARLES: French bacteriologist (1851-1908). Pupil and collaborator of Pasteur on the germ theory of disease. He built the first pressure steam sterilizer—known as "Chamberland's Autoclave."

1881 KOCH, ROBERT: German bacteriologist (1843-1910). Widely acclaimed as the "Father of Bacteriological Technic." He discovered the use of solid (liquefiable) culture media and investigated the etiology of infective diseases. He also discovered the cause of tuberculosis and advocated the use of bichloride of mercury as a germicide. Many important contributions to the field of sterilization and chemical disinfection originated in Koch's laboratory, with the able assistance of Wolffhügel, Gaffky and Loeffler.

1885 SCHIMMELBUSCH, CURT: German surgeon (1860-1895). He developed and evaluated the various details of aseptic technic. Also credited as the first to use the steam sterilizer for sterilization of surgical dressings. He advocated addition of sodium carbonate to boiling water to enhance its germicidal value and prevent corrosion of instruments. Published *Aseptic Treatment of Wounds.*

1888 VON ESMARCH, ERVIN: (1885-1915). Investigated the sterilizing efficiency of unsaturated or superheated steam. Also recommended the use of bacteriologic tests as proof of sterilization.

1888 KINYOUN, J. J.: American bacteriologist (1860-1919). He made important contributions to design of steam pressure chambers and first recommended the vacuum process to augment steam penetration of objects. He also studied gaseous disinfectants, particularly formaldehyde, and was largely responsible for development of steam-formaldehyde disinfector used in quarantine stations, hospital and municipal services.

1933 UNDERWOOD, WEEDEN: American engineer (1880-1946). Responsible for notable advances in design and application of pressure steam sterilizers. His investigations influenced the development of the modern temperature controlled sterilizer. He promoted the modern concept of sterile supply centralization for hospitals. Published *Textbook of Sterilization.*

REFERENCES

1. BRYAN, A. H., AND BRYAN, C. G.: *Principles and Practice of Bacteriology,* 3rd Ed. New York, Barnes & Noble, p. 2, 1942.
2. MACKAIL, J. W.: *The Odyssey* (Translated in Verse). London, Oxford, p. 474, Book XXII, 1932.
3. FORD, W. W.: *Clio Medica, Bacteriology.* New York, Hoeber, p. 34, 1939.
4. SPALLANZANI, L.: Saggio di osservazioni microscopiche relative al sistema della generazione di Signore Needham e Buffon. Modena, 1765. From: *A History of Science, Technology and Philosophy in the 18th Century,* by A. WOLF. New York, Macmillan, p. 474, 1939.
5. HAMILTON, J. B.: The Shadowed Side of Spallanzani. *Yale J. Biol. & Med.,* 7:151-170, 1934.
6. SCHULZE, F.: Vorlaufige Mittheilung der Resultate einer experimentellen Beobachtung uber Generatio aequivoca. *Ann. d. Physik u. Chemie,* 39:487-489, 1836.
7. SCHWANN, T.: *Ann. d. Physik u. Chemie,* 41:184-192, 1837.
8. TANNER, F. W.: *Bacteriology,* 3rd Ed. New York, Wiley, p. 9, 1937.
9. SCHROEDER, H., AND VON DUSCH, T.: Ueber Filtration der Luft in Beziehung auf Faulniss und Gahrung. *Ann. d. Chemie u. Pharmacie,* 89:232-241, 1854.
10. POUCHET, F. A.: Heterogenie ou traite de la generation spontanee, base sur des nouvelles experiences, Paris, 1859.
11. PASTEUR, L.: Memoire sur les corpuscles organises qui existent dans l'atmosphere, examen de la doctrine des generations spontanees. *Ann. de chimie et de physique, Paris,* 64:5-110, 1862.
12. FORD, W. W.: *Textbook of Bacteriology.* Philadelphia, Saunders, p. 22, 1927.
13. FORD, W. W.: *Clio Medica, Bacteriology.* New York, Hoeber, p. 88, 1939.
14. VALLERY-RADOT, R.: *The Life of Pasteur* (Trans. by R. L. Devonshire). New York, Doubleday, p. 255, 1926.

15. *Idem.*: p. 255.
16. METCHNIKOFF, E.: *The Founders of Modern Medicine* (Pasteur, Koch, Lister), New York, Walden Publications, p. 39, 1939.
17. VALLERY-RADOT, R.: *The Life of Pasteur.* p. 274.
18. TYNDALL, J.: On the Optical Deportment of the Atmosphere in Relation to the Phenomena of Putrefaction and Infection. *Phil. Trans. Royal Soc., 166*:27-74, 1876.
19. *Idem.*: Further Researches on the Deportment and Vital Persistence of Putrefactive and Infective Organisms from a Physical Point of View. *Phil. Trans. Royal Soc. 167*:149-206, 1877.
20. *Idem.*: *Selected Works of John Tyndall, Fragments of Science.* Westminster Ed., Vol.· II, Appleton, New York, p. 320.
21. *Idem.*: *Ibid.*, p. 323.
22. *Idem.*: *Ibid.*, p. 321.
23. LISTER, JOSEPH: On the Antiseptic Principle in the Practice of Surgery, *Brit. M.J., 2*:246-248, 1867. Also, *Lancet, 2*:353, 1867.
24. PELTIER, L. F.: A Brief Account of the Evolution of Antiseptic Surgery. *Journal-Lancet,* p. 442-444, Nov. 1950.
25. LISTER, JOSEPH: On the New Method of Treating Compound Fracture, Abscess, etc., with Observations on the Conditions of Suppuration. *Lancet, 1*:364, 1867.
26. LISTER, JOSEPH: An Address on the Effect of the Antiseptic Treatment upon the General Salubrity of Surgical Hospitals. *Brit. M.J., 2*:769-771, 1875.
27. ROBINSON, V.: *Story of Medicine.* From *Story of Sterilization,* by W. B. Underwood: *Surgical Supervisor, 6*:3-61, 1946.
28. KOCH, R., AND WOLFFHÜGEL, G.: Untersuchungen über die Desinfection mit heisser Luft. *Mitt. a. d. Kaiserl Gesund., 1*:301-321, 1881.
29. KOCH, R., GAFFKY, G., AND LOEFFLER, F.: Versuche über die Verwerthbarkeit heisser Wasserdämpfe zu Desinfektionszwecken. *Ibid.*: p. 322-340.
30. ZINSSER, HANS: *Textbook of Bacteriology,* Sixth Ed. New York, Appleton, p. 67, 1927.
31. WALTER, C. W.: *The Aseptic Treatment of Wounds.* New York, Macmillan, p. 18, 1948.
32. DAVIDSOHN, H.: Wie soll der Arzt seine Instrumente desinficirin? *Berl. Klin. Wchnschr., 25*:697, 1888.
33. VON ESMARCH, E.: Die desinficirende Wirkung des strömenden überhitzten Dampfes. *Ztschr. Hyg. u. Infektionskr., 4*:197, 1888.
34. RUBNER, M.: Zur Theorie der Dampfdesinfektion. *Hygienische Rundschau, 8*:721, 1898. *Ibid.*: *Modern Steam Sterilization,* Harvey Lectures, Harvey Soc. of New York, 1912-13, Philadelphia, Lippincott, p. 15-27.
35. WINSLOW, C. E. A.: Some Leaders and Landmarks in the History of Microbiology. *Bact. Rev., 14*:99-114, 1950.
36. STERNBERG, G. M.: Experiments to Determine the Germicide Value of Certain Therapeutic Agents, *Am. J. Med. Sc., 335* (April), 1883.
37. Personal Communication, Wilmot Castle Co., July, 1952.
38. Report on the Louisiana Quarantine, Abstract of Sanitary Reports, 1888.
39. KINYOUN, J. J.: *Public Health Rep.* Sept. 4, 1897.
40. SPRAGUE, E. K.: Formaldehyde Disinfection in a Vacuum Chamber. *Public Health Rep.,* XIV, Sept. 22, 1899.
41. UNDERWOOD, W. B.: The Story of Sterilization. *Surgical Supervisor, 6*, 3-61, 1946.
42. FROSCH, P., AND CLARENBACH, A.: Ueber das Verhalten des Wasserdampfes im Desinfektionsapparate. *Ztschr. Hyg. u. Infektionskr., 9*:183, 1890.
43. SCANLAN, S. G., LARSON, G. L., AND CLARK, P. F.: High Pressure Dressing Sterilizers or Autoclaves. *Modern Hospital,* Vol. XII, April 1919.

Chapter II

Thermal Destruction of Microorganisms

THE PROCESS by which bacteria are destroyed when subjected to heat is not clearly understood. The traditional theory is that death of bacteria at elevated temperatures is closely linked to the alteration of proteins involving some irreversible protoplasmic change within the bacterial cell. It is held by certain investigators[1, 2] that death is associated with the heat inactivation of vital enzymes or some enzyme-protein system in the organism. That other mechanisms may be operative when bacteria are destroyed by high temperatures was advanced as early as 1910 by Chick.[3, 4] Further studies have since led to the belief that the mode of action of heat on bacteria closely parallels the heat coagulation of proteins. Assuming this view to be correct, it is reasonable to conclude that the effect of moisture on the coagulation temperature of proteins must also bear some relationship to the temperatures at which bacteria are destroyed. To be sure, it is known that moist heat is a more efficient sterilizing agent than dry heat. When moisture is present bacteria are destroyed at considerably lower temperatures than when moisture is absent. This phenomenon has been explained on the basis that all chemical reactions, including the coagulation of proteins, are catalyzed by the presence of water.

Today it is generally accepted that death by moist heat is caused by the denaturation and coagulation of some essential protein within the bacterial cell (see Figs. 22 and 23), whereas death by dry heat is primarily an oxidation process. This theory is supported by experimental observations showing that the high temperature coefficients of bacterial death are also characteristic of protein coagulation; by the increase of death rate as the result of changes in the hydrogen-ion concentration of the medium; and by the fact that bacteria show a much greater resistance to dry than to moist heat.

ORDER OF DEATH

When a population of bacteria is exposed to a sterilizing influence the rate at which the individual organisms die is governed by definite laws. The order of death, as may be determined experimentally, follows a uniform and consistent course and it is commonly described as being logarithmic. This means that when a population of bacteria is in contact with a sterilizing medium the number of living cells decreases gradually, in such a manner that the logarithms of the numbers of the surviving cells at any one time, when plotted against this time, fall on a descending straight line.

Knowledge of the logarithmic order is highly important because it permits the bacteriologist to compute the death rate constant, designated "K." This term expresses by a single number the rate of death which bears a direct relationship to the efficiency of the sterilizing agent. The constancy of the death rate signifies that the number of bacteria that are killed each minute or per time unit is a constant percentage of the number of living

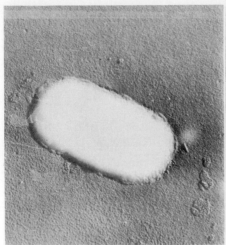

From Heden and Wyckoff[5]   *From Heden and Wyckoff*[5]

Fig. 22. Typical colon bacillus from a one-hour broth culture. Magnification 28,000 X. This shows the apparent uniformity of the cellular protoplasm.

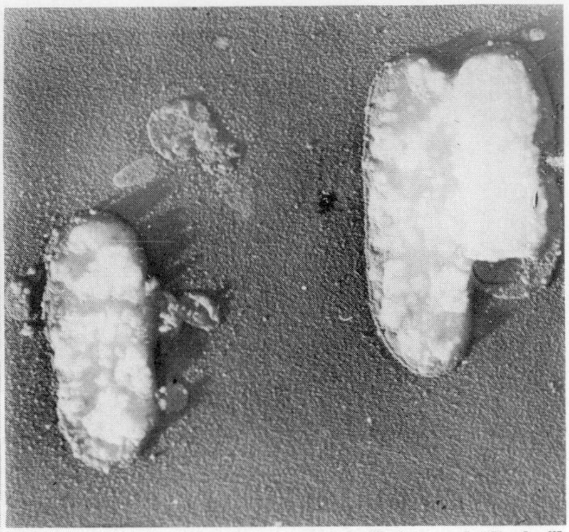

Fig. 23. Typical colon bacilli after being heated for ten minutes in saline at 50°C. Magnification 16,000 X. Heating the organisms in saline at temperatures above 50°C. granulates their protoplasm in an irreversible fashion.

bacteria at the beginning of each new minute. It is customary to compute the death rate constant, K, from the formula:

$$K = \frac{\log b - \log B}{t},$$

where b equals the number of living organisms at the beginning of the time unit; B equals the number of organisms surviving at the end of the time unit; and t equals the time unit or exposure period. The determination of death rates makes it possible to compare the heat resistance of different organisms at the same temperature, or the heat resistance of one particular organism at different temperatures.

It is important to note that the logarithmic order of death implies that the same percentage of living bacteria die every minute. Theoretically this means that complete sterilization is never attained. For example, the figures given in Table 1 are illustrative of a theoretical case, based upon the assumption that when a suspension of one million bacteria per ml. is subjected to a sterilizing influence, 90% of the bacteria are killed each minute of exposure. The figures near the end of the survivor column—0.1 or 0.01 bacteria per ml.—mean that only one bacterium remains alive in 10 ml. or in 100 ml. of the suspension. At the end of 12 minutes' exposure, one bacterium would still survive (theoretically) in 1,000,000 ml., equivalent to 1000 liters or approximately 250 gallons of the suspension.

As a practical measure, the above example shows the necessity of allowing a proportionately greater period of exposure for the sterilization of a liquid containing a high concentration of bacteria than for a liquid containing only a few bacteria. Rahn[6] has stated that this condition holds true for heat sterilization, chemical disinfection or pasteurization. Application of this principle is oftentimes overlooked in establishing minimum exposure periods for the sterilization of materials or products.

TABLE 1

A THEORETICAL EXAMPLE OF THE ORDER OF DEATH OF A BACTERIAL POPULATION

Minute	Bacteria Living at Beginning of New Minute	Bacteria Killed in One Minute	Bacteria Surviving at End of Minute	Logarithm of Survivors
First	1,000,000	90%=900,000	100,000	5
Second	100,000	= 90,000	10,000	4
Third	10,000	= 9,000	1,000	3
Fourth	1,000	= 900	100	2
Fifth	100	= 90	10	1
Sixth	10	= 9	1	0
Seventh	1	= 0.9	0.1	−1
Eighth	0.1	= 0.09	0.01	−2
Ninth	0.01	= 0.009	0.001	−3
Tenth	0.001	= 0.0009	0.0001	−4
Eleventh	0.0001	= 0.00009	0.00001	−5
Twelfth	0.00001	= 0.000009	0.000001	−6

THERMAL DEATH POINT AND THERMAL DEATH TIME

Some years ago the conception arose among bacteriologists that if a suspension of bacteria were gradually heated, a point would be reached on the ascending scale of temperature at which all of the cells in the suspension would be killed instantaneously. This gave rise to use of the expression "thermal death point" (the lowest temperature at which an aqueous suspension of bacteria is killed in 10 minutes), formerly the standard of comparison of heat tolerance of organisms of different species. Use of this term has been criticized by various investigators[7, 8, 9] on the grounds that it is misleading because it implies that a certain temperature is immediately lethal to a bacterial population, without regard to the exposure period, the environment surrounding the organisms or their physiological state.

In view of the evidence that death of bacteria under the influence of heat follows an orderly process, due to the irreversible coagulation of cellular protein, it must be admitted that there is no one temperature at which all of the cells in a suspension would be killed instantaneously. The process occurs chiefly as a function of time within a certain range of temperature. If the temperature is increased the time may be decreased or if the temperature is lowered the time must be lengthened. In other words, the killing of bacteria by heat is a function of the time-temperature relationship employed. For these reasons, the expression "thermal death point" has in recent years given way to a more practical measurement known as "thermal death time" or "thermal death time-temperature." This refers to a determination of the shortest period of time necessary to kill a known population of bacteria in a specific suspension at a given temperature.

When making thermal death time studies it is first necessary to prepare a standardized suspension of the test organism in a suitable medium. This is usually done in a sterile phosphate buffer solution at pH 7.0. The number of the organisms per ml. of the suspension may be determined microscopically by means of a Petroff-Hauser counting chamber. Quantities of the test suspension, usually 1-2 ml., containing 50 million organisms per ml. are transferred to special tubes or ampoules made from 9 mm. Pyrex tubing, approximately 12.5 cm. in length. The tubes are then sealed with the aid of an oxygen flame and immersed completely in a preheated oil bath maintained constant at the desired heating temperature. At the end of each time interval of heating, 5 minutes or less, four or more tubes are removed from the bath and plunged into ice water. The tips of the sealed tubes are then broken aseptically and the test suspension inoculated into sterile recovery culture medium. The cultures are then incubated at the optimum temperature for 30 days, following which colony counts are made to determine the number of survivors.

The nature of the medium in which the organisms are suspended has an important bearing on the thermal death time. Toxic substances, if present, become increasingly germicidal with slight increases in temperature. Also, products of metabolism show increased toxicity at higher temperatures. A pronounced acid or alkaline pH decreases the thermal death time, whereas the presence of oils or fats retards heat penetration and increases the time. At best, it is difficult to obtain consistent determinations of thermal death time values. Regardless of the precautions taken, certain inaccuracies may occur which are not easily controllable, such as variations in heat tolerance of organisms of the same species, number of cells, nature of suspending medium, etc. Comparable results can only be expected when conditions are standardized as to history and age of culture, number of cells or spores, pH of suspension, uniformity of suspension, size of test tubes, thermal conductivity and thickness of glass in test tubes. Table 2 gives the comparative resistance of vegetative cells and spores of certain aerobic sporeforming bacilli, expressed in terms of thermal death times.

Thermal death time studies are highly important in the field of applied bacteriology, as, for example, in the canning industry, where information is required on the resistances of food spoilage bacteria as a basis for developing adequate heating processes for canned foods. It should be remembered, however, that thermal death times are not precise values. In discussing this subject, Rahn[11] has stated, "all death time data have a cer-

TABLE 2

THE RESISTANCE OF VEGETATIVE CELLS AND SPORES OF AEROBIC SPOREFORMING BACILLI
(From Williams and Zimmerman[10])

Organism	Vegetative Cells Thermal Death Time In Minutes at 53° C.		Spores Thermal Death Time in Minutes at 99.5° C.	
	Lived	Died	Lived	Died
Bacillus brevis	2	4	14	16
Bacillus cereus	2	4	4	6
Bacillus subtilis, Sl	2	4	4	6
Bacillus subtilis, UT	10	12	10	12
Bacillus globigii	4	6	6	8
Bacillus mycoides, 420	4	6	10	12
Bacillus mycoides, SIII	4	6	6	8
Bacillus megatherium	4	6	4	6
Bacillus fusiformis	4	6	12	14
Bacillus mesentericus	20	22	10	12

tain range of possible error, the magnitude of which depends upon the spacing of the time intervals. The number of survivors is never zero, but becomes very small, e.g., 1 in 100 liters, 1 in 1000 liters, etc."

RESISTANCE OF MICROORGANISMS TO HEAT

Vegetative Forms: The resistance of microorganisms to heat covers a broad range of temperature. The extremes extend from approximately 122° F. (50° C.) for a few minutes' exposure to moist heat for the highly susceptible forms to 572° F. (300° C.) for 30 minutes' exposure to dry heat for the most resistant bacterial spores. Probably the yeasts and the yeast-like fungi are typical of the most readily killed forms of microbial life. In contact with moist heat at 122°-140° F. (50°-60° C.) vegetative yeast cells are usually killed in 5 minutes. However, in the spore stage these organisms require a temperature of 158°-176° F. (70°-80° C.) for killing in the same period of time. Beamer and Tanner[12] found that *Saccharomyces ellipsoideus* in dextrose bouillon (about 5 million cells per ml., pH 8.0) was killed at 140° F. (60° C.) in 15 minutes, and in grape-must with 8 million cells per ml., pH 2.6, at the same temperature in 20 minutes.

The vegetative forms of molds (fungi) are usually destroyed in 30 minutes' exposure to moist heat at 144° F. (62° C.), whereas certain spores may require a temperature of 176° F. (80° C.) for killing in the same period of time. Most of the organisms classified as the *Actinomyces* group are killed by moist heat at 140° F. (60° C.) in 15 minutes. According to Goyal[13] these organisms, including the spores, are killed by a time-temperature relationship of 30 minutes at 140° F. (60° C.) to more than one hour at 162° F. (72° C.). In contact with dry heat mold spores require a temperature of 230°-240° F. (110°-116° C.) for 90 minutes for their destruction.

In general, vegetative bacterial cells are killed by exposure to moist heat at 149° F. (65° C.) for 10 minutes or 176° F. (80° C.) for 5 minutes. Certain organisms may offer an exception to this rule. For example, *Streptococcus faecalis* is reputed to withstand a temperature of 140° F. (60° C.) for 30 minutes.[14] The staphylococci are among the most resistant of the nonspore-bearing species of bacteria. *Micrococcus pyogenes* var. *aureus* is not destroyed with certainty by exposure to a temperature of 140° F. (60° C.) for 30 minutes, but is destroyed at 149° F. (65° C.) within this time.[15] The great mass of evidence in support of a temperature of 140° F. (60° C.) for 30 minutes, such as is employed in the pasteurization of milk, leaves little doubt that this time-temperature relationship is fatal to all pathogenic nonsporulating bacteria, with the occasional exception of the staphylococci. It is of special interest to note, however, that the causative agent of Q fever, *Coxiella burneti*, was found by Ransom and Huebner[16] to survive temperatures as high as 145° F. (63° C.) when suspended in milk, sealed in vials and submerged for 30 to 40 minutes in water baths.

The tubercle bacillus (*Mycobacterium tuberculosis*) is one of the most difficult to destroy of all vegetative forms of bacteria. Although it offers approximately the same degree of resistance to heat as other nonsporing bacteria, it has a much higher resistance to chemical disinfectants, and it will remain viable for many months in polluted water, foods or in the dry state surrounded by organic matter. Smith[17] has stated that in books contaminated with the sputum of tuberculous patients the organisms remain viable from 2 weeks to 3½ months. According to Wilson,[18] the mammalian tubercle bacilli are completely destroyed by exposure to a temperature of 138° F. (58.9° C.) for 30 minutes, 140° F. (60° C.) for 20 minutes, 145° F. (62.8° C.) for 5 to 10 minutes, 150° F. (65.6° C.) for 2 to 5 minutes, or 160° F. (71.1° C.) for 12 seconds. In contact with dry heat they will withstand a temperature of 212° F. (100° C.) for 20 minutes but are destroyed in 45 minutes at this temperature. From studies on *Mycobacterium tuberculosis* var. *bovis*, strain No. 9805, Bundesen *et al.*[19] showed that this organism failed to produce tuberculosis in guinea pigs after exposure to temperatures of from 160° F. to 180° F. for periods of 15 to 30 seconds in chocolate drink, 12 per cent milk and 12 per cent ice cream mix.

Bacterial Spores: Spores are a normal resting stage in the life-cycle of certain groups of organisms, namely the *Bacilli* and *Clostridia*, and they constitute a phase of bacterial life in which the processes of the living cell are carried on at a minimum rate. It is commonly recognized that bacterial spores are the most resistant of all living organisms in their capacity to withstand external destructive agents. Anthrax spores, for example, dried on silk threads have been found viable after 60 years. Other viable spore-formers have been recovered from canned and hermetically sealed meat after a lapse of 115 years.[20] The magnitude of resistance to saturated steam

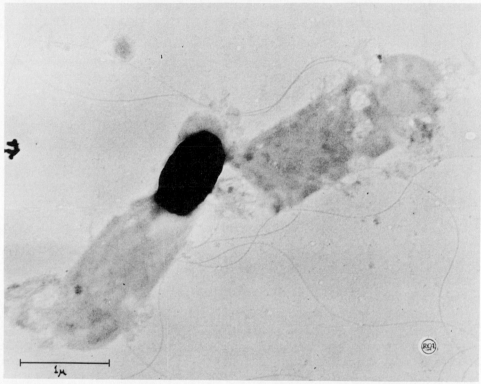

From Mudd and Anderson[11]

Fig. 24. Electron micrograph of *Clostridium sporogenes* cells from a three day culture. Only remnants or "ghosts" of the vegetative cells remain; in one "ghost" is a spore—a dense body of protoplasm.

is illustrated by the fact that certain spore cultures will withstand a temperature of 240° F. (116° C.) for over 3 hours, whereas the vegetative forms of most sporulating species are killed in a few minutes at temperatures ranging from 131° F. (55° C.) to 149° F. (65° C.).

From studies on the structure of bacterial forms by means of the electron microscope, it appears that spores are dense concentrations of bacterial protoplasm (Fig. 24). Just how this small mass of protoplasm differs in its chemical and physical properties from the protoplasm of vegetative cells is not clearly understood. However, the thermal resistance of spores is generally attributed to a low water content or to a relatively low salt content. Certain investigators hold that most of the water present in spores is bound (not in the free state), intimately associated with the colloids of the cell, and as such it is less reactive and more resistant to physical and chemical agents. Henry and Friedman[22] showed that spores of the *Bacillus* group have a bound water content of the order of 60 to 70 per cent, as compared with 3 to 21 per cent in the vegetative cells. The presence of lipoid material in the spore may also contribute to its heat resistance.

Spore resistance appears to vary widely from species to species and to a considerable extent within a species and within a given spore population. Williams and Harper[23] claim that luxuriance of growth and luxuriance of

TABLE 3

RELATIVE RESISTANCES OF BACTERIAL SPORES, MOLD SPORES, AND OF VIRUSES, REFERRED TO THE RESISTANCE OF E. COLI AS UNITY
(From Rahn[11])

Sterilizing Agent	Escherichia Coli	Bacterial Spores	Mold Spores	Viruses and Bacteriophage
Phenol	1	100,000,000	1–2	30
Formaldehyde	1	250		2
Dry Heat	1	1,000	2–10	±1
Moist Heat	1	3,000,000	2–10	1–5
Ultraviolet	1	2–5	5–100	5–10

sporulation are not governing factors in determining heat resistance of spores. Incubation at the optimum temperature favors increased thermal resistance. Most spores attain their maximum resistance several days after entering into the spore stage, whereas others, such as *Cl. botulinum* and *Cl. tetani,* appear to be more resistant when young.

In seeking an explanation of the mechanism of spore resistance Curran[20] has mentioned that the nature of the nutrients in the spore-producing medium is significant. Media deficient in certain metallic ions, such as phosphate, calcium, magnesium and iron yield spores of low thermal resistance. The higher the concentration of spores in a medium, the greater is their resistance, and proportionately more heat or a longer time is required to effect sterilization. The reaction of the medium is another important factor affecting heat resistance. The pH of maximum heat tolerance of different species may vary from 5.0 to 8.0. When spores are suspended in oily materials their heat resistance is markedly increased and the resistance of dry spores in strictly anhydrous fat approaches that of dry sterilization.

Rahn[11] has presented a summary of the relative resistances of bacterial spores, mold spores, and of viruses, based on the resistance of a vegetative organism *(E. coli)* as unity. These data are given in Table 3. The contrast between bacterial spores and the other forms is immediately apparent, where in the case of moist heat as the sterilizing agent, the death rate of *E. coli* is 3,000,000 times as great as that of spores.

From the literature it is evident that authorities are not always in agreement concerning the thermal death requirements of microbial life. Various time-temperature ratios have been recommended for moist heat sterilization, some of which carry a proportionately greater factor of safety than others in assuring the destruction of the most resistant spores. The data given in Table 4 are typical of recommended exposures to moist heat necessary to kill all life.

The commonly quoted statement that "no living thing can survive ten

TABLE 4

Time-temperature Relationship for Moist Heat Sterilization
(Compiled by McCulloch[9])

Authority	°Centigrade	°Fahrenheit	Time, Minutes
Jordan	120.0	248	5
Muir & Ritchie	120.0	248	7½
Gerard	115.5	240	10
Eyre	115.0	239	15
Beeson	115.0	239	20
Sternberg	115.0	239	25
Novy	110.0	230	15
McFarland	110.0	230	15

minutes' direct exposure to saturated steam at 121° C. (249.8° F.)" would seem to be reasonably close to a minimum standard of time and temperature required for sterilization. It is noteworthy, however, that Bigelow and Esty[24] reported the existence of thermophilic spores which required 23 minutes of direct exposure to saturated steam at 248° F. (120° C.) for their destruction. Also, Black and Tanner[25] found that certain aerobic thermophiles survived 100° C. for 24 hours, 115° C. for 1 hour, and 120° C. for 25 minutes. From the destruction times of bacterial spores subjected to moist heat given in Table 5, it is known that most resistant spores can rarely withstand 5 minutes' exposure to saturated steam at 121° C., while apparently none of the pathogenic organisms have been shown to be resistant to an exposure of even three minutes.

Heat Inactivation of Viruses: In terms of thermal resistance, the filtrable viruses are more closely related to the vegetative bacteria than the spore-bearing organisms. Whereas all appear to be inactivated by high temperatures, it is also evident that wide variations exist between different viruses. Moist heat at 131°-140° F. (55°-60° C.) for 30 minutes is fatal for most viruses, but when dried and in contact with dry heat they may withstand considerably higher temperatures. The vaccinia virus, for example, in dry

TABLE 5

Typical Destruction Times (In Minutes) of Bacterial Spores Subjected to Moist Heat

(From Perkins[26])

Organism	212° F 100° C	221° F 105° C	230° F 110° C	239° F 115° C	248-250° F 120-121° C	257° F 125° C	266° F 130° C	275° F 135° C	Investigator
B. anthracis	2								Schneiter & Kolb[27]
B. anthracis	5-15								Stein & Rogers[28]
B. anthracis	5-10	5-10							Murray[29]
B. cereus	6								Schneiter & Kolb[27]
B. stearothermophilus					12				Perkins[50]
B. subtilis	6-17								Schneiter & Kolb[27]
B. subtilis	10								Ecker[30]
Cl. botulinum	330	100	32	10	4				Esty & Meyer[31]
Cl. botulinum			30	10	4				Hoyt, Chaney & Cavell[32]
Cl. botulinum	300	120	90	40	10				Tanner & McCrea[33]
Cl. botulinum	300	40			6				Weiss[34]
Cl. oedematiens			10	4	1				Hoyt, Chaney & Cavell[32]
Cl. oedematiens			15						Ecker[30]
Cl. septicum			5						Ecker[30]
Cl. tetani	5-15	5-10							Murray & Headlee[35]
Cl. welchii	5-10								Headlee[36]
Cl. welchii		5							Ecker[30]
Putrefactive anaerobe 3679	780	170	41.6	15.6	5.6				McCulloch[37]
Thermophiles	834	405	100	40	11-12	3.9-4.6	1.7-2.2	0.7-0.9	Bigelow[24]
Soil bacilli	660			15					Ecker[30]
Soil bacilli	1020	420	120	15	6				Konrich[39]

form withstands a dry heat temperature of 212° F. (100° C.) for 10 minutes.[40]

The virus of poliomyelitis is quite susceptible to heat and according to Flexner and Lewis[41] it is inactivated at 122° F. (50° C.) for 30 minutes. However, a more recent reference[42] gives the thermal inactivation point of this virus at or below 167° F. (75° C.) for 30 minutes. According to the British Commission,[43] the virus of foot-and-mouth disease in defibrinated blood is rendered inactive in 20 minutes at 55° C., and in filtered, diluted vesicular fluid in 15 to 40 minutes. Other investigators[44] have shown that this virus is destroyed at 140-145.4° F. (60-63° C.) within 10 minutes. The virus associated with swine fever appears to be unusually resistant. In filtered blood it will withstand a temperature of 136.4° F. (58° C.) for 2 hours, but at 172.4° F. (78° C.) it is destroyed in 1 hour.[45] In a study involving six outbreaks of lethal infantile diarrhea in hospitals, Light and Hodes[46] determined that the infectious agent, a filtrable virus, was wholly inactivated by boiling for 5 minutes but it resisted heating at 158° F. (70° C.) for 1 hour.

During the past decade the causative agent of infectious hepatitis and/or homologous serum jaundice has been the subject of many investigations. Neefe[47] reported that this virus, in human albumin, was inactivated by heating for 10 hours at 60° C. Others[48] have stated that the agent withstands heating at 132.8° F. (56° C.) for 30 minutes, and it is unaffected by the normal concentration of chlorine added to drinking water. The usual germicidal solutions cannot be relied upon for killing of this virus. Murray[49] has reported that heating plasma containing the virus of serum hepatitis for 4 hours at 60° C. was found ineffective. It is believed that this virus is transmitted in certain instances by means of the single syringe multiple injection method. The commonly used methods of sterilization of syringes, needles and lancets by brief exposure in boiling water or immersion in chemical disinfectants are recognized as inadequate for the destruction of this virus, particularly in the presence of organic substances. The National Institutes of Health stipulate that apparatus and instruments capable of transmitting serum hepatitis from one person to another be heat-sterilized with minimum requirements as follows: "Heat sterilization shall be by autoclaving for 30 minutes at 121.5° C. (15 lb. pressure), by dry heat for 2 hours at 170° C., or by boiling in water for 30 minutes." Since the thermal resistance of this virus appears to be equal to that of bacterial spores it would seem unwise to attempt sterilization by any means other than the most reliable methods.

REFERENCES

1. ISAACS, M. L.: From F. P. Gay: *Agents of Disease and Host Resistance.* Springfield, Illinois, Charles C Thomas, Publisher, 1935, p. 228.
2. VIRTANEN, A. I.: On the Enzymes of Bacteria and Bacterial Metabolism. *J. Bact.,* 28:447-460, 1934.

3. CHICK, H.: The Process of Disinfection by Chemical Agencies and Hot Water. *J. Hyg.,* 10:237-286, 1910.

4. CHICK, H., AND MARTIN, C. J.: On the "Heat Coagulation" of Proteins. *J. Physiol.,* 40:404-430, 1910.

5. HEDEN, C-G., AND WYCKOFF, R. W. G.: The Electron Microscopy of Heated Bacteria. *J. Bact.,* 58:153-160, 1949.

6. RAHN, O.: Biochemistry of Disinfection. *Wallerstein Laboratories Communications,* IV: 107-111, 1941.

7. WILSON, G. S., AND MILES, A. A.: *Topley and Wilson's Principles of Bacteriology and Immunity,* 3rd Ed. Baltimore, Williams & Wilkins, 1946, Vol. I, p. 115.

8. TANNER, F. W.: *Bacteriology,* 3rd Ed. New York, Wiley, 1937, p. 158.

9. McCULLOCH, E. C.: *Disinfection and Sterilization,* 2nd Ed. Philadelphia, Lea & Febiger, 1945, p. 69.

10. WILLIAMS, O. B., AND ZIMMERMAN, C. H.: Studies on Heat Resistance. III. The Resistance of Vegetative Cells and Spores of the Same Organism. *J. Bact.,* 61:63-65, 1951.

11. RAHN, O.: Physical Methods of Sterilization of Microorganisms. *Bact. Rev.,* 9:1-47, 1945.

12. BEAMER, P. R., AND TANNER, F. W.: From A. Jorgensen: *Microorganisms and Fermentation.* London, Griffin, 1948, p. 262.

13. GOYAL, R. K.: From Topley and Wilson: *Principles of Bacteriology and Immunity,* 3rd Ed. Baltimore, Williams & Wilkins, 1946, Vol. I, p. 378.

14. TOPLEY AND WILSON: *op. cit.,* p. 601.

15. WILSON, G. S.: *The Pasteurization of Milk,* London, Edward Arnold & Co., 1942, p. 148.

16. RANSOM, S. E., AND HEUBNER, R. J.: Studies on the Resistance of Coxiella Burneti to Physical and Chemical Agents. *Am. J. Hyg.,* 53:110-119, 1951.

17. SMITH, C. R.: From Topley and Wilson: *op. cit.,* p. 419.

18. WILSON, G. S.: *op. cit.,* p. 148.

19. BUNDESEN, H. N., DANFORTH, T. F., WOOLLEY, H., AND LEHNER, E. C.: Thermal Destruction of Mycobacterium tuberculosis var. bovis in Certain Liquid Dairy Products. *Am. J. Pub. Health,* 43:185-188, 1953.

20. CURRAN, H. R.: Symposium on the Biology of Bacterial Spores. V. Resistance in Bacterial Spores. *Bact. Rev.,* 16:111-117, 1952.

21. MUDD, S., AND ANDERSON, T. F.: Pathogenic Bacteria, Rickettsias and Viruses as Shown by the Electron Microscope. *J.A.M.A.,* 126:561-571, 1944.

22. HENRY, B. S., AND FRIEDMAN, C. A.: The Water Content of Bacterial Spores. *J. Bact.,* 33:323-329, 1937.

23. WILLIAMS, O. B., AND HARPER, O. F., JR.: Studies on Heat Resistance. IV. Sporulation of Bacillus Cereus in Some Synthetic Media and the Heat Resistance of the Spores Produced. *J. Bact.,* 61:551-556, 1951.

24. BIGELOW, W. D., AND ESTY, J. R.: The Thermal Death Point in Relation to Time of Typical Thermophilic Organisms. *J. Infect. Dis.,* 27:602-617, 1920.

25. BLACK, L. A., AND TANNER, F. W.: A Study of Thermophilic Bacteria from the Intestinal Tract. *Zentralbl. Bakt.,* 75:360-375, 1928.

26. PERKINS, J. J.: Bacteriological and Surgical Sterilization by Heat. From Reddish, G. F.: *Antiseptics, Disinfectants, Fungicides, Chemical and Physical Sterilization.* Philadelphia, Lea & Febiger, 1954, p. 671.

27. SCHNEITER, R. AND KOLB, R. W.: Heat Resistance Studies with Spores of Bacillus Anthracis and Related Aerobic Bacilli in Hair and Bristles. *Public Health Repts., Supplement No. 207:1-24,* 1948.

28. STEIN, C. D. AND ROGERS, H.: Resistance of Anthrax Spores to Heat. *Vet. Med.,* 40:406-410, 1945.

29. MURRAY, T. J.: Thermal Death Point. II. Spores of Bacillus Anthracis. *J. Infect. Dis.,* 48:457-467, 1931.

30. ECKER, E. E.: Sterilization Based on Temperature Attained and Time Ratio. *Modern Hosp.,* 48:86-90, 1937.

31. Esty, J. R. and Meyer, K. F.: Heat Resistance of Spores of Bacillus Botulinus and Allied Anaerobes. *J. Infect. Dis., 31*:650-663, 1922.

32. Hoyt, A., Chaney, A. L. and Cavell, K.: Steam Sterilization and Effects of Air in the Autoclave. *J. Bact., 36*:639-652, 1938.

33. Tanner, F. W. and McCrea, F. D.: Clostridium Botulinum. IV. Resistance of Spores to Moist Heat. *J. Bact., 8*:269-276, 1923.

34. Weiss, H.: The Heat Resistance of Spores with Special Reference to the Spores of B. Botulinus. *J. Infect. Dis., 28*:70-92, 1921.

35. Murray, T. J. and Headlee, M. R.: Thermal Death Point. I. Spores of Clostridium Tetani. *J. Infect. Dis., 48*:436-456, 1931.

36. Headlee, M. R.: Thermal Death Point. III. Spores of Clostridium Welchii. *J. Infect. Dis., 48*:468-483, 1931.

37. McCulloch, E. C.: *Disinfection and Sterilization,* 2nd Ed. Philadelphia, Lea & Febiger, 1945, p. 138.

38. Bigelow, W. D.: Logarithmic Nature of Thermal Death Time Curves. *J. Infect. Dis., 29*:528-536, 1921.

39. Konrich, F.: Die bakterielle Keimtötung durch Wärme. From Jorgensen, A.: *Microorganisms and Fermentation.* London, C. Griffin, 1948, p. 113.

40. Topley and Wilson: *op. cit.,* p. 962.

41. Flexner, S., and Lewis, A. P.: The Transmission of Epidemic Poliomyelitis to Monkeys. *J.A.M.A., 53*:1913, 1909.

42. Breed, R. S., Murray, E. G. D., and Hitchens, A. P.: Bergey: *Manual of Determinative Bacteriology, 6th Ed.* Baltimore, Williams & Wilkins, 1948, p. 1258.

43. British Commission: Foot-and-Mouth Disease Research Committee, Ministry of Agriculture and Fisheries, London, 1927.

44. Zeller, H., Wedemann, W., Lange, L., and Gildemeister, E.: From Wilson, G. S.: *The Pasteurization of Milk,* London, Arnold, 1942, p. 148.

45. Topley and Wilson: *op. cit.,* Vol. II, p. 1964.

46. Light, J. S., and Hodes, F. L.: Studies on Epidemic Diarrhea of the Newborn: Isolation of a Filtrable Agent Causing Diarrhea in Calves. *Am. J. Pub. Health, 33*:1451, 1943.

47. Neefe, J. R.: Recent Advances in Knowledge of "Virus Hepatitis." *M.Clin. North America, 30*:1407, 1946.

48. Rhodes, A. J., and Van Rooyen, C. E.: *Textbook of Virology,* 2nd Ed. Baltimore, Williams & Wilkins, 1953, p. 291-295.

49. Murray, R.: "Razors and Homologous Serum Hepatitis." *J.A.M.A., 152*:656, 1953.

50. Perkins, J. J.: Unpublished data, 1955.

CHAPTER III

Principles of Steam Sterilization

MOIST HEAT in the form of saturated steam under pressure is the most dependable medium known for the destruction of all forms of microbial life. The bacteria-destroying power is composed of two factors, both of which are essential: moisture and heat. Atmospheric (flowing) steam has no value in surgical sterilization. Boiling water likewise is an inadequate microbicide and its use should be discouraged wherever pressure steam is available. Saturated steam possesses the following characteristics:

ADVANTAGES

1) Rapid heating and rapid penetration of textiles or fabrics.
2) Destroys most resistant bacterial spores in brief interval of exposure.
3) Quality and lethality may be easily controlled for various materials and supplies.

LIMITATIONS

1) Incomplete air elimination from sterilizer depresses temperature and prevents sterilization. Air is a stubborn opponent to the diffusion and expansion of steam.
2) Incorrect operation of sterilizer may result in superheated steam with diminished bactericidal power.
3) Not suitable for sterilization of anhydrous oils, greases, powders, etc.

In order to gain a clear conception of the functions of steam in sterilizing processes as well as an accurate working knowledge of the operation of sterilizers, it is essential to understand the physical and thermal properties underlying the production and control of steam. To the scientist or engineer it may appear superfluous to devote space and attention to the meaning and interpretation of such fundamental terms as heat, temperature, pressure, etc. However, it should be borne in mind that in the broad field of applied sterilization there are today many individuals responsible for the daily operation and care of sterilizers whose limited background of technical training and experience would hardly permit them to qualify as skilled sterilizer technicians. It is to this group primarily that the following details are directed:

HEAT AND TEMPERATURE

The usual conception of heat is that it comprises a basic form of energy produced by the vibratory motion or activity of the molecules of a body or substance. The hotter the substance or the more heat that is added to it, the more vigorous will be the activity of the molecules. Heat itself is not a substance because when it is added to or absorbed by a body there is no increase in weight. In one sense, heat may be likened to water in that it will only flow downhill, or rather, pass from the higher (hotter) range of temperature to the lower or colder level. The transfer of heat, upon which sterilization depends, involves an energy exchange between the sterilizing agent and the external object or receiver of heat. The process of heat transfer from one body to another may be accomplished by either conduction, convection or radiation.

If the transmission of heat from one part of a body to another or from one body to another in intimate contact occurs by molecular impact or agitation the process is termed conduction heating. For example, if one end of a bar of metal is heated, the other end also becomes hot. The molecular agitation set up in the heated end of the bar is transmitted from molecule to molecule until the opposite end is reached. The sterilization of instruments by means of dry heat is also an example of conduction heating.

Convection heating takes place only in liquids and gases. It implies a transference of heat from one point to another by means of a circulation of the liquid or gas itself. When a flask of solution, for example, is heated over a burner, the heated portion or bottom layer expands and rises through the entire volume. The bottom layer is replaced by a colder portion which also becomes heated and rises in its turn. Thus convection currents are set up and the heat is distributed throughout the solution by actual motion within the liquid itself.

The process of heat transfer by radiation involves the passage of heat from one object to another without warming the space between the objects. In other words, the heat is passed by means of a wave motion similar to that of light. In the strict sense, radiant heating is not used for sterilization purposes, although dielectric or induction heating utilizing radio frequency energy is employed to some extent for sanitization purposes in industry.

In distinguishing between heat and temperature, it should be understood that the latter term is used to define the hotness of a mass or body, according to some arbitrarily selected scale such as Fahrenheit or Centigrade. Temperature is not a measure of the quantity or amount of heat contained in a substance, but rather it gives an idea of the intensity or quality of heat present. For example, a glass of water at 140° F. (60° C.) is hotter, or at a higher temperature, than a pail of water at 60° F. (15.6° C.), but it does not contain as much heat because the quantity of heated substance is considerably less.

ATMOSPHERIC PRESSURE AND GAUGE PRESSURE

Since pressure is considered one of the fundamental properties of a working substance, it follows that atmospheric pressure, gauge pressure and vacuum must have a direct bearing on the behavior of a gas, vapor or liquid confined in a sterilizing chamber. Generally speaking, the average person is not inclined to recognize that he is living at the bottom of a great ocean of air which, by virtue of its weight, exerts upon the surface of the earth an enormous pressure of more than 300,000 million tons. The pressure of this great mass of air is commonly referred to as atmospheric or barometric pressure which, simply explained, means the weight of the column of air above the point or place in question.

Atmospheric pressure is known to diminish with elevation above the earth's surface because with increasing altitude there is a lesser quantity of air to exert a downward pressure. Also, atmospheric pressure varies from day to day due to atmospheric conditions, temperature changes, winds, etc. For these reasons, it is necessary to adopt some standard to which all variations of pressure can be referred. The standard accepted for this purpose is the weight of a column of the atmosphere at sea level which has been determined to be 14.7 pounds per square inch at a standard temperature of 32° F. or 0° C. It is also known that a column of atmosphere with pressure equivalent to 14.7 pounds per square inch will balance or support a column of mercury 29.92 inches (760 mm.) high. Since measurements of atmospheric pressure are made by means of a barometer it is customary to express the results in terms of the height (inches or millimeters) of a mercury column rather than in pounds or on a weight basis.

When a gas, vapor or liquid is confined in a container, the instrument commonly used for recording the pressure within the container is a pressure gauge. This device measures the difference between the pressure in the container and the external atmospheric pressure in pounds per square inch. The standard type of low pressure gauge used with steam sterilizers is shown in Figures 25 and 26. This is often referred to as a compound gauge because its construction permits a reading of both pressure in pounds per square inch and vacuum in inches of mercury. In the manufacture of pressure gauges the instruments are usually adjusted to indicate zero pressure at normal atmospheric sea level pressure which in reality is 14.7 pounds per square inch. Practically all steam and pressure gauges are initially set in this manner and the pressures indicated by the instruments are termed gauge pressures.

In scientific and experimental studies another pressure scale is employed. This scale is known as absolute pressure because zero on the scale indicates no pressure at all, or in other words, a perfect vacuum. To obtain a pressure reading relative to the true zero of pressure, the absolute zero, the pressure gauge reading must be added to the atmospheric pressure. This may be written as follows:

Abs. pressure = gauge pressure +14.7 pounds.

Also,

Gauge pressure = abs. pressure –14.7 pounds.

Vacuum gauges indicate the difference, expressed in inches of mercury, between atmospheric pressure and the pressure within the vessel or con-

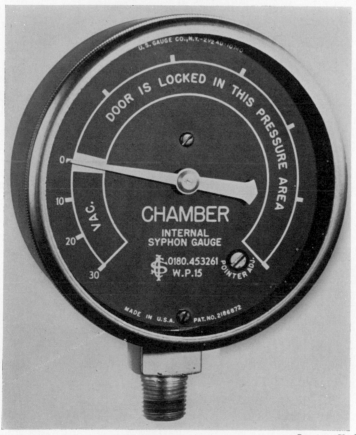

Courtesy U. S. Gauge Co.

Fig. 25. Low pressure gauge used on steam sterilizers. This permits reading of pressure in pounds per square inch and vacuum in inches of mercury.

tainer to which the gauge is attached. For all practical purposes, 2.04 inches height of mercury may be considered equal to a pressure of one pound per square inch. Hence for any reading of the vacuum gauge in inches, G, the absolute pressure for any barometer reading in inches, B, is: $\dfrac{B-G}{2.04}$.

For example, if a vacuum gauge on a sterilizer reads 15 inches and at the same time the barometer reads 29.4 inches of mercury, what would be the absolute pressure in pounds per square inch in the sterilizer?

Using the above formula:

$$\frac{29.4 - 15}{2.04} = 7.0 \text{ lb. per sq. in. abs.}$$

Figure 27 shows the relationship existing between atmospheric, gauge, absolute and partial vacuum pressures.

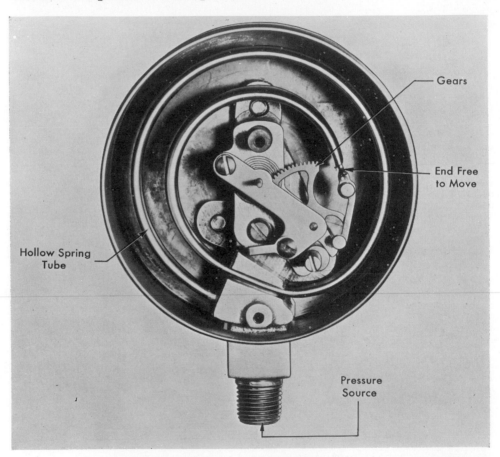

Fig. 26. Interior construction details of pressure gauge used on steam sterilizers. It consists essentially of a coiled brass tube closed at one end. The open end of the tube is connected to the pipe through which the fluid (steam) under pressure is admitted. When pressure is applied the tube tends to straighten out, moving a pointer to which it is connected by means of a gear arrangement.

SATURATED STEAM

Moist heat in the form of saturated steam under pressure is the most dependable medium known for the destruction of all forms of microbial life. Today, in every modern hospital, there may be found a variety of sterilizers or autoclaves, each performing a vital service in protecting the patient against infection, but all are dependent upon the application of certain fundamental principles allied with the use of steam as a sterilizing agent.

Steam is water vapor and, as such, it represents a physical state of water as truly as ice does, but as a gas it may be near or far away from its condensing or liquefying temperature. Saturated steam is water vapor in the

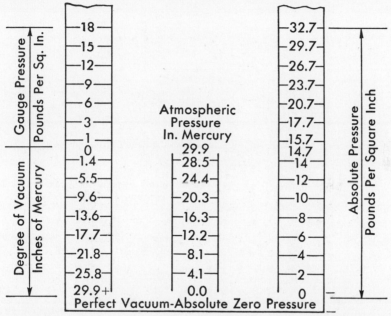

Fig. 27. Numerical relationship between gauge, atmospheric, absolute and partial vacuum pressures.

condition in which it is generated from the water with which it is in contact. Saturated steam cannot undergo a reduction in temperature without a lowering of its pressure, nor can the temperature be increased except when accompanied by a corresponding increase in pressure. Thus given the pressure of steam as it is ordinarily formed its temperature may be considered fixed or given its temperature the pressure may be, of course, as readily deduced, pressure and temperature being convertible terms. Therefore one may speak of saturated steam at a certain temperature or at a certain pressure.

It is a misnomer to state that "dry saturated steam" contains no water because all steam is a physical state of water. From a practical standpoint, saturated steam is always wet to at least some small degree as the result of some quantity of unvaporized water held in suspension or mechanically entrained with the steam. Dry saturated steam is a theoretical line of demarcation between the wet saturated and superheated steam phases. For sterilization purposes steam under pressure is used rather than atmospheric or flowing steam for the sole purpose of attaining higher temperatures. Pressure of itself has nothing whatsoever to do with the microbicidal

TABLE 6

SCALE OF PRESSURES AND EQUIVALENT TEMPERATURES OF SATURATED
STEAM FOR STERILIZATION PURPOSES

(From Perkins[1])

Gauge	Pounds Pressure Absolute	Temperature Degrees F	Degrees C	Sterilizing Application
80.3	95	324.1	162.2	
75.3	90	320.3	160.1→	Maximum pressure in steam supply lines.
70.3	85	316.3	158.0	(For pressure sterilizers)
65.3	80	312.0	155.6	
60.3	75	307.6	153.0	
55.3	70	302.9	150.6 →	Ideal pressure in steam supply lines.
50.3	65	298.0	147.8	
45.3	60	292.7	144.8	
40.3	55	287.1	141.9 →	Minimum pressure in steam supply lines.
				(For pressure sterilizers)
35.3	50	281.0	138.3	
30.3	45	274.4	134.6	
27.3	42	270.2	132.3 →	Emergency (high-speed) sterilization of instruments
25.3	40	267.3	130.7	
20.3	35	259.3	126.2	
19.3	34	257.6	125.3	
18.3	33	255.8	124.2	
17.3	32	254.1	123.4	Sterilization of hospital supplies—surgical instruments, dressings, solutions, etc.
16.3	31	252.2	122.3	
15.3	30	250.3	121.2	Sterilization of laboratory supplies. Commercial sterilization processes.
14.3	29	248.4	120.3	
12.3	27	244.4	118.0	
10.3	25	240.1	115.6 →	Sterilization of laboratory supplies. Commercial sterilization processes.
8.3	23	235.5	113.0	
6.3	21	230.6	110.3 →	Terminal heating of infant formulas.
4.3	19	225.2	107.1	
2.3	17	219.4	104.2	
0.0	14.70	212.0	100.0	Sanitization of instruments & utensils. Terminal heating of infant formulas. Streaming steam sterilization. Water boils @ sea level, New York City.
	14.13	210.0	98.8	Water boils @ altitude 1025 ft., Omaha, Nebr.
	13.03	206.0	96.6	Water boils @ altitude 3115 ft., Calgary, Alta.
	12.01	202.0	94.4	Water boils @ altitude 5225 ft., Denver, Colo.
	11.06	198.0	92.2	Water boils @ altitude 7381 ft., Laramie, Wyo.
	10.40	195.0	90.5	Water boils @ altitude 9000 ft., Quito, Ecuador
	8.95	188.0	86.6	Water boils @ altitude 12,700 ft., LaPaz, Bolivia

properties of steam. A scale of pressures and equivalent temperatures of saturated steam as employed for sterilization purposes is given in Table 6. Saturated steam at a temperature of 250°-254° F. (121°-123° C.) will destroy the most resistant forms of microbial life in a brief interval of exposure. These temperatures are not destructive of most materials and supplies and the necessary period of exposure is well within practicable limits.

SUPERHEATED STEAM

If saturated steam at any given temperature is subjected to a higher temperature, as for instance by passing it over heated surfaces or coils, it becomes superheated steam. By this process the steam is literally dried out and the peculiar advantages of a high moisture content, so necessary to sterilization, are dissipated. The properties of superheated steam approximate those of a perfect gas rather than of a vapor. It behaves much like dry hot air and takes up water with avidity. If superheated steam is used for sterilization purposes there is not only the likelihood of overheating the supplies, the abstraction of normal residual moisture from materials such as textiles or fabrics resulting in a reduction of tensile strength and premature disintegration, but also the ever-present danger of ineffective sterilization. With every degree of superheat added to steam its bactericidal properties are reduced until temperatures are attained which destroy bacteria by actual burning or oxidation, as occurs in the dry heat or hot air sterilizer.

HOW TO DETERMINE THE ULTIMATE TEMPERATURE OF SATURATED STEAM OR AIR-STEAM MIXTURES AT ANY PRESSURE

By consulting steam tables in engineers' handbooks, the temperature of pure saturated steam at various pressures may be determined. These steam tables can also be used to determine the ultimate temperature of any known mixture of steam and air at any gauge pressure. Air-steam mixtures do not develop the same temperatures characteristic of saturated steam at the same pressures—a fact rarely appreciated by those responsible for sterilizing technics. As a consequence, this condition is a contributing factor to many failures encountered in sterilizing processes. To determine the ultimate temperature of a known mixture of steam and air, apply the following formula:

$$Pl = Po - \left(\frac{30-V}{2} \right) \text{ (From Dalton's Law of Gaseous Pressures)}$$

in which

Pl = absolute pressure in pounds per square inch, the temperature of which is the desired factor. (Determine this by reference to steam tables.)
Po = absolute pressure applied to the sterilizing chamber = gauge pressure plus 14.7 pounds.
V = the degree of vacuum applied to the sterilizing chamber in inches of mercury.

The average operator of sterilizers need not make use of the above formula for other than a proper mathematical background for basic principles upon which sterilization depends. The actual temperatures attained in the sterilizer under ordinary conditions of proper and improper usage are given in Table 7.

REMOVAL OF AIR FROM STERILIZER BY MEANS OF PARTIAL VACUUM

The complete evacuation of air from a vessel or chamber defines a perfect vacuum. This is measured in terms of the height of a column of mer-

TABLE 7
STERILIZER TEMPERATURES WITH VARIOUS DEGREES OF AIR DISCHARGE

Gauge Pressure Pounds	Sat'd Steam Complete Air Discharge		Two-thirds Air Discharge (20" Vacuum)		One-half Air Discharge (15" Vacuum)		One-third Air Discharge (10" Vacuum)		No Air Discharge	
	°C	°F	°C	°F	°C	°F	°C	°F	°C	°F
5	109	228	100	212	94	202	90	193	72	162
10	115	240	109	228	105	220	100	212	90	193
15	121	250	115	240	112	234	109	228	100	212
20	126	259	121	250	118	245	115	240	109	228
25	130	267	126	259	124	254	121	250	115	240
30	135	275	130	267	128	263	126	259	121	250

cury which will be sustained under that condition. This column of mercury is 30 inches high. The combination vacuum-pressure gauges commonly used, as shown in Figure 25, are graduated for measurement of the degree of vacuum to this scale, in inches of mercury.

The usual vacuum type sterilizer is equipped with an ejector valve by means of which a maximum of about 10 inches vacuum can be attained. Occasionally a more powerful ejector is capable of creating a 15-inch vacuum, and in rare cases a 20-inch vacuum can be produced. Operating directions accompanying the vacuum type sterilizers usually instruct the operator to draw a partial vacuum of 10 to 15 inches as the initial step in sterilization. Such a procedure is useless because only one-third to one-half of the air is removed from the chamber and the residual amount is sufficient to seriously retard or prevent the attainment of proper temperature required for sterilization.

Admittedly there has been a great deal of misunderstanding relative to vacuum operation of sterilizers in the past. Operators have been led to believe that "vacuum" plays some mysterious part in sterilizing—that it is difficult to sterilize except by first creating some relatively minor degree of vacuum in the chamber. From the explanation given above it may be observed that a 10-inch vacuum means 10/30 of a perfect vacuum, or in other words the exhaust of only one-third of the air. A 15-inch vacuum exhausts one-half and a 20-inch vacuum two-thirds of the air. The temperatures resulting from such incomplete evacuation of air are not suitable for depend-

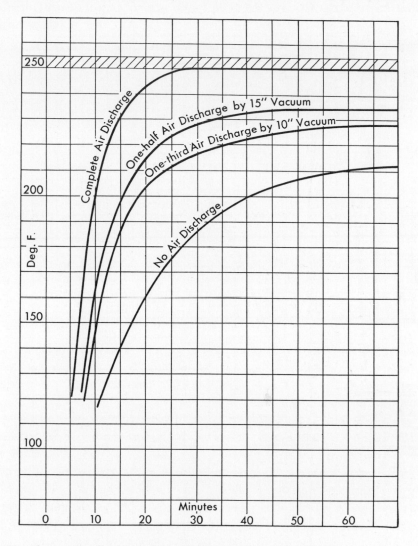

Fig. 28. The temperatures resulting from complete and partial air discharge from a sterilizing chamber operated at 15 pounds pressure.

able sterilization as indicated by the data in Table 7, and the temperature curves in Figure 28.

THE EFFECT OF GRAVITY ON AIR-STEAM MIXTURES IN A STERILIZING CHAMBER

When steam is admitted to a sterilizing chamber the relatively cool air present is much heavier than the steam at the normal sterilizing temperature. Steam has a density of 0.07 pounds per cu. ft. as compared with 0.12 for air under the same pressure and temperature and they show a marked disinclination to mix. This means that when steam is forced by pressure

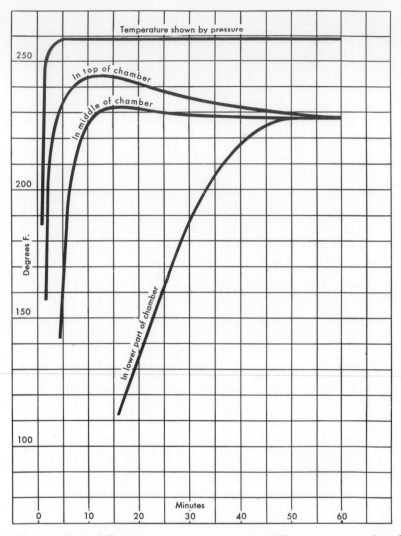

Fig. 29. These radical differences in temperature for different areas in the chamber are representative of a sterilizer from which air has not been discharged. Measurements were made with potentiometer and three thermocouples, one located near the top, the second in the middle and the third close to the bottom of the chamber.

into a sterilizing chamber containing air, the steam will literally float to the top of the chamber, compressing the air at the bottom. It is known, however, that the air and steam will eventually mix, resulting in a uniform gas made up of steam and air, in which a part of the heat contained in the steam will have been absorbed by the air.

This mixing process which results after a long period of time in a uniform temperature throughout the chamber is a most uncertain condition. The period required for this mixture to occur is affected materially by the character of the load and under no condition can it ever be determined precisely except by actual temperature measurements. However, the important details for consideration are:

1) The presence of air greatly reduces the ultimate temperature of the steam below that of pure saturated steam at the pressure maintained.

2) Throughout the normal period of sterilization, the temperatures in the lower areas of the chamber will be substantially lower than in the upper areas, due to differences in specific gravities and reluctance of steam and air to mix.

This latter fact accounts for radically misleading tests which are often noted in an attempt to prove the adequacy of a sterilizing process. For example, a culture test consisting of a sample of contaminated material placed in the upper part of a sterilizing chamber from which very little air has been removed will frequently show complete sterilization because the test material will have been subjected, for at least a brief interval of time, to nearly pure saturated steam at the operating pressure. Similarly, sterilization indicators located in the upper part of a poorly air-evacuated chamber will often incorrectly indicate sterilizing conditions. Tests made in imperfectly air-evacuated chambers, at the bottom, will invariably show failure in any reasonable period of exposure.

To further illustrate the importance of gravity or stratification of air-steam mixtures in a sterilizing chamber, the reader's attention is called to the temperature curves, Figure 29. They demonstrate effectively the differences in temperature encountered in different areas of a sterilizer from which air has not been evacuated. It is easily conceivable that tests made in the upper portions of the load might have indicated satisfactory conditions for sterilization, but it is certain that any test made in the lower areas must have failed.

HOW STEAM STERILIZATION IS ACCOMPLISHED

Steam sterilization as normally conducted in the autoclave is a product of heat plus moisture in which the moisture factor plays an exceedingly important part. It is generally accepted that the thermal destruction of microorganisms closely parallels the heat coagulation of proteins. Various workers who have investigated this phenomenon have concluded that death occurs as the result of the heat denaturation of the proteins which make up the bacterial cell. When moisture is present this coagulation process takes place at relatively low temperatures but when moisture is absent a considerably higher temperature is required for bacterial destruction.

Steam possesses the singular property of being able to heat materials, and particularly to permeate porous substances by the relatively rapid process of condensation, as opposed to the very slow process of heat absorption as in the case of hot air or any other gas used as the heating medium. Steam gives up its heat in sterilizing only by the process of condensing back into the water from which it came. Specifically this means that every fibre or particle of any porous article undergoing sterilization will abstract, absorb or contain a quantity of moisture from the steam in exact proportion to the amount of heat absorbed by the article. Knowledge of this principle is of great importance to the student because it explains in many instances how various supplies should be prepared for steam sterilization, i.e., an arrangement of the materials that will provide for thorough, rapid and complete permeation with steam. If the steam can permeate any mass of materials such as gowns, sheets, towels or other porous supplies, it will heat that mass through condensation and leave in it the finely dispersed moisture required for sterilization.

The condensation process of heating makes use of the latent heat of steam. The heat required to convert a unit mass of water into steam at the same temperature is called the latent heat of vaporization of water or simply the latent heat of steam. For example: Heating one pound of water from room temperature of 70° F. and converting it into steam at 212° F. requires first the expenditure of $(212°–70°) = 142$ heat units, to bring the temperature of the water to 212° F. Then there must be added for each pound of water 970 heat units to convert that pound of water at 212° F. into steam at 212° F. This factor of 970 heat units is known as latent heat. Then to heat each pound of steam at 212° F. into steam at 250° F. (15 pounds gauge pressure), the normal sterilizing range, requires only 13.5 heat units. It is obvious that a high percentage of the energy stored in steam, actually over 80 per cent, is accounted for in the latent heat.

In abstracting heat from steam, for every pound that is condensed into water, surrounding objects absorb that latent heat. This feature is highly important in its application to the permeation of dry goods, fabrics or textiles. As steam contacts the outer layer of fabric, the cooler substance immediately causes a film of steam to condense, leaving in the fabric a minute amount of water, that moisture so necessary for the destruction of microbial life. The next film of steam immediately fills the space created by the volume collapse of the previous film (99 per cent decrease in volume), but it does not condense in the outer layer; rather it passes through and attacks the second layer of fabric—condenses and heats it. So on until the entire mass of fabric has been heated, after which the package will contain an amount of moisture (condensate) exactly equivalent to the amount of heat abstracted from the steam. Continuation of the process will cause no further condensation, but the temperature of the fabric will remain constant at the temperature of the surrounding steam.

Since all steam sterilization is based upon "direct steam contact," it follows that the same process of condensation and heating applies to instruments, utensils or other articles undergoing surface sterilization. With these supplies there is no permeation of steam through the metal, the object being only to heat and sterilize the surface. In this case the cold metal condenses the steam until the article is heated to the temperature of the steam.

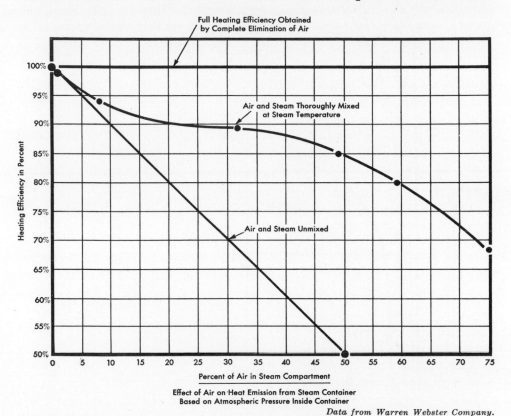

Data from Warren Webster Company.

Fig. 30. The effect of air on the heating efficiency of a steam chamber, based on atmospheric pressure inside chamber.

Throughout sterilization the metal surfaces are bathed with an abundance of moisture as compared with porous fabrics, which greatly facilitates sterilization. Because of the rapid heating effect and the abundance of moisture, it becomes possible to prescribe a shorter exposure period for instruments than for fabrics which require time for permeation.

THE ADVERSE EFFECTS OF AIR UPON THE PENETRATING POWER OF STEAM

It has been explained how steam heats porous materials by its peculiar process of condensation. The great opponent to the diffusion of steam is air, and all fabrics as they are placed in the sterilizer have their interstices filled with air at the surrounding temperature and at atmospheric pressure. Unless the steam is able to displace this air it cannot permeate the material

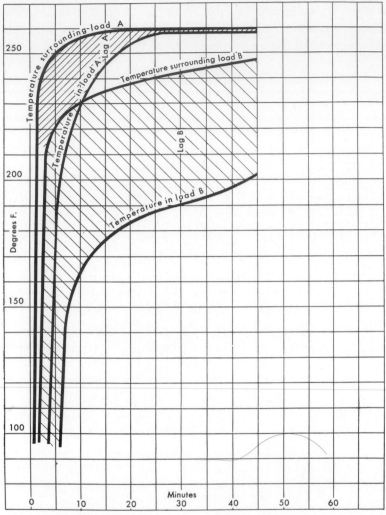

Fig. 31. These temperature curves are typical of the lag in steam penetration to be expected in a sterilizer from which air has not been discharged. The load consisted of a large package of Hampton pads. Pressure was maintained at 20 pounds. When the air was completely discharged from the chamber the temperature in the package [Lag A] rapidly approached that of the surrounding steam [Load A]. When only a small amount of air was discharged, the temperature in the package lagged approximately 50°F. [Lag B] that of the surrounding steam [Load B] throughout a 45-minute exposure.

and its behavior will then be similar to that of hot air under the same operating pressure. When air is mixed with the steam, obviously only the steam content of the mixture heats by the condensing process. The air has no useful penetrating power. The heating or penetrating power of the mixture is reduced in accordance with the proportion of air present. This point is illustrated graphically in Figure 30.

If the sterilizing chamber is well exhausted of air so that the free spaces all about the load are promptly filled with pure steam, then the air pockets within a bulky package of fabrics will dissipate rapidly by gravity to the bottom of the chamber from which a correctly designed gravity discharge system will permit escape. If, however, the chamber has not been evacuated of air, then there will be no material difference in density between the air pockets within the package and the air which has gravitated to the areas below the package. These air pockets will therefore remain in the load and greatly retard the entrance of steam.

The temperature curves shown in Figure 31 illustrate this point rather convincingly. Also, they further emphasize the necessity for placing any sterilization indicator in the center of the package undergoing study rather than near the surface.

The presence of air in the sterilizer is a grave handicap to effective sterilization for several reasons; first, because it reduces the ultimate possible temperature of steam at any pressure; second, because of reluctance of steam and air to mix, resulting in great variations in temperature in various parts of the chamber; third, the ultimate reduced temperature can be attained only after prolonged periods of exposure; finally, because of its adverse effect upon steam penetration of porous supplies.

AUTOMATIC AIR ELIMINATION FROM STERILIZING CHAMBERS

The first essential requirement for an efficient steam sterilizer is that some means must be provided for the automatic removal of air and condensate from the chamber without reliance upon skillful manipulation of hand valves or any other precise and confining attention to the sterilizer. To this end, it is generally true that all modern sterilizers are equipped with a thermostatic valve for the automatic control of air and condensate discharge from such chambers, with excellent results. Prior to the introduction of thermostatic valves on sterilizers it was necessary to control the air and condensate discharge by hand regulation of a drainage valve located near the front bottom of the sterilizing chamber. The obvious fault of that system was the necessity for complete reliance upon the individual, the close attention required, and the degree of safety being largely a matter of the care and skill of the operator.

Thermostatic valves are of the general classification commonly known as steam traps. They contain flexible metallic elements filled with a volatile liquid which expands under heat or contracts when cool, opening or closing the discharge orifice of the valve. A sectional diagram depicting the functional parts of a thermostatic valve is given in Figure 32. It should not be assumed that the usual steam trap, available from the nearest supply store, can be applied satisfactorily for this delicate operation of automatic air removal. The discharge orifice of the usual steam trap is so small that an abnormal period of time is required to evacuate a sterilizing chamber. Still more objectionable is the fact that some of these traps are designed to shut off before air discharge is complete.

The more sensitive thermostatic valves, specially designed for use with sterilizers, permit rapid and complete evacuation of air. The proper appli-

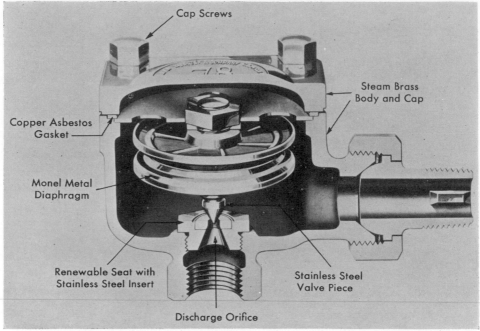

Courtesy Warren Webster Co.

Fig. 32. Sectional diagram of thermostatic valve used on steam sterilizers.

cation of such valves affords the opportunity for the automatic discharge of all air from the sterilizing chamber, so that the maximum possible temperature throughout the chamber can be attained quickly. Fortunately these better grades of valves are fairly dependable, not readily subject to structural changes in use which interfere with their performance. The best of them, however, do fatigue after long service and it is always necessary to check their performance to avoid the hazards of attempted sterilization with a chamber badly clogged with air. No valve will remain permanently accurate.

METHOD FOR DETERMINING THE EFFECTIVENESS OF AIR DISCHARGE FROM STERILIZING CHAMBER

From the foregoing the reader will have observed that for safe operation some dependable method must be adopted for determining the degree of air discharge from a sterilizing chamber. That has now been made possible by the simple method of measuring the temperature in the chamber discharge line. It has been shown that air or any mixture of steam and air will gravitate to the lower areas of the chamber. It follows as an obvious physical fact that if the discharge line is clogged or if the thermostatic valve is not working properly there will be no material advance in temperature in the discharge line, but if the line is free, the temperature will advance after the air has been eliminated and replaced by steam to the temperature of the steam. Only when this has occurred will the indicated temperature advance to the sterilizing range. Even then this temperature will always lag one to two degrees behind the actual temperature of the medium surrounding the load. The thermometer reading will be, without exception, a measurement of the coldest medium within the sterilizing chamber. A partial clogging of the system will simply retard the movement or clearance of air, all of which will be indicated by the thermometer.

At this point the student might well pose the question as to why is it not desirable to measure temperature within the sterilizing chamber instead of in the discharge system. The purpose is, to measure the effectiveness of air discharge which under all conditions is the fundamental requirement, and to indicate promptly if there is an interruption which must be cleared. A thermometer bulb placed at any fixed point within the sterilizing chamber would measure merely the temperature at that point. It would also reflect the temperature of circulating currents of steam and would not be so clearly indicative of the condition which the operator needs to know. In addition, the bulb of such a thermometer would necessarily be installed permanently at some point close to the steam jacket wall, out of the way of the load—giving free access to the chamber. In this position, the thermometer bulb would always respond to some extent to the temperature of the hot steam jacket surrounding the chamber.

STERILIZING CONDITIONS ARE BASED UPON TEMPERATURE RATHER THAN PRESSURE

In spite of all that has been written on this subject during the last fifty years the tendency still prevails to think of steam sterilization in terms of pressure rather than temperature. Moist heat is the sterilizing agent. Pressure is only incidentally significant. The common practice of measuring the sterilizing period from the instant that the pressure gauge shows 15 pounds, perhaps 20 pounds, with little regard for anything else, should definitely be discouraged. Often such observations are made with sterilizers from which little air has been exhausted.

Under the presently established system of effective steam sterilization the period of exposure is measured, without immediate regard for pressure, from the instant that the thermometer in the discharge line shows temperature of 250° F. (the equivalent of saturated steam at 15 pounds gauge pressure), the minimum range considered safe for sterilization. This indication also means that the temperature of the steam surrounding the load will range from one to two degrees higher in every part of the chamber.

It is obvious, of course, that pressure must be regulated at the prescribed range in order that suitable temperature can be attained, and for each kind of heat (steam, electricity or gas) it is a simple matter to provide automatic pressure regulation about which the operator of the sterilizer need not be greatly concerned. The immediate and constant interest of the operator should be centered in the maintenance of "discharge line temperature" which is indicative of these essential factors:

1) That the air discharge system is or is not functioning properly.

2) Measurement of the temperature of the coldest medium surrounding the load—maintaining that temperature within the prescribed safe range.

THE MOST PRACTICABLE RANGE OF STEAM PRESSURE FOR STERILIZERS

Due to the deficiencies of many sterilizers with respect to the attainment of sterilizing temperature in a brief interval of time, there exists an all too prevalent tendency to increase the operating pressure range and the periods of exposure beyond those actually needed. Whereas the pressure carried for the sterilization of surgical supplies in the average hospital sterilizer is usually in the range of 15-20 pounds, it is also known that in more than a few instances considerably higher pressures are employed, notwithstanding the fact that the sterilizers themselves were not designed for use with steam pressures greater than 20 pounds gauge. In the sterilization of heat sensitive supplies, rubber gloves and glucose solutions particularly, temperatures higher than those of pure steam at 15-17 pounds are needlessly destructive. It is also true that various fabrics show a greater rate of deterioration when sterilized repeatedly under steam pressures higher than the optimum range.

When pressure sterilizers are used in areas or localities of high altitude, it becomes necessary to employ proportionally greater steam pressures in order to attain the minimum standard range of temperature required for sterilization, namely, 250-254° F. The data given in Table 8 clearly shows that the boiling point of water varies with the barometric pressure at various altitudes. Hence it becomes necessary to compensate for this reduction in temperature by increasing the pressure when steam is admitted to a sterilizing chamber; otherwise the minimum standard range of temperature could not be maintained at high altitudes. As an approximation, the boiling point of water is reduced 2° F. (1.1° C.) for each 1000 feet increase in altitude above sea level. From the figures given in the last column of

Table 8 it may also be observed that for each 1000 feet elevation above sea level the pressure in the sterilizing chamber should be increased approximately 0.5 pound per square inch gauge. When these factors are taken into consideration there is little excuse for not operating surgical supply steri-

TABLE 8

Boiling Point Water °F.	Altitude Above Sea Level Feet	Atmos. Pressure Lbs./Sq. In.	Barometer Reduced to 32° F. Inches	Steam Pressure Required Lbs./Sq. In. Gauge
212	Sea Level	14.7	29.9	15-17
210	1025	14.1	28.7	15.6-17.6
208	2063	13.5	27.6	16.1-18.1
206	3115	13.0	26.5	16.7-18.7
204	4169	12.5	25.4	17.2-19.2
202	5225	12.0	24.4	17.7-19.7
200	6304	11.5	23.4	18.2-20.2
198	7381	11.0	22.5	18.7-20.7
196	8481	10.6	21.6	19.1-21.1
194	9579	10.1	20.7	19.6-21.6
192	10685	9.7	19.8	20.0-22.0
190	11799	9.3	19.0	20.4-22.4
188	12934	8.9	18.2	20.8-22.8

lizers under proper physical conditions to assure the maintenance of minimum standards for sterilization.

This chapter has dealt with the basic principles or engineering fundamentals of pressure steam sterilization. The factors discussed are those which govern precise, dependable performance. There are other factors equally as important relating to the preparation of materials for sterilization and the loading of supplies in the sterilizer. Without due regard for these elements the sterilization process in the most perfect of sterilizers can easily remain uncertain.

REFERENCES

1. PERKINS, J. J.: Bacteriological and Surgical Sterilization by Heat. From Reddish, G. F.: *Antiseptics, Disinfectants, Fungicides, Chemical and Physical Sterilization*, Philadelphia, Lea & Febiger, 1954, p. 664

CHAPTER IV

Minimum Standards for Sterilization

DOWN THROUGH the years various standards have been proposed and established for the sterilization of surgical supplies. Certain of these standards were obviously based upon expediency, taking into consideration the often extreme inaccuracies resulting from the use of highly inefficient sterilizers. For many years the common practice for sterilizing bulk loads of supplies was "20 pounds pressure for 1 hour." This was a purely arbitrary rule which had little or no scientific background, for which apparently no one could formulate a logical excuse or reason—except in average usage it seemed to suffice. It must be remembered, however, that the old style sterilizers were operated with "pressure" as the sole indication of regulation. There was no means for measuring the degree of air evacuation, other than the vacuum gauge, and there was no means for measuring the temperature developed by the steam in the chamber.

With the introduction of temperature control for sterilizers which occurred in 1933, it became immediately apparent that detailed investigations were needed to more clearly define minimum requirements and exposure periods for adequate sterilization without waste of time and undue destruction of fabrics from oversterilization. W. B. Underwood,[1] a leading investigator in the field of sterilization, was largely responsible for the initial attack on this problem. He frequently demonstrated by means of potentiometer tests on sterilizers in daily use in hospitals that far better sterilizing influence in 30 minutes' exposure could be attained with a temperature-controlled sterilizer than was shown in routine performance under pressure control in one full hour exposure. The results of these early studies by Underwood are shown in Figure 33. That such hazardous conditions continue to exist through the use of highly inefficient sterilizers has recently been the subject of an investigation by the Advisory Committee on Sterilization for Queensland hospitals.[2]

If, in using the modern surgical supply sterilizers, we continue to sterilize bulk loads at 20 pounds pressure for 1 hour, the common practice under the older system, many of the supplies such as textiles and rubber goods will show marked evidence of premature destruction. In addition, a great amount of time will be literally wasted, thereby affecting the daily output of the sterilizers. It is unwise to establish any standard for surgical sterilization without due regard for the economic factors involved. A comparison between the old style pressure-controlled sterilizer and the modern (automatic) temperature-controlled sterilizer may be likened to the prescribing of some drug at known concentration as opposed to the use of the same

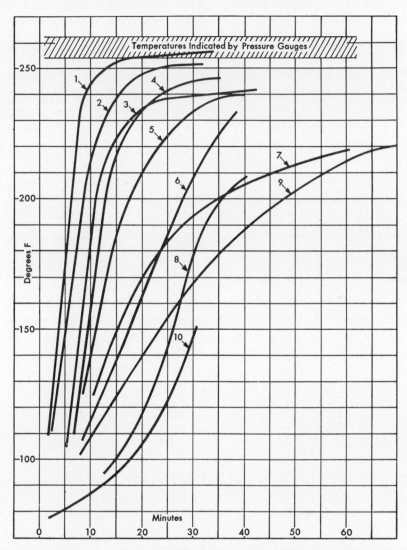

Fig. 33. These curves record the actual temperatures attained within the loads of ten surgical supply sterilizers found in six hospitals. The sterilizers were operated under pressures of 17-22 pounds, with no means of measuring the degree of air elimination or the true temperatures developed. The shaded area denotes the temperatures which were indicated by the pressure gauges for saturated steam.

drug of unknown dilution. In the temperature-controlled sterilizer steam of maximum lethal effect is employed, but with any pressure-controlled sterilizer it is always uncertain as to the degree that the steam may have been diluted with air.

MINIMUM REQUIREMENTS OF TIME AND TEMPERATURE

One of the most difficult problems encountered in attempting to define safe sterilization is to determine from reliable data the minimum time-temperature relationship needed to insure destruction of the most resistant forms of microbial life. Unless this relationship can be stated positively, it is useless to attempt to discuss the subject intelligently or to make specific recommendations on the preparation and sterilization of various materials and supplies. Much of the information written on the subject is either vague in meaning, inconclusive or avoids the issue entirely. Certain of the standards proposed for surgical sterilization have been based upon a time-temperature relationship adequate for the destruction of pathogenic spores but not entirely adequate for the destruction of nonpathogenic spore-bearing organisms. Others propose the use of a time and temperature sufficiently great to cause unnecessary destruction of materials and to be wasteful of time and fuel.

In establishing minimum standards for surgical sterilization, careful attention must be given to the prescribing of exposure periods for the various types of loads that will insure a time-temperature relationship adequate for the destruction of the most resistant forms of microbial life. Any exposure period that is selective in its lethality to microorganisms is not in keeping with the concept of absolute sterility—the goal of all surgical sterilization. In other words, it should be expedient always to prescribe a performance which carries a reasonable factor of safety in terms of temperature or time or both, based upon reliable experimental data relating to the destruction of the pathogenic spores, but also great enough to provide for the destruction of the still more resistant nonpathogenic spore-bearing organisms.

In developing a safe minimum standard for surgical sterilization, several workers have proposed the use of garden soil which contains a variety of heat resistant aerobic and anaerobic spore-bearing and nonspore-bearing organisms as a control. Walbum,[3] for example, in using soil as a control in the steam sterilization of supplies, gives the following times and temperatures as necessary for sterilization of materials loaded in the autoclave:

> 222.8° F. (106° C.) .... 4-5 hours
> 233.6° F. (112° C.) .... 1 hour
> 249.8° F. (121° C.) .... 30 minutes
> 273.2° F. (134° C.) .... 10 minutes
> 291.2° F. (144° C.) .... 5 minutes

In a similar study, Ecker[4] determined that one-gram samples of air dried and powdered garden soil inserted in the center of laparotomy sets, and maternity supplies, were found to be sterile after exposure at 240° F. (116°

C.) in the autoclave for periods of 60, 45, 30 and 15 minutes. When samples of the same soil were placed in carefully packed dressing drums it was found that an exposure of 45 minutes at 240° F. (116° C.) was necessary for sterilization. Ecker also found in a long series of experiments that the spores of pathogenic anaerobes are destroyed at 240° F. (116° C.) for 15 to 20 minutes, whereas a temperature of 250° F. (121° C.) for 30 minutes is sufficient to destroy the highly resistant nonpathogenic spore-bearing organisms of garden soil. The spores of *Cl. novyi* survived 5 minutes at 230° F. (110° C.) but were destroyed in 10 minutes at this temperature. The spores of *Cl. welchii* survived exposure of 15 minutes at 215° F. (101.7° C.) but were destroyed at 220° F. (104° C.) in 5 minutes. Spores of *B. subtilis* were killed at 215° F. (101.7° C.) in 10 minutes. These results relating especially to the resistance of soil seem to agree with the recent work of Bang and Dalsgaard,[5] who observed that when garden soil was autoclaved at 248° F. (120° C.) for 20 minutes effective sterilization took place, but when heated for only 10 minutes the bacterial content was 200,000 organisms per gram of soil.

In an attempt to accurately define the minimum limits of saturated steam temperature requirements for surgical sterilization, Underwood[6] conducted a long series of tests by planting dried spores of *Cl. welchii* and *B. subtilis* in gauze packs, approximating actual conditions of surgical sterilization. His findings revealed that an exposure period of 5 minutes to saturated steam at 225° F. (107° C.) gave evidence of sterility in all test packs upon incubation of the cultures. These data were apparently confirmed by the work of Ecker, referred to above.

Walter[7] has made the recommendation that 13 minutes' direct exposure to saturated steam at 250° F. (121° C.) is a safe minimum standard for surgical sterilization. This time and temperature conform closely to the thermal death time of the most resistant bacterial spores, and in the opinion of this writer it represents one of the safest and most practical standards that has yet been developed for reliable routine sterilization.

Generally speaking, authorities are in agreement that in direct contact with saturated steam at a temperature of 250° F. (121° C.), a period of 5 to 10 minutes is sufficient to insure destruction of most resistant forms of microbial life. (See Table 5, page 42.) However, to define minimum standards of time and temperature required for steam sterilization of the wide variety of surgical supplies used in hospitals today is a difficult matter. The time-temperature relationship selected must not only be bacteriologically safe, but it must also permit the prescribing of practical exposure periods for the various supplies, including reasonable margins of safety, with due regard for economic factors. On the basis of carefully conducted studies strengthened by experience in many hospitals and laboratories, it has been shown that minimum standards of time and temperature substan-

tially greater or less than the following are either incompatible with modern
sterilizer design (requiring steam pressure in excess of maximum operating
pressure) and unnecessarily destructive of materials or unsafe from the
standpoint of effective sterilization:

° F.	° C.	Time (Minutes)
270	132	2
257	125	8
250	121	12
245	118	18
240	116	30

*The times and temperatures given above do not denote prescribed expo-
sure periods for the sterilization of the various kinds of surgical supplies.*
Rather, they indicate the absolute minimum standards of time and temperature to be maintained throughout all portions of a load in direct contact with saturated steam in order to accomplish effective sterilization. They
do not provide the additional time factor required for steam penetration
of porous supplies such as fabrics nor do they attempt to compensate for
the rate of heat transfer through solution containers.

DEFINING THE PROPER RANGE OF TEMPERATURE AND PRESSURE

In establishing precise standards for surgical sterilization, it becomes
necessary to define the most suitable range of temperature and pressure
for the sterilization of all types of supplies. This means that we must pre-
determine and measure within fairly close limits the quality of steam maintained in the sterilizer, to the end that any sterilizing process can be reproduced repeatedly, with the least possible variation. With the one exception
of the high-speed (emergency) sterilization of instruments, there is little
justification for maintaining steam temperature higher than 250°-254° F.
(121°-123° C.), equivalent to 15-17 pounds pressure, because sterilization
normally occurs within a brief period at this range. Another reason for
limiting the temperature to this range is that 250° F. (121° C.) may be
considered as the critical temperature for most surgical supplies. Exposure
to temperature substantially beyond this range results in more or less rapid
deterioration of materials, such as textiles, rubber goods, etc., not to mention the needless waste of fuel. Discolored muslin wrappers, brownish in
appearance, are many times the direct indication of oversterilization, a
detail of unnecessary expense to the hospital.

The use of one range of pressure and temperature is a thoroughly logical
procedure. With modern sterilizing equipment featuring automatic control of pressure, it is normally not difficult to maintain the prescribed range

with a total variation of no more than 1-2 pounds. There is the mistaken supposition that steam at 20-22 pounds pressure permeates (heats) the load much faster than steam at 15-17 pounds pressure. To be sure, the higher pressure will result in a correspondingly higher temperature in any modern sterilizer, but the rate of heating to the desired range of 250°-254° F. (121°-123° C.) is not sufficiently greater to justify serious consideration. Furthermore, most sterilizers today are designed for a maximum operating pressure in jacket and chamber of 20 pounds per square inch. To meet the requirements of standard engineering (ASME Code) practice, this pressure permits the setting of the safety (blow-off) valve at no more than 10 per cent higher pressure than the maximum design pressure of the sterilizer. For this reason, it is obvious that the average sterilizer should not be operated at a pressure much greater than 19 pounds if the proper tolerance is to be maintained between maximum jacket pressure and the point of blow-off of the safety valve.

Experience has long since demonstrated the inconsistency and impracticability of using one range of temperature for one class of supplies and another range for some other class, because presumably the same organisms may be encountered in any of the supplies. The most practical reason for one fixed range of temperature and pressure for all supplies is the ability to standardize procedures, to have all pressure sterilizers controlled in exactly the same manner. In many hospitals this has been done most effectively and to the marked advantage of the institutions.

STANDARDIZATION OF STERILIZING TECHNICS

. . . the primary requisite for reliable routine steam sterilization. This can be accomplished through the applied integration of four factors, namely: 1) Regulation of the sterilizer so as to maintain temperature of 250°-254° F. (121°-123° C.); 2) correct methods of preliminary cleaning, arranging and packaging of supplies to insure direct steam contact; 3) proper loading of sterilizer; and 4) adequate exposure period that will provide for complete penetration of the load and insure destruction of microbial life with a liberal margin of safety.

Developments of the past twenty years have provided, in the modern (automatically-controlled) pressure sterilizer, a precision instrument, but its value will be minimized or perhaps lost altogether unless hospitals cooperate to the extent of prescribing and maintaining equally high standards with respect to preparation of materials and supervision of loading methods. In the standardization of sterilizing technics there is no substitute for intelligent, painstaking supervision.

Of the various factors upon which effective sterilization of surgical supplies depends there is no one more important than the exposure period. This does not mean that other factors are less important, but rather that for every item undergoing sterilization there is a minimum period of exposure based upon adherence to a specific procedure for the preliminary preparation of the item, the method of packaging or wrapping and the manner of placing the item in the sterilizer. Unless the principles of correct technique are rigidly enforced the exposure period becomes little more than an attempt toward sterilization. With intelligent application of these requirements the following exposure periods at 250°-254° F. (121°-123° C.) provide minimum time for heat penetration and sterilization:

	Minutes
Surgical packs, normal size in muslin covers	30
Dressing drums, with muslin liners	45
Instruments in trays, with muslin covers	15
Instruments, wrapped for storage	30
Utensils in muslin covers	15
Rubber gloves in muslin wrappers	20
Treatment trays with muslin wrappers	30
Dressing jars, loosely packed, on sides	30
Glassware, empty, inverted	15
Syringes, unassembled, in muslin or paper covers	30
Sutures, silk, cotton or nylon	15

All supplies requiring a common exposure period may be safely and economically sterilized in the same load, with the exception of rubber gloves and solutions. In fact, for all bulk loads of supplies a continuous exposure to saturated steam at 250°-254° F. for 30 minutes provides a technique which is practicable, safe and does not destroy the materials. Rubber gloves should always be sterilized separately in order to avoid the possibility of retarding the immediate passage of steam to the gloves. Solutions must also be sterilized separately, never in mixed loads, because the method of exhausting pressure and cooling of solutions after sterilization is not applicable to the drying of fabrics and other supplies.

REFERENCES

1. UNDERWOOD, W. B.: *A Textbook of Sterilization,* 2nd Ed. Chicago, Lakeside, Donnelley 1941, p. 2.
2. JOHNSON, D. W.: *Handbook of Sterilization Procedures.* Brisbane, Australia: A. H. Tucker, Govt. Printer, 1953, p. 9-11.
3. WALBUM, L. E.: *Sterilization of Surgical Instruments. Hosp.—Tid.,* 76:57, 1933; *Zeitschr. Hyg. u. Infektionskr. 112:281,* 1931.
4. ECKER, E. E.: Sterilization Based on Temperature Attained and Time Ratio. *Mod. Hosp., 48:86,* 1937.
5. BANG, O., AND DALSGAARD, A. T.: Symposium on Sterilisation, *Arch. Pharmaci og Chemi., 25:699,* 1948. From *Pharmaceut. J., 162:236,* 1949.
6. UNDERWOOD, W. B.: *op. cit.,* p. 3-4.
7. WALTER, C. W.: *Aseptic Treatment of Wounds,* New York, Macmillan, 1948, p. 76.

Chapter V

The Modern Surgical Supply Sterilizer

THE TERMINOLOGY used in describing the modern surgical supply sterilizer is frequently misleading. The more common expressions noted in designating equipment of this type are "autoclave," "dressing sterilizer," "pressure steam sterilizer" and "steam pressure sterilizer." The term "autoclave" naturally takes precedent over all other names because of its historical background. However, by way of definition the word "autoclave" means self-closing, as in the case of a vessel made close by the pressure of steam within against the lid. To use the word "autoclave" indiscriminately when speaking of the various types of pressure steam sterilizers being manufactured today, steam jacketed chambers as well as the single wall sterilizers commonly used in the laboratory, is inaccurate and confusing to say the least. Basically, there are two distinct kinds of pressure steam sterilizers—the steam jacketed or double wall type, which constitutes the almost universal standard for sterilization of surgical supplies, and the single wall (non-jacketed) sterilizer used only in the laboratory or in highly specialized industrial applications.

STRUCTURAL FEATURES

A typical steam heated pressure steam sterilizer of the surgical supply type, equipped with "Cyclomatic" control for automatic operation, is shown in Figure 34. The structural and valving features as provided by different manufacturers will vary to some degree but the essential elements of control are the same. Although this sterilizer is properly designated a "pressure steam sterilizer," its performance is gauged not by pressure but by temperature as measured by a thermometer. Pressure gauges are provided, one for the jacket that surrounds the chamber and another for the chamber in which supplies are sterilized. These gauges are, however, of minor significance because the sterilizing power of steam is a function of its temperature rather than its pressure.

In Figure 35 is shown a longitudinal cross-section of the same sterilizer as illustrated in Figure 34. The body of the sterilizer consists of the cylindrical sterilizing chamber surrounded on the sides by a steam jacket which is enclosed by the outer shell covered on the sides by a finishing jacket. The standard material of construction for the inner chamber, outer chamber, backhead and door frame is Monel metal joined by fusion welding into a seamless unit without the use of rivets or solder. This feature of all-welded

73

construction is a comparatively new method of fabrication of the industry and it provides greater structural strength, smooth surfaces devoid of crev-

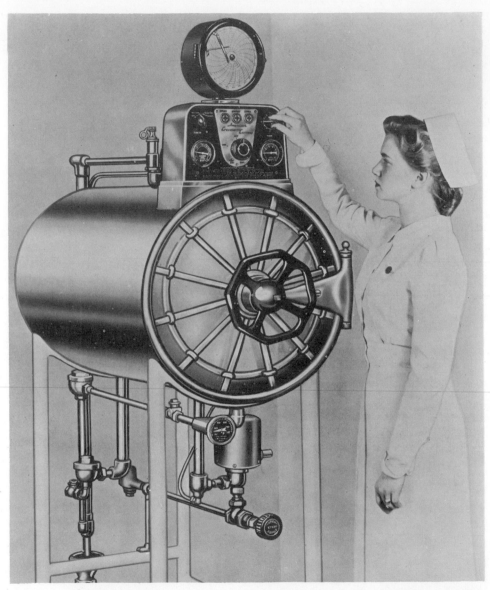

Fig. 34. Cylindrical pressure steam sterilizer, surgical supply type, steam heated, equipped with "Cyclomatic" control for automatic operation.

ices and long-time resistance to the corrosive and erosive action of steam, water and solutions. The exterior of the steam jacket is covered with air-cell asbestos for insulation (not shown) which is confined by a finishing jacket of polished stainless steel. A safety steam-locked door closes the front end of the chamber and it is made steam tight by compression through the door mechanism against a flexible heat-resistant gasket. The

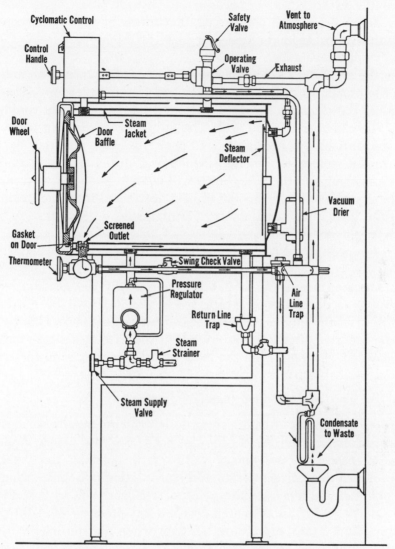

Fig. 35. Longitudinal cross-section diagram of sterilizer shown in Figure 34.

gasket is held firmly in place by means of a dove-tailed groove around the periphery of the door.

PURPOSE OF THE STEAM JACKET

In Figure 35 it may be seen that the sterilizing chamber has a steam jacket which surrounds the side walls of the chamber only, does not cover the backhead. Pressure is first generated in the jacket space prior to the admission of that steam to the chamber, and this pressure is maintained throughout the performance. This means that the walls of the sterilizing chamber are heated by the steam jacket, no condensate forms on them, and they are always dry. It is not necessary to provide jacketing for the back-head or door because the condensate that forms on these surfaces drains directly downward behind a deflector plate to the bottom and is then discharged from the chamber.

When the sterilizer is set in operation, steam is first turned on until pressure at the proper range has been developed in the jacket only. Then, with the load in the chamber, steam is admitted and it promptly contacts the walls of the chamber and the load. The only condensate that contacts the load is that formed by heating the load itself. After the materials have been heated to the temperature of the surrounding steam, no more condensate will form in them and the entire mass will contain finely diffused moisture, the exact equivalent of the amount of heat abstracted from the steam. Even though the load is distinctly moist, it contains no excess moisture, and as such, drying is not difficult.

When the pressure in the chamber is then suddenly exhausted, the heat that has previously been transferred to the load begins to take effect in drying. The moisture in the fabrics is vaporized by the residual heat and if this vapor is permitted to escape freely the load will be satisfactorily dried within a brief interval of time. This drying effect is possible only with the steam jacketed sterilizer. Otherwise, in the case of a single wall sterilizer, the vapor escaping from the load would recondense on the chamber walls and be reabsorbed by the load.

THE SAFETY DOOR

From the standpoint of engineering design the potentially weakest point on a pressure steam sterilizer is the door. Far too few people responsible for the purchase and operation of sterilizers in hospitals today recognize the importance that correct design and construction play in insuring safety of the operator. To illustrate the point, a sterilizer such as that shown in Figure 34, 20 inches in diameter, has a total pressure of 4700 pounds, approximately 2.3 tons, exerted on the door when the sterilizer is operated under 15 pounds per square inch pressure. Knowledge of this fact alone should command the respect of the most careless of operators and also stress the importance of a pressure-locked safety door to prevent explosive or premature opening while the chamber is under pressure.

The locking mechanism of a truly pressure-locked safety door should be a positive one, automatically actuated when chamber pressure is applied, unlocked only by exhaust of pressure. A sectional view of this type of door is shown in Figure 36. On the inside of the door there is an opening through, which is closed by a flexible diaphragm about 5 inches in diameter, shaped like a shallow pan and made of corrosion-resistant metal. This diaphragm expands outward under internal pressure and causes the engagement of two clutch plates which, when engaged, prevent the turning of the center plate that controls the movement of the radial locking arms from the locked position to the unlocked position. The internal pressure of

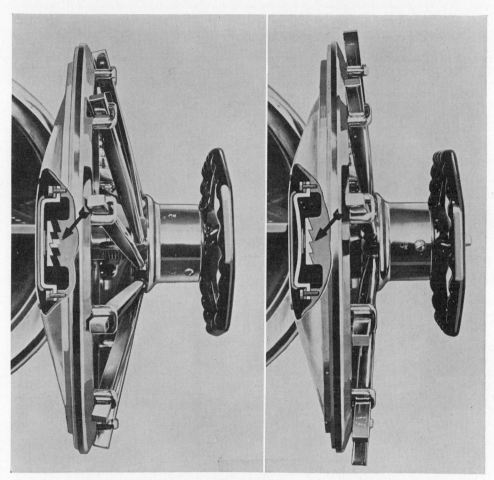

Fig. 36. Detail of the locking mechanism of a typical pressure-locked safety door for sterilizers.

the sterilizer holds these two clutch plates engaged through the action of the flexible diaphragm.

THERMOSTATIC VALVE (STEAM TRAP) IN CHAMBER DISCHARGE SYSTEM

This valve designated "air line trap" in Figure 35 controls the flow of air and condensate from the sterilizing chamber automatically. When the valve is cool, the thermostatic element inside contracts, leaving the orifice wide open for free discharge. When steam is admitted to the chamber for sterilizing, air is forced out by way of the screened outlet leading to the discharge line and then through the thermostatic valve by the pressure of the incoming steam. The valve remains open until steam following the air heats the valve, then the element gradually expands and closes the orifice. The thermostatic element is extremely sensitive and throughout sterilization, as condensate or air pockets gravitate to the valve, it will open slightly until the cooler fluid has been discharged.

Occasionally the thermostatic valve may become clogged with lint or

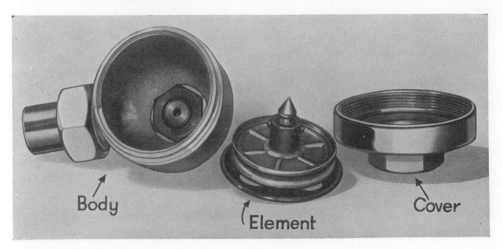

Fig. 37. Disassembled thermostatic valve showing component parts. The thermostatic element contains a fluid which expands under heat to close the orifice in the body.

sediment so that it cannot function properly. Also, after long service the thermostatic element (Fig. 37) may fatigue or lose its fluid content upon which it depends for thermostatic action. In either case the valve will close off entirely or in part, slowing down or completely interrupting air and condensate discharge.

If the sterilizer becomes sluggish or lags appreciably in attaining the proper temperature, the chamber drain line should be flushed out with a hot solution of tri-sodium phosphate. Should the sluggishness persist it is advisable to remove the thermostatic element and check it for clogging. If the orifice is unobstructed, shake the element to check the fluid content. If there is no fluid in the element, it should be replaced by a new element at once. Usually this procedure will be found to remedy the difficulty.

One should not confuse the thermostatic valve which controls the chamber discharge system with the return trap from the jacket of steam heated sterilizers. Usually these two valves have the same bodies but the orifices and the thermostatic elements are different. The chamber discharge valve is adjusted primarily for the rapid discharge of air and condensate while the jacket trap is adjusted primarily for condensate drainage. The orifice in the chamber discharge valve is much larger than in the jacket (return line) trap. It is standard practice to place on the cover of each valve an identifying number which should be used when requisitioning new elements for use with any make of sterilizer.

THE RETURN SYSTEM

For all pressure steam sterilizers of the jacketed type it is necessary to provide a "return" system for the purpose of receiving the discharge from the steam jacket, a more or less continuous flow of condensate which is controlled by the return line trap shown in Figure 35. This trap is also thermostatic in its action and when cool its orifice will remain open for free discharge. The thermostatic element responds to heat and it will close off nearly, but not quite completely, when contacted by steam following the water or condensate discharge. Directly back of the return line trap is located a check valve. It opens freely for the discharge of condensate from the jacket but closes against any back pressure which may occur in the return line system. This feature is necessary because occasionally the return line piping beyond the sterilizer is so small that appreciable back pressure may be developed from other equipment located on the same line. If steam were to back up to the location of the trap, the heat might cause the trap to close off and thus interfere with the performance of the sterilizer.

A point which many people fail to comprehend is that no steam jacket can function properly unless the return system is so controlled that condensate is disposed of just as rapidly as it forms. Interference with this discharge is always a serious matter. Primarily the discharge is controlled by the trap, but obviously the trap cannot function unless the piping into which it feeds is not closed off or restricted. Oftentimes sterilizers are unjustly criticized when the fault lies entirely with the steam supply or the return system.

THE PRESSURE CONTROL VALVE

Before the initial operation of the sterilizer, the automatic pressure control valve should be carefully adjusted to insure that it will deliver to the jacket the prescribed amount of pressure, i.e., 15-17 pounds. The valve (Fig. 38) is strictly a pressure regulator. It is so constructed that an internal expansion diaphragm (flexible bellows) expands or contracts, as pressure varies in the jacket of the sterilizer, reacting against a regulating spring, thereby opening and closing the orifice in the valve proper. Regulation for any desired pressure in the range of 15 to 30 pounds is accomplished by a handwheel at the side which, when turned, increases or lessens the tension on the valve spring.

As previously stated, a pressure of 15-17 pounds should be maintained in both jacket and chamber of the sterilizer. While the pressure gauge must be used for the initial adjustment to this range, it should be borne in mind that commercial pressure gauges at best are highly inaccurate. After use they frequently become distorted due to fatigue, often reading several pounds high. For this reason, it becomes necessary to regulate the sterilizer

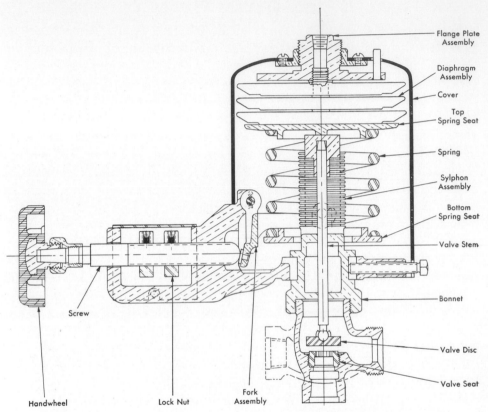

Fig. 38. Cross-section diagram of pressure control valve used on sterilizers.

pressure with direct reference to the temperature produced in the chamber. This may be accomplished as follows:

With or without a load in the sterilizer, turn steam to the jacket, and wait until the pressure has become stable at the maximum range. Then turn steam to the chamber and wait until the temperature as indicated by the thermometer has become stable at its maximum range. If the stabilized temperature is below 250° F., turn the regulating handle on the pressure control valve clockwise half a turn or so, wait until the temperature has become stable again at the higher range. If the maximum temperature is still too low, repeat the procedure until the temperature remains constant at slightly above 250° F.

If the temperature is above 254° F., reverse the process, turn the regulating handle counter-clockwise a little at a time until the maximum temperature is within the prescribed limits. Once adjusted, the valve should require no further regulation unless the steam supply line pressure fluctuates badly. If this does occur, the maintenance engineer should be consulted so that proper arrangements can be made to stabilize the supply line pressure.

OPERATION OF THE STERILIZER

In tracing the course of steam through the sterilizer, the reader should keep in mind that the same essential features will apply to any modern surgical supply sterilizer, providing the principles of gravity air discharge and thermometric control are incorporated. Steam from the main supply line or source is admitted at the bottom of the steam jacket. In the diagram (Fig. 35), the sterilizer is heated by direct steam from the supply line and the pressure is reduced to the proper range by initial adjustment of the pressure control valve. If the sterilizer is heated by electricity or gas, a steam generator or boiler is mounted under the sterilizer, and steam is delivered directly to the jacket from the generator. Control of pressure then is governed by automatic regulation of the heat.

In beginning operation with a cold sterilizer, steam is first admitted from the source to the jacket, with the connection to the chamber closed, until the jacket pressure becomes constant at 15-17 pounds. This constitutes the reservoir from which the chamber steam will be drawn. In sterilizing, the load is placed in the chamber and the door locked immediately after the jacket has attained the correct pressure. Then the operating valve is turned to "Sterilize" which permits the jacket steam to flow through the multi-port valve and piping on top of the sterilizer and into the chamber at the top center of the back end. At this point the steam is deflected upward by means of a baffle to prevent undue wetting of the load.

It is important to remember that when steam is admitted to the chamber, the chamber and the load of more or less porous supplies are filled with air. This air must be evacuated in order to attain the sterilizing temperature and to facilitate thorough permeation of the load with steam. The method of evacuation is accomplished as follows:

Air is more dense than steam, and as steam enters the chamber it gravitates above the air, fills the upper areas of the chamber and compresses air at the bottom. Since steam is admitted under pressure, air in the lower areas is forced out through the screened outlet at the extreme bottom near the front end, through the thermometer case and the pipe that leads to the thermostatic (air line) valve, then on to the vertical pipe which is vented to the atmosphere at the top and drained to the waste through the open (sanitary) funnel at the bottom. This air break above the open funnel leading to the drain connection is highly important. It prevents possible back flow of contaminated waste to the sterilizer.

When the sterilizer is cool, the thermostatic (air line) valve is open, offers no restriction to the flow of air and condensate to the vent or waste. Only when air evacuation is complete and steam finally contacts the thermostatic valve does it close, interrupting the discharge. Thereafter it will open intermittently to discharge condensate as it accumulates. This method of air evacuation is known as the "gravity" system and it has been almost universally employed on pressure steam sterilizers produced since 1933.

From the foregoing, it is obvious that some method must be provided for definite measurement of the degree of air discharge and quality of steam

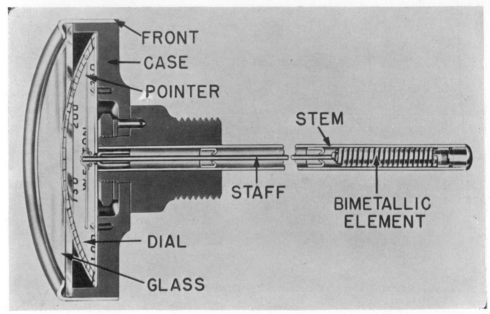

Fig. 39. Sectional view of bimetallic, dial-type thermometer used on sterilizers.

in the chamber. This is the specific function of the thermometer which, located in the discharge line that drains air and condensate from the chamber, will immediately respond to any interruption of air discharge from the chamber. Under any condition of performance, the thermometer will indicate never less than the temperature of the coolest medium surrounding the load. This is due to the fact that air or any mixture of steam with air will invariably gravitate below pure steam. The thermometer, therefore, when properly located in a correctly designed discharge system serves as a reliable means of measuring the sterilizing quality or lethality of the steam in contact with the load.

The majority of pressure steam sterilizers in use today are equipped with a bimetallic (dial type) thermometer. Occasionally mercury thermometers are used but wide experience has shown the mercury column to be difficult to read and it also responds more slowly to temperature changes than the bimetallic type. With the bimetal thermometer the circular dial and pointer method of indicating temperature permits the use of easily read, widely spaced scale graduations. The temperature sensitive element (Fig. 39) employed consists of a strip of bimetal wound into a continuous multiple

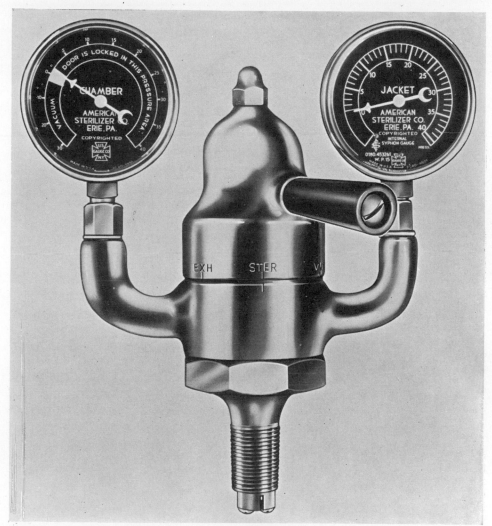

Fig. 40. Dialed top operating valve for controlling the progressive phases of the sterilizing cycle.

helix. Thermometers of this type are consistently accurate to within ±1° F. in the sterilizing temperature range.

When the sterilizer is functioning properly, temperature will advance to 250° F. within five to ten minutes, at which point the period of exposure is timed. When the sterilizing period is complete, steam is exhausted from the chamber, but the jacket pressure is maintained, by turning the operating valve to the "Exhaust" position. The steam then escapes through the venting system.

DIALED TOP OPERATING VALVE

The device shown in Figure 40, widely known as a dialed top operating valve, first appeared on surgical supply sterilizers in 1928. It possesses this highly advantageous feature—the one valve controls all the functions, admits steam to the chamber, exhausts steam from the chamber, creates a mild degree of vacuum for drying the load following sterilization. It facilitates the work of the unskilled operator by simplifying the manual control operations. Sterilizers not equipped with a top operating valve require at least two and sometimes three individual valves to accomplish the same control. With standard procedure, the valve operates as follows:

In starting the sterilizer from cold, the operating valve is first turned to "OFF" and in that position there is no connection between the jacket and the chamber, but a very small port is opened to the exhaust line. To admit steam from jacket to chamber, the valve handle is turned to "STER," steam then flows through the valve and through a connecting pipe which leads to the rear of the chamber where the steam enters behind a deflector plate. At the close of the sterilizing period the valve is turned to the "EXH" position. This opens up an outlet to the exhaust piping and cuts off the flow of steam from the jacket to the chamber.

When the chamber pressure has been exhausted to zero gauge, the valve is turned to the "DRY" position, thereby permitting steam from the jacket to escape through an ejector built into the top operating valve. This exerts a slight degree of suction or vacuum on the chamber to expedite the escape of vapor which is discharged to the vent. To further enhance the drying of the load, a small stream of filtered air is admitted to the chamber through the air filter as the result of the influence of the ejector. As this air stream circulates through the chamber it entrains vapor and carries it to the vent. From 15 to 20 minutes is usually sufficient to dry the load adequately for storage or immediate use. The singular advantage gained by this procedure is the almost complete elimination of residual vapor, steam and odors from the chamber when the door is finally opened.

AUTOMATIC CONTROLS FOR PRESSURE STERILIZERS

During the past few years sterilizer manufacturers have made a valuable contribution toward advancement of the art through development of automatic control mechanisms designed to minimize the human element in sterilizer operation. Sterilizers equipped with efficiently designed automatic controls overcome many of the problems and inaccuracies attendant with the manual method of control. Typical of the class of automatic controls is the instrument shown in Figure 34, mounted on top of the sterilizer. Its principal function is not limited to automatic timing of the selected exposure period, but rather it extends to all phases of the sterilizing process, to the end that all steps in the cycle normally carried out manually by the operator are conducted automatically according to a predetermined pattern. This means that when the control is set for operation, it times the exposure period at the correct temperature, exhausts steam from the chamber, governs the process of drying, and finally sounds an alarm announcing completion of the process.

The mechanical means responsible for the sequence of operations is a motorized multi-port valve located on top of the sterilizer in back of the instrument control case. A small electric motor inside of the case or housing is connected to the multi-port valve by means of a shaft and an arrangement of small gears for the transfer of movement from one station of the valve to another. The feature of automatic time-temperature control is accomplished through the use of a sensitive and accurate thermoswitch located in the chamber discharge line of the sterilizer, adjacent to the indicating thermometer. The thermoswitch, in turn, is connected to an automatic reset timer by means of electrical connections leading to the rear of the control box on top of the sterilizer.

The details of the instrument panel on one type of automatic control are shown in Figure 41. The two pressure gauges, one for the jacket and the other for the chamber, are of the conventional type and they are placed in the same relative positions as the corresponding gauges on any modern sterilizer equipped with a top operating valve. The control handle located in the center of the panel is easily recognized because of the circular arrows descriptive of its movement in a clockwise direction. The various stations of the motorized valve are made known to the operator by means of the leading arrow on the control handle which, at any time during the sterilizing process, coincides with the corresponding station on the dial.

Above the control handle there are four signal lights designated "Steam," "Exhaust," "Timing," and "Sterile." The first light (red) designated "Steam" comes on as soon as steam is admitted to the chamber and it remains on during the entire exposure period. The second light (yellow) designated "Exhaust" appears immediately upon exhausting steam from the chamber and it also remains on during the drying process. The third light (white) designated "Timing" remains on during the period that the timer is in operation. The fourth light (amber) designated "Sterile" appears only upon completion of the entire cycle of operation. Thus each light functions as a "telltale" indicator of the proper sequence of events during the sterilizing process.

The "Selector" switch located in the upper right of the panel serves as the individual control for either fast or slow exhaust of steam from the chamber, the drying process, and also for "Manual" operation of the sterilizer should this be desired at any time. When the load consists of fabrics or wrapped supplies the "Selector" should be turned to the "F. Exh. & Dry" position. Then, following the exposure period, the control will automatically exhaust steam from the chamber and proceed to dry the load by means of the vacuum drier system. When sterilizing glassware or utensils, or whenever the drying process is not required, the "Selector" should be turned to the "Fast Exh." position.

The method of operation in solution sterilization differs somewhat from

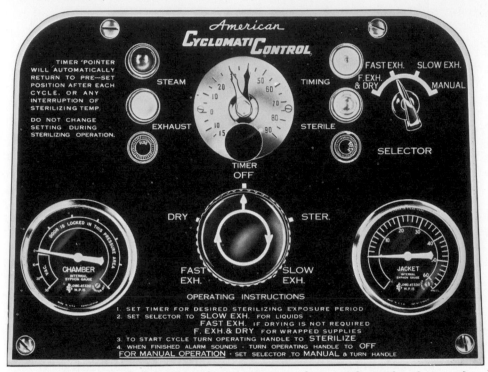

Fig. 41. This is typical of the class of automatic controls currently employed on modern surgical supply sterilizers.

that of dry goods, instruments, utensils, etc. Here it becomes necessary to turn the "Selector" to the "Slow Exh." position. While the solution is being heated and as long as exposure continues there will be no boiling of the liquid, even though the temperature may be far in excess of the normal (atmospheric) boiling point of water. This is due to the steam pressure maintained in the chamber, at all times equal to or in excess of the pressure possible to develop from the heat of the liquid. After sterilization, when the chamber pressure is reduced, the condition reverses, and unless pressure is exhausted slowly the liquid will boil so violently that stoppers may be blown out of the flasks and some of the solution may escape into the chamber. It is essential, therefore, that the rate of exhaust be accurately controlled to insure that the liquid will dissipate its heat at about the same rate as the pressure is reduced in the chamber so that violent boiling will not occur. This requirement is automatically taken care of when the "Selector" switch is set at the "Slow Exh." position. When the pressure in the chamber has been reduced to atmospheric, a sensitive pressurestat,

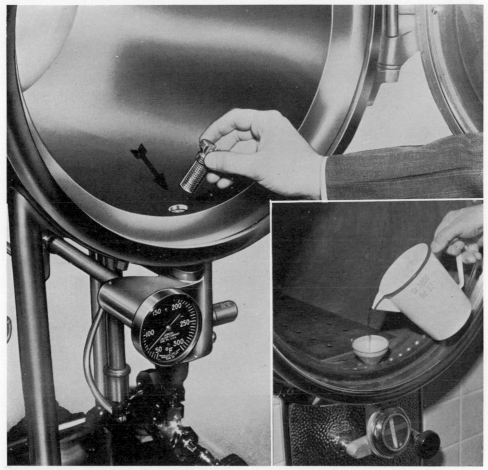

Fig. 42. Remove this plug screen daily before operating the sterilizer. Clean the strainer thoroughly so that the openings are entirely free from lint and sediment.

Fig. 43. Method of cleaning chamber drain line.

built into the control, closes a circuit to an alarm which sounds, announcing completion of the cycle.

The "Timer" located near the top center of the instrument panel is graduated from zero to 90 minutes in intervals of 5 minutes. Since the "Timer" is controlled by the thermoswitch located in the chamber discharge line it will operate only when the sterilizing temperature of 250° F. is reached and maintained in the chamber. If, at any time, during the sterilizing period the temperature in the chamber discharge line should fall below 250° F., the "Timer" will stop, reset itself to the beginning of the selected exposure time, and it will not resume its timing operation until the temperature again rises to 250° F. This feature of automatic recycling assures continuous exposure of the load to saturated steam at the correct temperature. The sub-zero graduations on the "Timer" dial refer to the time consumed in drying of the load, normally a minimum of 15 minutes, by means of the vacuum drier system.

DAILY CARE OF STERILIZERS

It should be the routine duty of someone to clean the interior of the sterilizer every day, before it is heated. This may be easily accomplished by washing the surfaces with water containing a mild detergent such as Calgonite. If this is not done the walls of the chamber often become coated with greasy substances originating from the materials sterilized and also due to the entrainment with steam of volatile compounds used in the treatment of boiler water. The tray in the bottom of the chamber and any other wire-mesh or perforated metal shelves used in the sterilizer should be cleaned in a like manner.

All modern sterilizers have a freely removable plug screen or strainer located in the opening to the chamber discharge line. This screen should be removed daily (Fig. 42) before operating the sterilizer, while it is cool, and thoroughly cleaned so that the pores are free from lint or sediment. If this detail is neglected the sterilizer cannot be depended upon for prompt and efficient performance.

At intervals of one week it is excellent practice to clean out the chamber discharge system as suggested in Figure 43. The procedure only involves removing of the plug screen as indicated above, inserting a funnel into the opening and then pouring into the line one to two liters of hot trisodium phosphate solution, containing about one ounce of the trisodium phosphate per liter of hot water. The periodic flushing of the discharge system will keep the line free from clogging substances which, if allowed to accumulate, may offer some retardation to free discharge of air and condensate from the chamber.

OPERATING INSTRUCTIONS
FOR STERILIZERS EQUIPPED WITH "CYCLOMATIC" CONTROL

1) DAILY BEFORE HEATING STERILIZER

Remove plug screen from bottom of chamber and clean lint and sediment from pores of strainer.

2) TO HEAT JACKET

A) FOR DIRECT STEAM HEATED STERILIZERS (Fig. 44A): With Valve Handle (located in center of "Cyclomatic" Control) at "Off" position, open "Steam Supply" valve. Do not attempt to sterilize until "Jacket "Gauge" shows 15 to 17 pounds pressure.

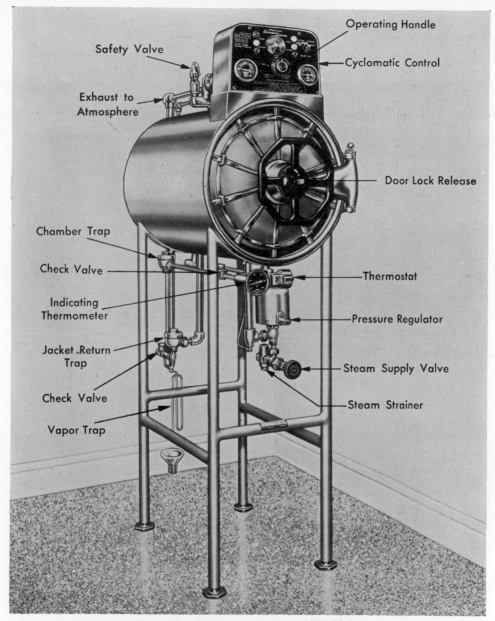

Fig. 44A. Direct steam heated sterilizer.

B) For Electrically Heated Sterilizers (Fig. 44B): Open "Hot Water Supply Valve" to fill generator until indicator shows "Full." Do not fill beyond "Full" line. If too much water is admitted, open "Waste Valve" until indicator shows "Full." With "Valve Handle" (located in center of "Cyclomatic" Control) at "Off" position, turn "Switch Handle" to "On." Do not attempt to sterilize until "Jacket Gauge" shows 15 to 17 pounds pressure.

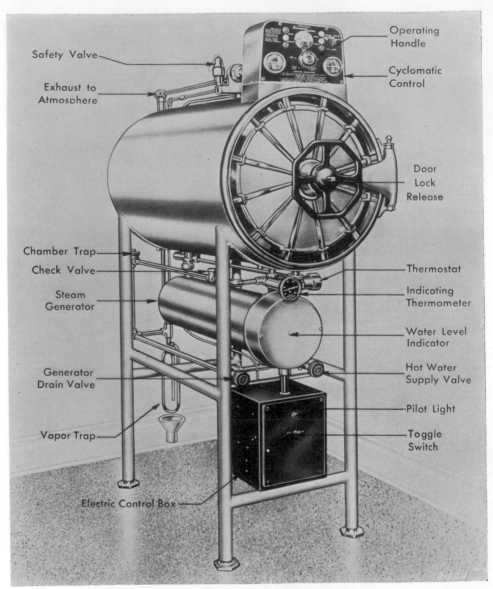

Fig. 44B. Electrically heated sterilizer.

C) FOR GAS HEATED STERILIZERS (Fig. 44C): Open "Hot Water Supply Valve" to fill generator until indicator shows "Full." Do not fill beyond "Full" line. If too much water is admitted, open "Waste Valve" until indicator shows "Full." With "Valve Handle" (located in center of "Cyclomatic" Control) at "Off" position, turn "Gas Supply Valve" on full. Pilot light will ignite gas. Do not attempt to sterilize until "Jacket Gauge" shows 15 to 17 pounds pressure.

ARRANGEMENT OF LOAD

Place flat packs of supplies on edge. If there are several tiers of such packs, place alternate tiers crosswise of each other to assure adequate steam circulation. Do not permit crowding of packs into tight masses. Do not sterilize rubber gloves with heavy loads of general supplies. Under no condition atempt sterilization of solutions with other supplies.

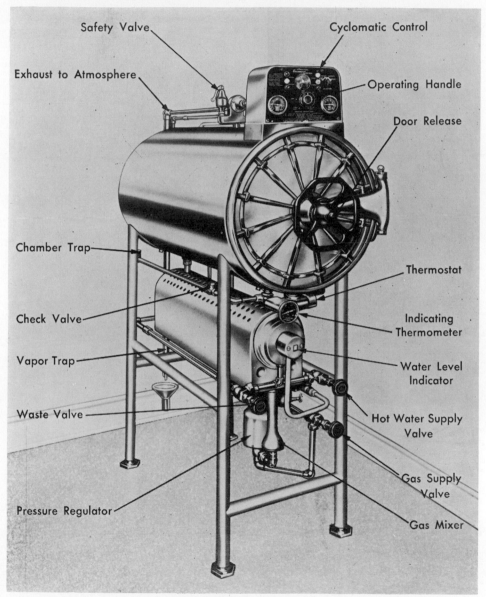

Fig. 44C. Gas heated sterilizer.

3) TO STERILIZE ALL MATERIALS

With load in sterilizer and door locked, turn "Timer" to desired exposure period. Then turn "Selector" switch to the appropriate position of
"Slow Exh." for liquids.
"Fast Exh." if drying is not required.
"Fast Exh. and Dry" for surgical packs, wrapped supplies, etc.

Turn "Valve Handle" (clockwise only) to "Ster." Operator may now leave sterilizer and return only when cycle has been completed.

RECOMMENDED PERIODS OF EXPOSURE
At 250° F. (121° C.)

	Minutes
Instruments in trays with muslin covers	15
Utensils in muslin covers	15
Rubber gloves in muslin wrappers	15-20
Surgical packs, dressings in muslin covers	30
Solutions (aqueous) in Pyrex flasks	30
Drums with muslin liners	45

With "Valve Handle" turned to the "Ster." position, the red signal light (designated "Steam") will come on, indicating that steam is entering the chamber. When the temperature in the chamber drain line reaches 250° F., the "Timer" will begin to operate and count back to zero. The white light indicates when "Timer" is operating. At completion of timed sterilizing period, the valve automatically moves to the selected "Exhaust" position. Then the red light goes out and the yellow ("Exhaust") light comes on.

If "Selector" has been set on the "F. Exh. and Dry" position, the valve will automatically move to "Dry" after the chamber pressure has been reduced to zero.

When the load is completely processed, the amber ("Sterile") signal light will come on and alarm will sound until "Valve Handle" is turned manually to "Off." The load may now be removed from the sterilizer.

4) MANUAL OPERATION

In the event of electrical current failure, the sterilizer may be operated manually by simply turning "Selector" to "Manual," and then turning "Valve Handle" (clockwise only) to that position on the dial which corresponds to the proper sequence of operations in the sterilizing cycle.

5) TO TURN OFF HEAT

A) For Direct Steam Heated Sterilizers: Unless sterilizer is to be used again within a short time, close "Steam Supply Valve" and permit sterilizer to cool.

B) For Electrically Heated Sterilizers: Unless sterilizer is to be used again within a short time, turn "Switch Handle" to "Off" and permit sterilizer to cool. Drain water from generator by opening "Generator Drain Valve."

C) FOR GAS HEATED STERILIZERS: Unless sterilizer is to be used again within a short time, close "Gas Supply Valve" and permit sterilizer to cool. Drain water from generator by opening "Waste Valve."

CAUTION: If the sterilizer is electrically or gas heated and if it is to be used for two or more successive sterilization cycles, the generator must be filled to the "Full" line with water after *each* complete cycle.

CHAPTER 6

Preparation and Sterilization of Dressings
And Dry Goods

SURGICAL PACKS

E FFECTIVE STERILIZATION of surgical supplies is not only dependent upon conscientious operation of the sterilizer but also upon correct methods of packaging and proper arrangement of loads in the sterilizer. Operators should constantly bear in mind that reliable performance
demands complete permeation of every strand and fibre of the materials
with the moisture and heat of the steam. This permeation will occur rapidly
or slowly, depending upon the size and density of the pack and upon the
arrangement or positioning of the load in the sterilizer.

Movement of Steam in Sterilizer: The movement of air and steam
through the sterilizer has a direct bearing on the preparation of packs for
sterilization. All modern sterilizers employ the gravity system for air elimination in which steam enters the chamber at the back end, floats promptly
to the top of the chamber, compresses air in the bottom areas, forcing the
air from the chamber through an opening in the extreme front bottom. This
assures movement of steam from one end of the chamber to the other and
from top to bottom.

Except during the initial stage of the sterilizing process, there is no rapid
movement of steam or air. When the free air in open spaces surrounding
the load has been eliminated, there is an approach to a static condition of
the gases. Since the pressure is uniform, the only movement of gases will
be occasioned by the slow release of air from the load itself. This is brought
about by gravity. Air being heavier than steam will gravitate downward out
of the packs, and steam will replace it as rapidly as the air can escape. This
movement will be fast or slow depending upon the density and depth of the
mass through which the discharge must occur.

It is obvious that a pack 6 inches in depth will present twice as much
resistance as a similar pack 3 inches in depth. With the same reasoning, if
two packs each 6 inches in depth are placed in the sterilizer in close contact,
one immediately above the other, the effect will be the same as if both
were wrapped in one package 12 inches in depth. On the other hand, if the
upper pack is separated from the lower one by a short distance, steam will
quickly fill the intervening space and permeate the lower pack essentially
the same as if the two were placed side by side in the sterilizer.

It is important to remember that the vital discharge of air from the load always occurs in a downward direction, never sidewise. Knowledge of this condition provides the background for this basic rule:

Prepare all packs and arrange the load in the sterilizer so as to present the least possible resistance to the passage of steam through the load, from the top of the chamber toward the bottom.

Assume for analysis a simple package consisting of ten pieces of muslin cut into 10 inch squares and wrapped together without folding. If this pack were placed in the sterilizer flat side down as in Figure 45, air within

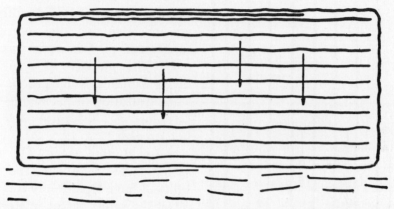

Fig. 45. Packs made up of many layers of fabric placed in the sterilizer horizontally, as shown, are difficult to sterilize because air within the pack must travel downward through the many layers of fabric to escape. Each horizontal layer adds to the resistance and as the outer layers become moist from steam, the resistance is further increased.

the pack would have to pass through 10 layers of muslin, plus the cover, in its downward passage. The resistance of the dry pack will be increased by the moisture of the steam in contact with the outer layers, further retarding the evacuation of air. Also, the closer the weave of the fabric, the greater the resistance. If this same pack is now placed in the sterilizer vertically (on edge) as shown in Figure 46, even though the pack be wrapped fairly tight, there will remain minute spaces between layers through which air can gravitate toward the bottom with comparative freedom.

The above rule should guide the operator in preparing every pack or drum of bulk supplies to be subjected to sterilization and also in the arrangement of the load which will normally consist of several packs. This point can not be overemphasized, especially when heavy packs are encountered as illustrated by the two temperature curves in Figure 47. The pack tested in this case (Fig. 48) was abnormally large and dense, but it serves as a good example to show the importance of proper positioning in the sterilizer and to indicate the hazards encountered when packs are too large and dense.

HAZARDS OF ABNORMALLY LARGE OR DENSE PACKS

While the temperature curve in Figure 47 shows that 33 minutes exposure at 250° F. (121° C.) would have been adequate for sterilization of the pack when placed on edge in the sterilizer, this by no means justifies acceptance of the pack as suitable. The day of the old-fashioned laparotomy set containing far more materials than actually required for the surgical procedure and with little consideration for the internal arrangement of the pack should be over. The practice of using large dense bundles is hazardous. Rigid standardization of packaging should be enforced. The largest pack should not exceed 12 x 12 x 20 inches in size for routine work. The factors which seem to indicate the desirability of huge laparotomy sets do not offset the safety factor in sterilizing.

When tests show that any pack, sterilized by itself, requires more than 30 minutes for sterilization, or is barely sterilized in 30 minutes, resting either vertically or horizontally in the sterilizer, that indicates the pack is too large and it should be broken down into smaller packs. Reliable routine sterilization of surgical supplies correctly prepared can be accomplished in 30 minutes exposure to saturated steam at 250° F. (121° C.). Many operating room supervisors and central supply department supervisors have long since discovered this fact, but the practice of using abnormally large or dense packs still persists in many hospitals. With all of our refined knowledge of the subject of sterilization, it still is not unusual to find recording thermometer charts on surgical supply sterilizers showing exposure periods ranging from 30

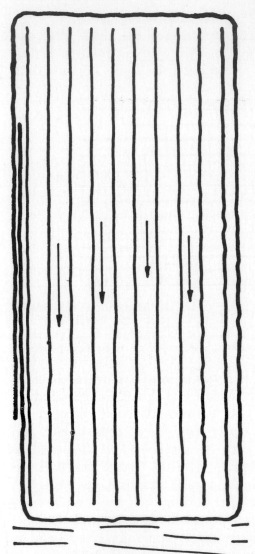

Fig. 46. If the pack shown in Figure 45 is placed on edge with layers of fabric in a vertical position as shown here, air will escape quickly through the minute spaces between layers.

to 90 minutes. The hospital pays heavily for such inconsistencies. Substantially more than 30 minutes exposure for sterilization hastens deterioration of fabrics. The economic factor can not be ignored because

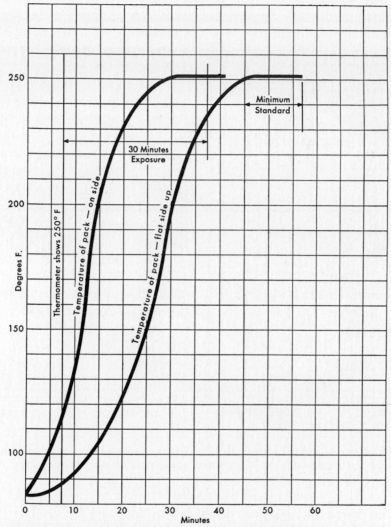

Fig. 47. These two curves show load temperatures attained with the pack illustrated in Figure 48. With the pack flat side up, 50 minutes exposure is required for sterilization. When the pack is placed on edge in the sterilizer, 33 minutes exposure is required to meet the minimum standard for sterilization.

any hospital has a considerable investment annually in replacement of such supplies. It is indeed possible to effect a substantial savings on supplies subject to repeated sterilization simply by establishing standardized methods for the preparation and sterilization of supplies. If the operating room or central supply room blindly persists in preparing large, over-stuffed packs such as shown in Figures 48 and 49, then the periods of exposure must be prolonged to 45-60 minutes, with resultant deterioration of outer fabrics.

To further explain the hazardous element involved in the use of abnormally large or dense packs, suppose there are several of these to be sterilized in one load. If through carelessness the load is arranged as in Figure 50,

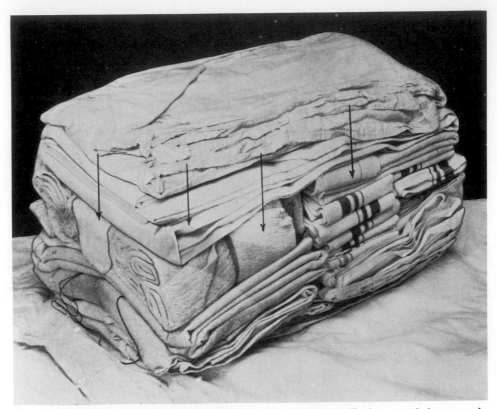

Fig. 48. This is the pack referred to in Figure 47, an abnormally large and dense pack. The practice of using such large and heavy packs should be discouraged.

the upper packs would retard passage of steam to the lower packs so seriously that 60 minutes exposure might not be adequate for sterilization. But if these packs are broken down into moderate sizes, some degree of carelessness in loading could be tolerated without jeopardizing the end result in a 30-minute exposure period. By establishing methods of packaging that permit safe sterilization in 30 minutes, definite economies will be effected. More work can be done with the sterilizers in a given time. Less steam and fuel will be required. Materials will need to be replaced less frequently.

PROTECTIVE COVERING FOR SURGICAL PACKS

The protective covering or wrapper for surgical packs logically precedes any discussion on what constitutes the ideal pack from the standpoint of

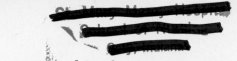

bulk and density. The wrapper must provide protection against contact contamination in handling, guard against the entry of insects or vermin (cockroaches, ants, silverfish, etc.) and it must also serve as a dust filter. When packs or porous supplies are removed from the sterilizer they are more or less filled with vapor and as this vapor condenses it creates a negative pressure condition within the goods. This results in a definite

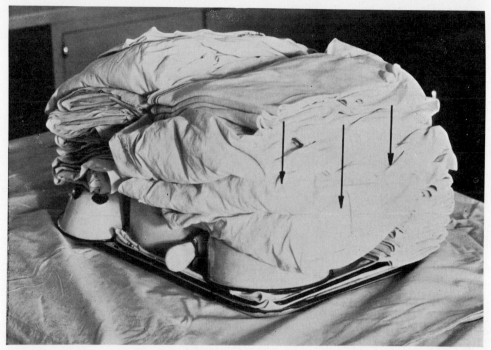

Fig. 49. Another example of faulty arrangement of the individual pack. The inclusion of basins with fabrics in one package should not be permitted. The basins seriously interfere with steam permeation and retard drying following sterilization.

intake of room air from which dust particles must be removed in the covering envelope or the contents may be contaminated.

Broad experience has shown that a minimum of two thicknesses of good quality muslin serves ideally as wrapping material. Two thicknesses are used to guard against possible minute flaws in the muslin. Badly worn muslin should not be used because the thin portions may not filter out dust particles effectively. Some hospitals prepare covers for surgical packs from two ordinary bed sheets (63 x 90 inches), folded crosswise so as to form four thicknesses of fabric. With this procedure the finished wrapper is about 63 inches long and 45 inches wide. It will serve to cover adequately a large pack with dimensions of about 22 x 15 x 8½ inches.

Canvas covers or other heavy woven fabrics should not be used because the tightly woven structure seriously retards the passage of steam. For the

same reason canvas should not be used for table covers or any other requirement where sterilization is necessary. Heavy woven fabrics should be
wrapped individually for sterilization, never with other goods.

Paper Wrappers as a Substitute for Muslin: During the last few years
there has developed a fairly widespread usage of paper products as a substitute for muslin in the wrapping of supplies. Coarse, brown wrapping
paper (30 or 40 lb. Kraft) is used rather extensively in hospitals for the

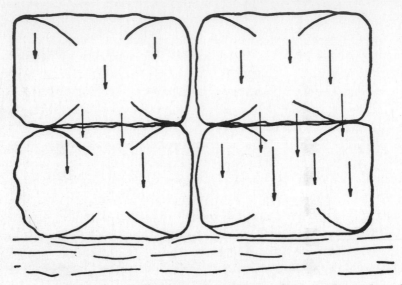

Fig. 50. Abnormally heavy packs arranged in the sterilizer as shown here become
doubly hazardous. In effect, the pack is double its normal depth and an exposure
period of 60 minutes or longer might still be inadequate for steam penetration through
the lower packs.

wrapping of gloves. This type of paper will pass steam quite freely, but not
as rapidly as muslin. Assuming that it is devoid of holes it will also filter out
dust particles satisfactorily. The principal objection to its use for surgical
supplies is the obvious hazard of contamination through rupture in handling. Many institutions use small paper bags for packaging cotton balls,
small dressings, syringes, etc. for floor use with apparent success and economy. In this case the application is not as critical as for the supplies used
in the operating room.

Beck, Shay and Purdum[1] recently examined 55 samples of paper to
determine their value as a wrapping material for articles to be sterilized
by means of steam under pressure or by hot air. The results of this study
showed that the Kraft-type papers were the most suitable and most economical. The conclusions drawn in this study have been criticized by
Walter[2] on the basis that the—"data is not valid because conditions of the
test were not critical."

Whittenberger[3] has reported on the steam sterilization of paper-wrapped packages by comparing the effectiveness of standard muslin wrapping with "Sterilwraps."* Measurements were made in terms of the temperature attained at the core of a 10-inch cube of muslin. The results showed that layer for layer the barrier to steam was about the same for both materials, but for standard wrapping procedure the "Sterilwraps" were significantly superior in terms of the time required to reach a given temperature. No mention was made of the economic virtues of "Sterilwraps" as compared to muslin wrappers.

As a substitute for muslin, certain hospitals are using the vegetable parchment paper known as "Patapar, 27-2T." Available evidence on this product indicates that it will permit passage of steam at a useful rate through a single layer. It possesses high wet strength and does not tear easily. The results of bacteriological tests[4] on objects wrapped in "Patapar" indicate that it is safe to use with the normal period of exposure required for sterilization. It is advisable, however, to add an additional 5 to 10 minutes to the drying time following sterilization because the water vapor transmission rate of the parchment is slower than that of muslin.

At the present time there is insufficient evidence to warrant the use of paper as a substitute for muslin, especially for the wrapping of those supplies destined for use in the operating room. The principal objection to the use of paper is that one never knows when the wrapper may develop holes or cracks not grossly visible, but still sufficiently large to permit contamination to gain access to the interior of the package. A striking example of this condition was noted recently by the writer during a routine inspection of sterile supplies in a leading hospital. The paper wrappers from several packs were removed and grossly examined for holes or tears. Two of the wrappers from packs destined for the operating room contained holes about ⅛ inch in diameter. The indiscriminate use of paper may also interfere with present day standards for sterilization of supplies. The repeated use of paper wrappers is certainly not safe practice. In contrast, double thickness muslin, of good quality, retains its characteristics for a long period of time. It is probably the safest material that can be used for the wrapping of surgical supplies. If a hospital anticipates substituting paper for muslin as a wrapping material reliable information should be obtained beforehand on the steam and air transmission characteristics as well as the economic virtues of the product.

CORRECT METHODS OF PACKAGING

In developing correct methods of packaging, the first requirement is to restrict the size and density of the individual pack so that 30 minutes

---

* A product of Meinecke & Co., New York City.

exposure will insure uniform steam permeation with an adequate margin of safety in sterilization. This can be accomplished by limiting the largest pack to dimensions of 12 x 12 x 20 inches in size for routine work. Do not attempt to mix trays or basins with fabrics, all in one package, as in Figure 49. The basins interfere with air removal and also retard effective drying of the fabrics following sterilization.

The major laparotomy pack shown in Figure 51, arranged for muslin

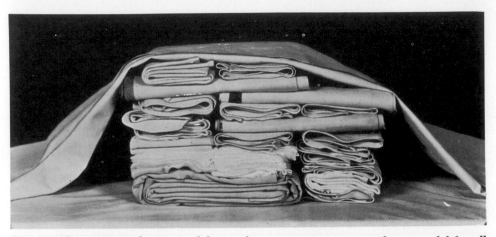

Fig. 51. This major pack, arranged for muslin wrapping, is suggested as a model for all heavy packs. Note how alternate layers are crossed to promote steam permeation. The table drape is folded once and spread out to form ultimately an inner covering of the pack. This provides a convenient method of draping the table as the pack is opened. After the pack has been covered with the table drape, an outer double thickness muslin cover is put on and held in place with cord.

wrapping, is suggested as a model for all heavy packs. The materials are ideally arranged in this pack to promote rapid and complete permeation of steam through the mass. The pack includes:

22 hand towels	4 applicators
2 skin towels	24 sponges, 4″ x 4″
1 lap sheet	12 sponges, 4″ x 8″
1 Mayo table drape	6 large abdominal sponges
1 cautery cover	1 package tonsil sponges
1 tongue depressor	

To facilitate the work when this pack is opened in the operating room, the table drape is folded once only and spread on the work table in two thicknesses only. It will be used to form the inner covering of the pack. More than two thicknesses of the table cover over the rest of the pack should not be permitted because of the resistance of heavier covering to the intake of steam. The gauze sponges are located near the center of the pack to break up the close contact between the other more closely woven fabrics. Gauze being light and porous admits steam through the center of the pack for prompt contact with the heavier articles on either side. All other articles are folded flat and each succeeding layer is placed crosswise of the one below, to promote free circulation of steam through the mass.

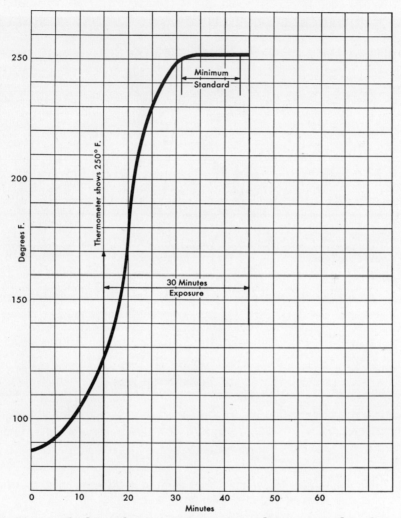

Fig. 52. This graph shows the time-temperature conditions attained in the center of the model pack illustrated in Figure 51, when subjected to 30 minutes exposure at 250° F. in a fully loaded sterilizer.

When the materials are all assembled as shown, the extended sides of the table drape are used to cover the pack, then the double thickness muslin cover is applied. The covers should not be drawn up too tightly, only enough to hold the materials together. The outer cover and package can be tied with a substantial cord, preferably a No. 1 awning cord, or tie strings (spool tape) can be sewed on the muslin cover to simplify the procedure. Figure 52 shows the sterilizing effect attained in the center of the pack illustrated in Figure 51 when subjected to 30 minutes exposure at 250°-254° F. in a fully loaded sterilizer.

The use of pins for holding wrappers in place should be discouraged on

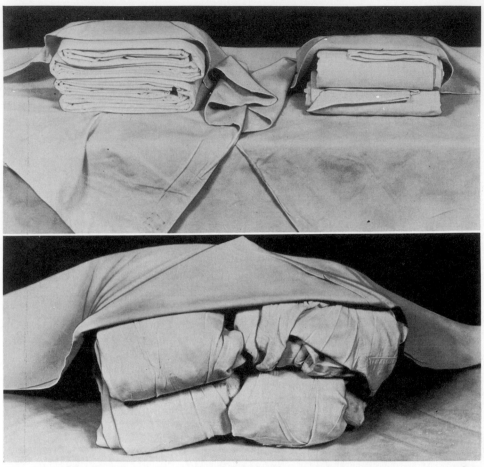

Fig. 53. Table drapes may be wrapped separately in packs containing no more than two drapes each.

Fig. 54. When it is necessary gowns may also be wrapped separately in units of four, with muslin covers as shown.

all surgical supplies. Pins shorten the life of fabrics, increase the tendency of tearing or tight wrapping, and the holes may permit contamination to the interior. Pressure-sensitive tape* may also be used for the sealing of packs and other wrapped supplies. It will withstand autoclaving and offers a convenient means for labeling or identification of the individual packs. A soft pencil ("Venus" 6B) will be found satisfactory for labeling packages.

---

* Tyloc-Tape, Johnson & Johnson, New Brunswick, N.J.

Walter[5] has described another highly efficient method for the preparation of a laparotomy kit. He recommends the use of a wooden trough with dimensions of 22 x 13 x 8½ inches to serve as a guide in limiting the size and shape of the package to standard dimensions which permit uniform steam penetration. In this procedure the wrapper consists of two sheets (63 x 90 inches) folded crosswise and interleaved pamphletlike to form four thicknesses 63 inches long and 45 inches wide. The sheets are then draped in the trough as the first step in preparing the package.

Table Drapes, Sheets and Gowns: Of the various kinds of dry goods encountered in the operating room the table drapes and sheets are the most difficult to sterilize. These fabrics are closely woven with few interlacings and when they are ironed, folded together several times and again ironed, the result is an exceedingly compact mass through which steam can permeate only very slowly. If such materials are wrapped with other supplies, the interference in the passage of steam to other articles may constitute a hazard. For this reason, it is advisable wherever possible to wrap such articles separately or in packs containing no more than two drapes or sheets each, as shown in Figure 53. Such packs are easily sterilized within 30 minutes and they may be included in the same load with the major packs. Towels, on the contrary, present no special problem when included in the major pack. The towel fabric is relatively coarse and even when ironed it offers little resistance to the passage of steam.

When it is found necessary to reduce the size and density of large packs, gowns may also be removed and wrapped separately. The arrangement shown in Figure 54 is suggested. The gown pack includes four rolled gowns in a muslin wrapper. These packs can also be sterilized with the major load in 30 minutes exposure, with a liberal margin of safety. As a rule, it is not necessary to remove gowns from a major pack, providing all of the other articles have been properly arranged in the pack. The loose arrangement of the gown fabric, even when folded, offers little resistance to the passage of steam.

USE OF DRESSING DRUMS, JARS OR CANS

It has long been known that the use of drums in sterilizing necessitates considerably greater exposure time, particularly when the drums are heavily loaded—as they almost invariably are. Regardless of the number and arrangement of portholes in the drum, passageways for the escape of air and intake of steam are restricted far more than when goods are put up in packs. To illustrate this point see Figure 55. The older forms of drums with sliding bands for closing and opening ports are definitely hazardous. Operators are prone to forget to open the ports prior to sterilization. Also the idea that closure of the ports following sterilization will render the drum essentially dust-proof is erroneous. The loose fitting cover will always admit air and dust quite freely. Modern drums have no sliding bands but do have more and better distributed portholes around the walls for the escape of air and the entrance of steam. Even with these improvements the metal surface of the drum still very seriously retards passage of steam to the contents, espe-

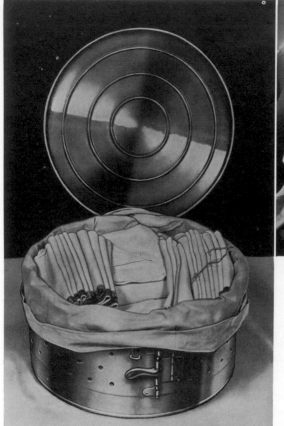

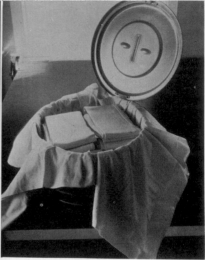

Fig. 56. If drums are used, the load must be carefully arranged as shown here, to avoid filling in the open spaces around the walls of the drum. The drum should be placed on edge in the sterilizer to facilitate steam penetration.

Fig. 55. This is typical of the hazardous condition encountered in the use of drums. The compact arrangement of materials, crowded against the ports in the sides, necessitates prolonged exposure. This load was sterilized in half the time when removed from the drum.

cially when the drum is fully loaded. For these reasons the use of drums can not be recommended.

If drums must be used, it is of extreme importance to limit the size and density of the load. Under no condition is it safely permissible to crowd the contents against the inside walls of the drum. Figure 56 illustrates the proper technique of loading. Place the flat packages of sheets, table covers, towels, etc., in the drum as shown, but do not fill it completely. Do not attempt to fill in the open spaces at the sides, rather leave them open for steam circulation. When the cover is closed, it must not compress the goods. The contents are completely surrounded by two thicknesses of muslin covering. This covering of muslin serves as an air filter to eliminate dust when air is drawn in following removal of the drum from the sterilizer. Loaded in this manner, sterilization should occur in 30 minutes exposure. However, because of the ever-present possibility of tight packing, it is recommended that the exposure period be extended to 45 minutes at 250° F. (121° C.).

Stainless steel, enamelware or other metal jars and cans are commonly used in hospitals for containing gauze squares, cotton balls and small

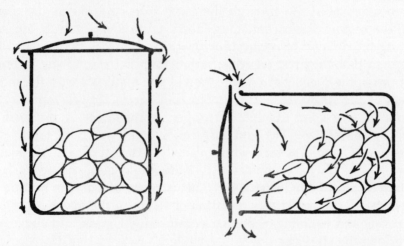

Fig. 57. The incorrect and correct way to place metal jars or cans containing dressings in the sterilizer. Right side up, even with the cover removed, air is trapped in the container. Resting on its side, with the cover held loosely in place, air will drain out and steam will promptly take its place as indicated by the arrows.

dressings for floor use. This type of container is suitable only for loose dressings and it should never be filled with tightly compressed materials. Figure 57 shows the correct and incorrect way to place jars or other non-porous containers of dry material in the sterilizer. When placed in the sterilizer upright, with or without the loose fitting cover in place, air cannot escape, and it will be difficult, if not impossible, to effect sterilization in any reasonable period of exposure. By placing the jar on its side in the sterilizer, with the cover removed or held loosely in place by means of pressure-sensitive tape, the air will drain out slowly and steam will take its place as indicated by the arrows in Figure 57. Tightly wrapped articles should never be placed in jars or other non-porous containers because the admission of steam during sterilization is retarded by having to enter at the open end and traverse the depth of the jar.

The problem of jar sterilization furnishes the background for another important principle governing sterilization of several articles, e.g., delicate instruments or hollow needles placed in test tubes. If the tube or jar is closed, steam cannot enter, and the only sterilizing effect will be that of dry heat developed from the surrounding steam. *An excellent rule to follow when sterilizing any dry material in a jar or test tube is to imagine that the container is filled with water. Then place it in the sterilizer in a horizontal position so that the water would drain out freely.*

ARRANGEMENT OF LOAD IN STERILIZER

The fundamental rule in loading the sterilizer is to prepare all packs and arrange the load in such a manner as to present the least possible resistance to the passage of steam through the load, from the top of the chamber toward the bottom. Packs containing sheets, table covers, towels, etc., which constitute the difficult-to-permeate-with-steam group must be placed in the sterilizer so that they rest on edge, rather than flat side down, in order to permit prompt and complete permeation of the materials with the moisture and heat of the steam.

Figure 58 is a good example of proper arrangement of the load for a moderate size sterilizer. The load has been laid out on a table top in exactly the position it would assume when placed in the sterilizer. All packs are resting on edge, in loose contact with each other; also, the upper layer is placed crosswise of the lower layer. This is recommended as routine practice in order to promote free circulation of steam to the lower packs. Avoid compressing and jamming of the packs into a tight mass, and above all, do not overload the sterilizer.

In loading small cylindrical or square-shaped sterilizers with bulk goods, the operator should be aware of the purpose of the perforated or wire-mesh tray in the bottom of the chamber. As air is released from the load, it gravitates downward to the space underneath the tray and then flows into the chamber discharge outlet. If this tray is omitted or if it becomes flattened so that it conforms to the shape of the sterilizer, the back end of the chamber will become air clogged. Sterilization will then be seriously retarded and, in addition, the goods resting on the bottom will become saturated with water. Examine the tray frequently and make sure that it does elevate the load slightly above the bottom of the chamber.

Another example of good loading practice for a large bulk sterilizer is shown in Figure 59. Here it will be observed that there are no oversized packs and all are placed on edge, without crowding, to facilitate free access for steam penetration. Properly arranged loads in large sterilizers can be sterilized just as effectively as in small chambers. In some respects, the large chamber equipped with shelf-type loading car does not present the problem apparent in small sterilizers. The shelves automatically provide an open space between tiers or layers of packs as a passageway for steam.

The size of the sterilizer or the amount of material placed in it is not the determining factor in fixing the period of exposure. The exposure must be

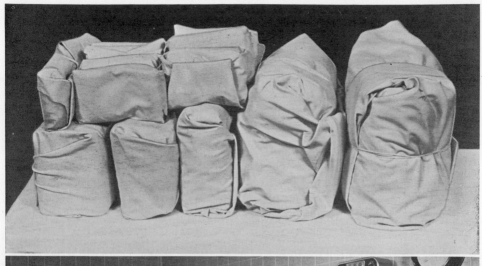

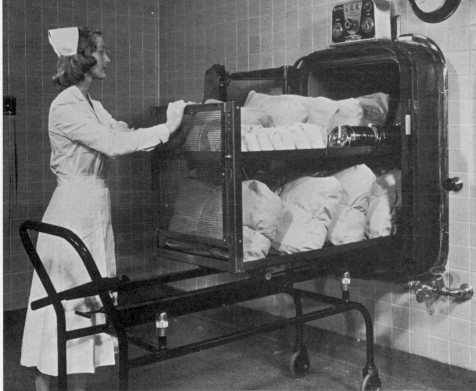

Fig. 58. A good example of proper arrangement of the load for a moderate size sterilizer. All packs rest on their sides in loose contact with each other. This arrangement promotes rapid steam permeation. The upper layer of packs should be placed crosswise of the lower layer as shown.

Fig. 59. Another example of good loading practice for the large surgical supply sterilizer. The large packs are all resting on edge with adequate space between them for free circulation of steam.

determined initially by the size of the largest and most compact pack in the load. Then if these packs are arranged properly, it matters not whether the sterilizer contains one pack or fifty. The only factor subject to change under that condition will be the time required for the temperature to reach the sterilizing range, as indicated by the thermometer. With heavy loads, the temperature will rise more slowly.

SUPERHEATING OF FABRICS DURING STERILIZATION

The effect of steam sterilization on dessicated fabrics or textiles produces a condition known as superheat, causing rapid deterioration of fabrics. This subject is little understood by those responsible for the sterilization of surgical supplies. Before explaining the causes of this condition, it is necessary to define the meaning of superheat. It comes from our knowledge of the properties of steam. *Superheated steam is steam the temperature of which exceeds that of saturated steam at the same pressure.* It is produced by the addition of heat to saturated steam which has been removed from contact with the water from which it was generated. A similar condition occurs when dehydrated or thoroughly dried fabrics are subjected to steam sterilization. The temperature of the fabric exceeds that of the surrounding steam, frequently rising 25°-50° F. higher than the temperature of the steam in the sterilizer. When this occurs, it exerts a destructive effect on the tensile strength of the cloth fibres which, of course, hastens deterioration of the fabric.

Freshly laundered fabrics, if sterilized promptly, do not undergo superheating. The reason for this is that the fibres are in a relatively normal state of hydration prior to sterilization. On the other hand, if fabrics are stored in areas of low humidity for even short periods of time, they give up some of their normal residual moisture content to the atmosphere. Then, when subjected to sterilization, the fibres adsorb additional water from the steam, thereby releasing excess latent heat which results in superheating of the fabrics.

The cumulative effect of superheating of textiles has been carefully studied by Walter.[6] His findings showed that samples of freshly laundered (hydrated) textiles lost 50% of their tensile strength after 70 trips through the laundry and sterilizer, while identical samples which were repeatedly sterilized without laundering lost 73% of their tensile strength. The control samples which were laundered only, lost 20% of their tensile strength. Johnston[7] has presented further evidence on this subject to the effect that fabrics which were sterilized 20 times without laundering lost 50% of their tensile strength. The charred muslin wrappers and cloth liners in drums, commonly observed in many hospitals, are typical of extreme superheating.

To effectively guard against the problem of superheating, the hospital should institute control measures to insure that:

- Freshly laundered fabrics are used only for supplies undergoing sterilization.
- Freshly laundered fabrics are not subjected to storage in areas of low humidity prior to sterilization.
- Surgical packs and other wrapped supplies are not subjected to preheating in the sterilizer, with steam in jacket only, prior to sterilization.
- Sterilizers are not operated with steam at a higher pressure and temperature in the jacket than in the chamber.

DRYING OF LOAD FOLLOWING STERILIZATION

While dressings are undergoing sterilization, the fabrics become saturated with moisture, the condensate left in the goods as heat is absorbed from the steam which permeates them. This moisture, finely distributed through the load, is at the same temperature as the surrounding steam, namely 250° F. (121° C.). The same condition prevails at the close of exposure time, but immediately when pressure reduces, with the exhaust of steam, the moisture flashes into steam or vapor, brought about by the residual heat in the goods—above the boiling point of water—and the heat conducted to them from the hot steam jacket. The real drying process then resolves itself into the detail of getting rid of the vapor as fast as it forms.

For years operators were trained to believe that creation and maintenance of some minor degree of vacuum would bring about satisfactory drying of the load. That method has long since been proved to be faulty, because, with rare exceptions, the greatest degree of vacuum possible to attain in conventional sterilizers is 10 inches of mercury as indicated by the chamber gauge. That would mean 10/30 or one-third of the vapor eliminated from the chamber, and maintaining this degree of vacuum after it is attained is an utter waste of power and time. There are three well known systems of drying in common use, any one of which will give good results if performed correctly:

A) The simplest method known is to exhaust the steam from the chamber to zero gauge pressure, leaving the jacket pressure on to keep the walls of the chamber hot. When chamber pressure has been exhausted, unlock the door and open it slightly, about ¼ inch, just enough to permit vapor to escape. This will provide a chimney effect in which room air will enter at the bottom of the door, while vapor mixed with this air will escape at the top of the door. An interval of 15-20 minutes will usually suffice to dry the load satisfactorily. Objectionably, this method permits all vapor to escape into the room.

B) The second method is a combination of the old so-called vacuum system and the "cracked-door" process described above. Pressure is exhausted from the chamber to zero, then the operating valve is turned to the vacuum position for a short time only, about 5 minutes. In this period the vacuum valve will exhaust about all the vapor it is capable of handling.

Then the vacuum is broken, the door unlocked and cracked just enough to permit the remainder of vapor to escape. By this method only two-thirds of the vapor will escape into the room as compared with the simple "cracked-door" method. Otherwise the results will be identical.

C) The third system involves the principles of both the older methods

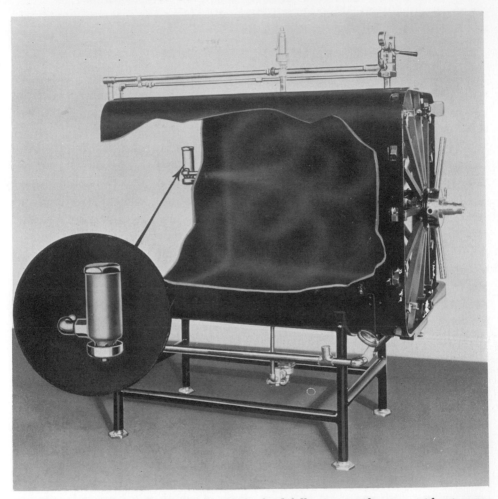

Fig. 60. Vacuum dryer device for drying the load following sterilization, without opening door of sterilizer. The device functions as a pump to circulate filtered air to the chamber where it entrains with the vapor and both are then discharged to the vent.

but it exhausts practically all vapor to the vent. The system employs a vacuum dryer (ejector) device in conjunction with the operating valve on the sterilizer. It is used in this manner: Following sterilization, pressure is exhausted to zero, then the operating valve is turned to the vacuum or dry position. Instead of creating a partial vacuum the device functions as a pump to circulate filtered air to the chamber where it entrains with the vapor and both are then discharged to the vent (see Fig. 60). Under this system, when the door is opened, there is no noticeable escape of vapor. The minimum drying time is 15 minutes for the average load.

There is very little difference in drying efficiency by either the "cracked-door" method or the vacuum dryer process. However, the latter system possesses the advantage of preventing vapor from escaping into the room—a detail worthy of consideration, especially in the interests of air conditioning.

It has been determined experimentally that a large surgical pack, weighing approximately 12 pounds, retains 9 ounces of moisture as condensate from the steam in the normal sterilizing process. This figure of 9 ounces, representative of a 5% increase in weight of the package, was determined immediately after the steam in the sterilizer had been exhausted to atmospheric pressure. In 10 minutes drying by the "cracked-door" process 35% of the residual moisture was removed, in 20 minutes drying 50%, and in 30 minutes 65% of the initial 9 ounces of moisture. Obviously there would be no purpose in extending the drying time beyond 30 minutes because the residual moisture in the average pack would represent less than 2% increase over the original weight.

CAUSES OF WET DRESSINGS

Dressings delivered from the sterilizer in a wet or soggy condition present a definite hazard and they should never be sent to the operating room. Even when dressings are well dried out in the sterilizer sufficient vapor remains in the goods so that sudden cooling may result in condensate forming objectionably—perhaps dangerously. It is unwise to place freshly sterilized packs or other wrapped supplies on any cold surface such as a metal table top. The sweating that occurs on the cool table top will accumulate in little pools of water which may pick up contamination. In turn, this contaminated water may be reabsorbed by the fabric rendering it unsterile. Probst[8] has demonstrated clearly that once sterile cloth becomes damp, even if the water source is sterile, it allows contamination to take place provided it is in contact with an unsterile object. Beck and Collette[9] also proved that bacteria readily pass through two layers of wet cloth whereas two layers of dry cloth prevent such migration.

The proper handling of sterilized packs as they are removed from the sterilizer demands that they never be stacked up in close contact with each other, but rather maintained in such a position that air can circulate freely around them, on all sides. When loading carriages are used, it is good practice to leave the load on the carriage, after removing from the sterilizer, for 15 or 20 minutes. If no loading carriage is used, the packs should be laid out on edge, preferably on a wire mesh or slatted wooden surface covered with several layers of muslin to absorb the sweating moisture.

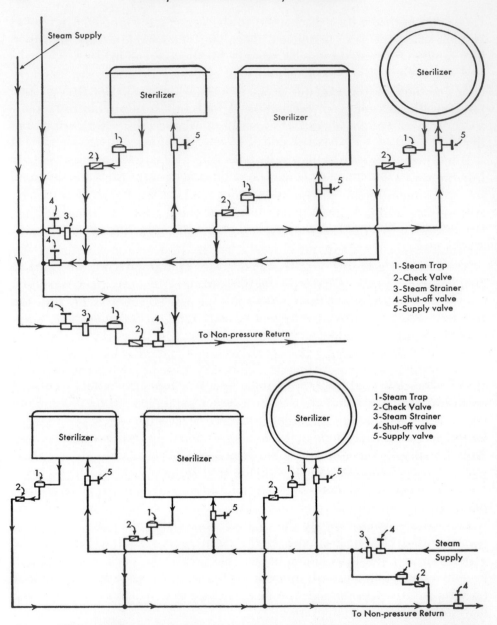

Fig. 61. When sterilizers are fed from adjacent steam supply risers, application of suitable traps as indicated in this diagram will keep the risers filled with dry steam. The supply system should be protected by a steam strainer and accessible shut-off valves as shown. Lacking this or some equally effective method of draining condensate from supply lines, they will fill up with water and seriously interfere with sterilization and drying.

Fig. 62. When sterilizers are fed from long horizontal runs of supply steam piping, the line can be kept free from condensate by the trapping method indicated in this diagram.

In addition to faulty methods of packaging and loading, there are other conditions responsible for wet dressings. Most of these require the attention of a trained serviceman or maintenance engineer for correction. Those of major importance are:

1) *Clogging of chamber discharge line on sterilizer.* If the air and condensate discharge line becomes clogged with sediment and lint, or if the thermostatic valve or check valve fails to open properly, water will collect in the bottom of the chamber and the lower portion of the load will not dry satisfactorily. This fault will be indicated by the presence of water in the bottom of the chamber when the door is opened. If no water is found in the chamber, but if the lower portion of the load is perceptibly wet, that will indicate sluggish performance of the discharge system. In either case, the remedy is to clean out the line and check the operation of the thermostatic valve.

2) *Improperly drained steam supply line.* An improperly drained steam supply line may deliver water to the sterilizer instead of steam. If this fault is pronounced, both jacket and chamber will fill with water and the load will be saturated. There is only one remedy for this difficulty. The steam supply line must be adequately drained before it reaches the sterilizer by a correctly trapped bleeder line, as shown in Figures 61 and 62. An indication of water in the supply line or a clogged return trap from the jacket of the sterilizer is a loud hammering noise which occurs when steam is turned on to the sterilizer.

3) *Overfilling steam generator with water.* On electric or gas heated sterilizers, wet dressings are sure to occur as the result of overfilling the boiler or steam generator with water. This usually occurs through carelessness of the operator in not shutting off the filling valve when the proper level has been reached. It may also occur by slow leakage of the water filling valve.

4) *Faulty sterilizer installation.* An occasional cause of wet dressings is the incorrectly installed sterilizer with the back end lower than the front end. In this case, condensate will drain to the rear and the vapor forming from it will saturate the goods. This can be easily corrected by adjusting the supports on the sterilizer so that the front end is slightly lower than the back end.

Summary of Factors Governing Steam Sterilization of Surgical Supplies

PACKAGING

1) Use freshly laundered fabrics to guard against superheating.
2) Limit the size and density of the individual packs to insure uniform steam permeation with a liberal margin of safety for sterilization.

3) Use double thickness muslin or its equivalent as wrapping material for surgical supplies.

LOADING OF STERILIZER

4) Place all packs on edge and arrange the load in the sterilizer so as to present the least possible resistance to the passage of steam through the load, from the top of the chamber to the bottom.

5) Place all jars and other non-porous containers of dry material on their sides in the sterilizer so as to provide a horizontal path for the escape of air.

EXPOSURE PERIOD

6) Establish a standard exposure period for all bulk supplies that will provide for complete penetration of the load and insure destruction of all microbial life with a liberal margin of safety.

7) Time the sterilizing period from the moment that saturated steam at 250° F. (121° C.) fills the chamber as indicated by the thermometer in the chamber discharge line.

DRYING OF LOAD

8) Establish a minimum drying period of 15 minutes for all bulk loads of supplies.

9) Guard against the placement of freshly sterilized packages on cold surfaces.

REFERENCES

1. BECK, C. E., SHAY, D. E., AND PURDUM, W. A.: An Evaluation of Paper Used for Wrapping Articles to Be Sterilized. *Bull. Am. Soc. Hosp. Pharm.*, 10:421-427, 1953. (See also *Bull. Am. Soc. Hosp. Pharm.*, 12:511, 1955.)
2. WALTER, C. W.: *Bull. Am. Soc. Hosp. Pharm.*, 11:317, 1954.
3. WHITTENBERGER, J. L.: *Steam Sterilization of Paper-Wrapped Packages.* New York, Meinecke.
4. Bio-Research Laboratories: Report on Sterility Tests of Objects Wrapped in Patapar, Oct. 7, 1950, San Francisco, Calif.
5. WALTER, C. W.: *Aseptic Treatment of Wounds.* New York, Macmillan, 1948, pp. 97-98.
6. WALTER, C. W.: *Aseptic Treatment of Wounds.* New York, Macmillan, 1948, p. 64.
7. JOHNSTON, L. G.: Personal Communication, June 3, 1947.
8. PROBST, H. D.: The Effect of Bactericidal Agents on the Sterility of Surgical Linen. *Am. J. Surg.*, 86:301-308, 1953.
9. BECK, W. C., AND COLLETTE, T. S.: False Faith in the Surgeon's Gown and Surgical Drape. *Am. J. Surg.*, 83:125, 1952.

Chapter VII

Preparation and Sterilization of Rubber Goods

THE HANDLING, washing and sterilizing of rubber goods presents special problems to the hospital. As a rule, rubber goods do not wear out—they are destroyed. Rubber will deteriorate with age, exposure to light, heat and chemicals, but the life of any rubber article is materially shortened by abuse and careless handling. With the exception of the synthetic products, rubber is of vegetable origin, and sunlight, heat, oils, greases and solvents are natural enemies of rubber. While contact with these substances, including light, cannot be avoided in normal hospital routine, it is suggested that care be exercised to remove any oils, greases, or solvents thoroughly and as soon as possible.

RUBBER GLOVES

Before new gloves are put into use, they should be washed to remove any talcum powder which may be on them. The irritants occasionally present in rubber gloves can be removed by soaking in a 5% solution of sodium carbonate for 15 minutes, followed by rinsing and sterilization. The life of the gloves can be prolonged by permitting them to rest for 48 hours after sterilization and before the next period of use.

Immediately following an operation, the gloves should be washed off in cold water before removing them from the hands. This step can be accomplished most conveniently in the scrub sink with the aid of a brush to loosen any adhering particles of dried blood. This detail is often neglected, adding to the difficulties of thorough washing later. After removing the gloves from the hands, the fingers should be pulled out, then place them in a container of water until the time of final washing. From this point onward the processing of gloves involves the following operations:

1) Washing.	5) Powdering.
2) Drying.	6) Packaging.
3) Testing.	7) Sterilization.
4) Sorting.	8) Storage.

The manual washing of gloves, one at a time, hanging them individually on racks or glove trees to dry, and powdering each one inside and outside, by hand, are elements of an outmoded technique which is rapidly giving way to a mechanized process, utilizing labor-saving machines and devices.

Today most hospitals are aware of the advantages of mechanical aids in the processing of gloves. Automatic washers, glove conditioners and dryers are used in many hospitals with a high degree of efficiency and economy. Some of the larger institutions send all of their gloves to the main hospital laundry for processing. However, experience has shown that the key to a successful mechanized operation for the average hospital is the establishment of a glove processing room as a part of the central supply department. All of the above operations can then be performed in a centralized area

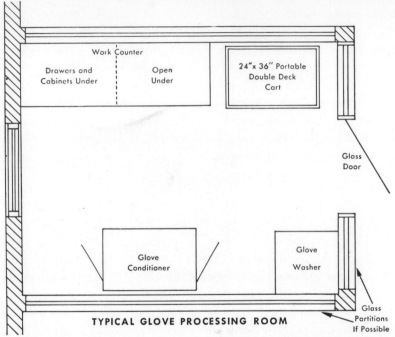

Fig. 63. Typical layout for a modern glove processing room. The plan requires an area of about 80 square feet and is considered adequate for hospitals of 125-300 beds.

and the various related tasks can be turned over to non-professional workers. A typical layout for a modern glove processing room is shown in Figure 63. The individual mechanical equipment items shown on this plan include an automatic washer, domestic type, glove conditioner for drying and powdering and a surgical glove tester. Utilizing this layout under actual hospital conditions, Prickett[1] has reported a savings of $1.75 of direct labor cost per 100 gloves processed by the mechanized method, when compared with a representative manual method.

Following the washing and drying process, the gloves are tested for holes or defects. Each glove is inflated with compressed air supplied by the glove tester. When holes are found they are marked with a red wax pencil for later identification in patching. Gloves found to be punctured are separated from the others, and after mending with liquid glove patch, they are retained for use on the wards for lumbar punctures, rectal and pelvic exami-

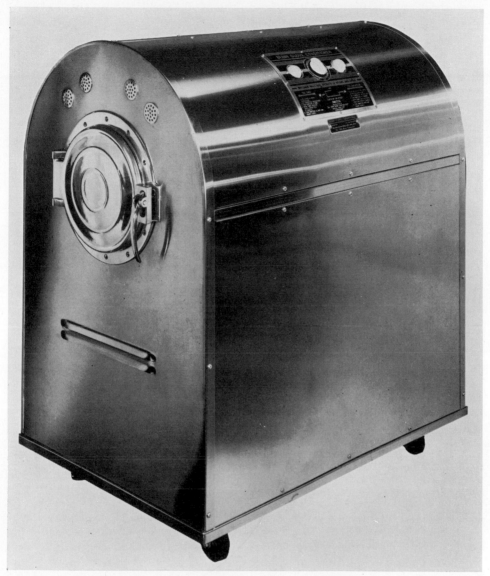

Fig. 64. Glove processing apparatus for the drying, powdering and conditioning of rubber gloves.

nations, etc. The gloves are then powdered in an automatic glove conditioner such as the type shown in Figure 64. To avoid unnecessary handling of the gloves after they are powdered, Lehmann[2] recommends that they be paired and clipped together with colored, plastic, spring-type clothespins before putting them in the powdering unit. Different colored clothespins are used to designate the various sizes. Talcum powder is no longer recommended as a lubricant for gloves because of its demonstrated irritating properties which may result in granulomatous reactions in tissues.[3, 4, 5, 6] The commercial product known as "Biosorb," which is a mixture of amylose and amylopectin, derived from corn starch, has largely replaced talc as a surgical glove lubricant. According to Lee, Collins and Largen,[7] "the fact that starch powder is biologically 'nonirritating' and absorbable, when

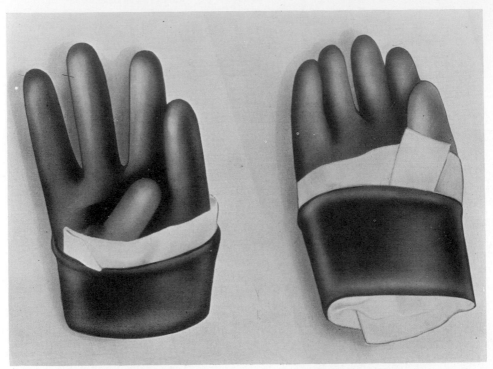

Fig. 65. In wrapping gloves for sterilization, it is good practice to insert a band of gauze or muslin in the wrist fold as shown here, to permit free contact of steam to the folded-over surfaces. It is also suggested that a pad of gauze or muslin be inserted in the palm of the glove, as far in as the fingers, to hold the apposing surfaces apart and to permit steam to effectively contact the interior.

finely dispersed, does not mean that the basic surgical principles of avoiding contamination of wounds with foreign material may be abandoned. Air contamination should be kept at a minimum and gloves should be thoroughly washed as free of powder as possible before the operation is begun. If a glove is torn or punctured, it should immediately be replaced and the fresh glove should be washed before the wearer returns to the surgical field."

Although not commonly recognized, rubber gloves constitute one of the most difficult of all items to be sterilized in the hospital. The reason is obviously not one of steam penetration through successive layers of material but rather ineffective air removal from the fingers of the gloves. Care

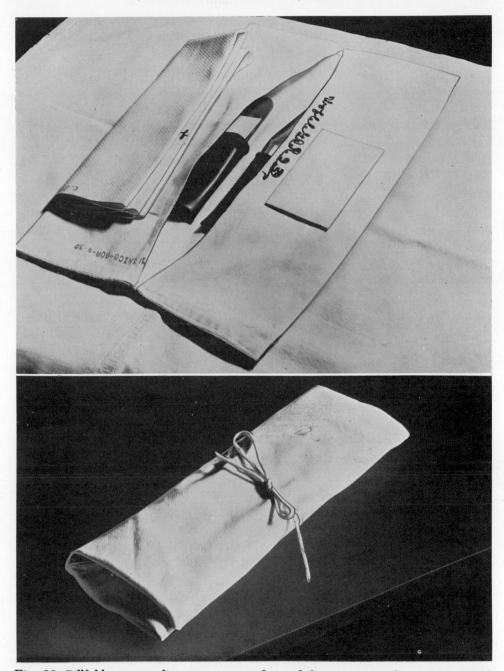

Fig. 66. Billfold type muslin cover commonly used for wrapping gloves. The paired gloves are inserted, with thumbs up, into the pockets of the muslin envelope. A small quantity of powder ("Biosorb") in a small steam-permeable paper envelope or in a gauze sponge can be included as shown.

Fig. 67. The envelope shown in Figure 66 should be wrapped in this manner. The outer covering is designed for the purpose and includes tie strings.

must be used in the packaging and wrapping of the gloves to insure that all surfaces shall be freely exposed to the steam as shown in Figure 65. Where the wrist section of the glove is folded back to form the cuff, it is important to keep the two surfaces separated from each other. This can be done by placing a band of gauze or muslin under the fold when the wrist section is turned back. It is also suggested that a pad of gauze or muslin be inserted in the palm of each glove, as far in as the fingers, to hold the apposing surfaces apart and to promote egress of air and intake of steam. The chief factor to keep in mind in packaging is to prepare the glove so that no pressure is applied which might force any two surfaces into tight contact with each other.

Covers for gloves should be of the billfold type, with a pocket for one glove on either side of the median line as shown in Figure 66. Each glove should be placed in its respective pocket carefully with the thought in mind that when the package is later placed in the sterilizer the thumbs should be resting up in order to assist air clearance. A small amount of "Biosorb" powder (1cc.) can be folded in a gauze sponge or placed in a small, steam-permeable paper envelope and included in the wrapper as shown. A folded towel may also be placed between the leaves of the envelope when they are folded together. Although the billfold type envelope is often used with no further covering, this is not considered good practice. An outer muslin wrapper should be used for additional protection as illustrated in Figure 67.

Gloves are preferably sterilized alone, not in combination with other bulk loads of supplies. The packs should rest on edge in the sterilizer, with the thumbs up, well away from the sidewalls of the chamber. A large instrument tray with wire-mesh or perforated bottom makes an ideal container for them (Fig. 68). It is imperative that the gloves be stacked loosely, never more than one tier deep. The trays should always be placed in the upper two-thirds of the sterilizer, not on the bottom shelf. Residual air present in the lower portion of the chamber, even as little as 0.1%, will hasten the rate of deterioration of rubber. For sterilization, an exposure period of not less than 15 minutes and no longer than 20 minutes at 250°-254° F. is recommended, followed by a minimum of 15 minutes drying. After sterilization the gloves should be held in storage for a period of 24 to 48 hours before dispensing for use. This will help the rubber to regain its tensile strength, prevent tackiness and the useful life will be prolonged.

RUBBER CATHETERS, DRAINS AND TUBES

All articles made of rubber, especially latex and red rubber, are highly susceptible to attack and deterioration by chemical agents. No rubber article should be subjected to cleaning agents made of or containing hydrocarbons, oxidizing acids or oils. The following substances are known to cause deterioration and they will destroy the usefulness of all articles made of rubber:

1) Mineral and vegetable oils, such as petroleum jelly and mineral oil, cause swelling and tackiness.

2) Hydrocarbon solvents, ethers and esters, such as acetone, benzene, and cleaning fluid cause swelling and rapid deterioration.

3) Oxidizing acids, such as sulfuric and hydrochloric, cause rapid deterioration.

4) Copper and manganese cause rapid catalytic decomposition.

5) Phenols and cresols, such as Lysol, carbolic acid, hexachlorophene, and soaps containing phenol or phenyl compounds, cause stickiness and disintegration.

6) Quaternary ammonium compounds, such as benzalkonium chloride, cause tackiness and decrease resistance to steam sterilization.

7) Volatile amine compounds, such as morpholine, benzylamine and cyclohexylamine, will contribute to rubber deterioration. Some hospitals add volatile amine compounds to their steam boilers to protect the supply lines against corrosion. Since the compounds are volatile they will be present in the steam during sterilization and thereby contribute to deterioration of rubber.

Prior to sterilization, rubber catheters should be cleaned with an alkaline detergent such as tri-sodium phosphate or Oakite, followed by copious rinsing with water. This permits the rubber to become hydrated and if sterilized promptly superheating will not occur. A dry catheter upon contact with steam will undergo deterioration as the result of superheating. Catheters may be packaged in cellophane tubing or in long paper envelopes, several of which are commercially available. When sterilized by saturated steam under pressure the exposure period should be 15 minutes at 250° F. These same conditions regarding preparation and sterilization of rubber catheters apply equally to vinyl catheters and tubes.

WOVEN CATHETERS, BOUGIES AND FILIFORMS

Woven catheters are used primarily for either diagnostic or treatment purposes. The coating on the catheters is composed of synthetic resinous materials which absorb water, especially in the presence of heat.[8] The principal chemical agents which cause deterioration of woven catheters are: alcohol, cresols, phenols, glycerin and *alkali detergents*.

Before sterilization, the catheters should be thoroughly cleaned in a solution free from alkali or organic solvents. Water containing a mild liquid soap is recommended. Green soap containing glycerin or phenol or solutions of tri-sodium phosphate should not be used. The cleaning agent should be forced through the lumen either by means of a syringe or siphon. Copious

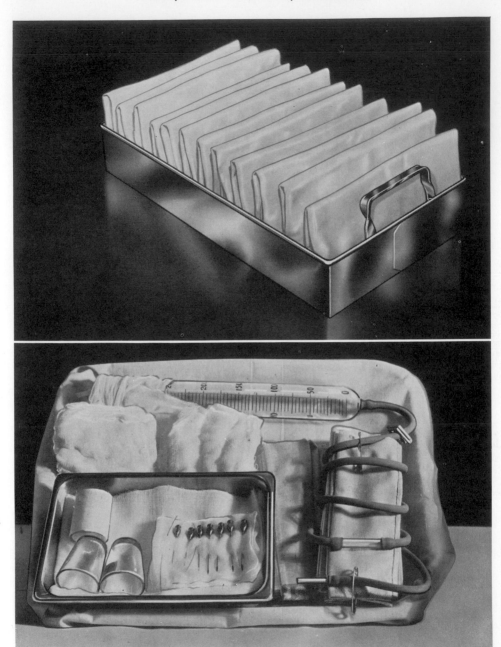

Fig. 68. The instrument sterilizer tray or its equivalent with wire-mesh bottom makes an ideal container for gloves. The glove packs should rest on edge in the sterilizer, stacked loosely, never more than one tier deep.

Fig. 69. When it is required to sterilize a long length of tubing attached to a bottle or burette, the entire assembly should be flushed with freshly distilled water just before wrapping, and the interior surfaces left moist. The tubing should be carefully coiled but not kinked in the package.

rinsing should be avoided because of the possibility of forcing too much moisture into the catheter surface. After cleaning, the catheter should be wrapped in muslin, without bending or coiling, and sterilized with steam under pressure at 250° F. for 15 minutes. After the catheter has been used for the first time, it should again be cleaned and thoroughly dried out before being sterilized the second time. This may be accomplished by placing the catheter in a warm dry area and leaving it there for 3 or 4 days, or by drying it out in the sterilizer with steam to jacket only for 15 minutes. Once a catheter has been properly dried out after the first sterilization and use, the physical structure of the coating changes so that subsequent sterilizations will not develop blisters or cracks.

RUBBER TUBING

Sterilization of rubber tubing is difficult, yet no possible contamination can be tolerated because of its frequent use in intravenous therapy or for other equally critical applications. Thorough preliminary cleaning is essential for safe preparation of new tubing to remove impurities and also for used tubing which may contain traces of blood, residual drugs, etc. In the case of transfusion tubing, the practice should be rigidly enforced of thorough rinsing in cold water immediately after use to prevent blood from drying in the lumen. Effective cleaning may be accomplished by immersing the tubing in a large basin containing a 0.5 per cent solution of sodium hydroxide or 5 per cent sodium carbonate and boiling for 15 minutes. The tubing should be coiled slowly into the solution to avoid the formation of air pockets, or better yet, the alkali solution should be circulated slowly through the tubing during the period of boiling. A large irrigating syringe may be used for this purpose or a reservoir of the alkali solution may be attached to a ring stand above the basin, connected to the tubing, and the solution slowly trickled through the lumen. After cleaning, the tubing should be rinsed with freshly distilled water until all traces of alkali have been removed.

For sterilization, assemble the tubing with required connectors or attachments, and just before wrapping, flush out the entire assembly with distilled water, but do not drain completely. Rather leave the interior distinctly moist and wrap in double thickness muslin. The tubing should be carefully coiled but not kinked in the package (see Fig. 69). The residual moisture in the tubing plus the heat of the steam conducted to the interior will be sufficient for sterilization when exposed for 30 minutes to a temperature of 250° F. (121° C.).[9]

REFERENCES

1. PRICKETT, E. A.: *A Study of the Operating Room.* Sect. II, School of Nursing, Univ. of Pittsburgh, 1954, p. 9-20.

2. LEHMANN, E. E., AND BISHOP, F. W.: We Streamlined Our Glove Technic. *Am. J. Nursing,* 52:176-177, Feb. 1952.
3. SEELIG, M. G.: The Talcum Powder Evil. *Am. J. Surg.,* 76:272-273, 1948.
4. GERMAN, W. M.: Dusting Powder Granulomas Following Surgery. *Surg., Gynec., & Obst.,* 76:501-507, 1943.
5. LEE, C. M. JR., AND LEHMAN, E. P.: Experiments with Nonirritating Glove Powder. *Surg., Gynec. & Obst.,* 84:689-696, 1947.
6. POSTLETHWAIT, R. W., HOWARD, H. L., AND SCHANKER, P. W.: Comparison of Tissue Reaction to Talc and Modified Starch Glove Powder. *Surgery,* 25:22-29, 1949.
7. LEE, D. M., COLLINS, W. T., AND LARGEN, T. L.: A Reappraisal of Absorbable Glove Powder. *Surg., Gynec. & Obst.,* 95:725-737, 1952.
8. OUTWIN, E. S.: *Care and Sterilization of Catheters, Drains and Tubes.* C. R. Bard, Inc., Summit, New Jersey, (1955).
9. UNDERWOOD, W. B.: *New Method of Preparing Rubber Tubing for Sterilization.* The Surgical Supervisor, July, 1944.

CHAPTER 8

Preparation and Sterilization of
Surgical Instruments

THE ESTABLISHMENT of high quality standards for the care and sterilization of surgical instruments should be of vital concern to every hospital. The practice of aseptic surgery demands safe, rapid and effective methods for the sterilization of instruments and other supplies. This requirement can best be met initially through the medium of intelligent and efficient planning of the operating suite with special attention given to the necessity of providing adjunct sterilization facilities to serve each pair of operating rooms. An approach to the ideal arrangement is shown in Figure 70. The basic equipment for the substerilizing room consists of an instrument washer-sterilizer for post-operative washing and terminal sterilization of instruments from septic cases, and a high-speed pressure instrument sterilizer for routine or emergency sterilization of instruments. The usual pair of water sterilizers is not shown, since this equipment is rapidly becoming outmoded in favor of the flask method for supplying sterile water or isotonic fluids directly to the operating room from the central supply or solution preparation room. When this procedure is used, a blanket and solution warming cabinet occupies the space devoted to water sterilizers. A small dry heat sterilizer for cutting edge instruments is also a useful item of equipment for the substerilizing room.

THE SELECTION OF QUALITY INSTRUMENTS

The skill of the surgeon may frequently be impaired as the result of the quality and condition of the instruments at his command. No instrument is better than the steel from which it is made. For perfect instruments the tempering and workmanship are of great importance and care should be exercised in the selection of a reliable brand of instrument. Because of the superior properties of certain alloys of stainless steel, the majority of present-day instruments are made from this metal. Several kinds of stainless steel are used and the difference lies in the formulas of the steel, providing a different quality for different purposes.

The term "stainless" is a relative one in that metallurgical science has not yet developed any steel which is completely stainless under all conditions. Basically, stainless steel contains much less carbon than ordinary steel and, in addition, it also contains other metals such as chromium and nickel in order to produce corrosion resistance. With surgical instruments it is far more important to have the proper hardness and elasticity than to have absolute corrosion resistance, providing the corrosion resistance is kept sufficiently high. The carbon content is of vital importance. If the percentage of carbon is too low, then the resulting steel is too soft. If it is

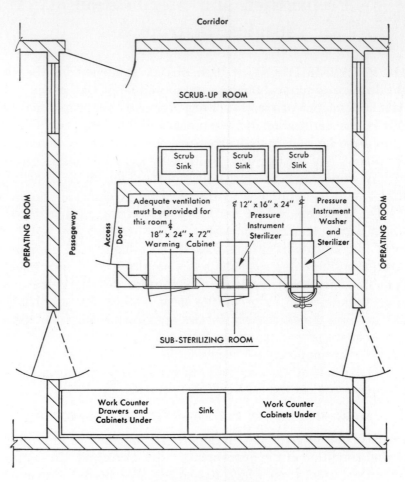

SURGERY SUB-STERILIZING ROOM

Fig. 70. Sub-sterilizing room. This is an approach to the ideal arrangement of providing adjunct sterilization facilities for each pair of operating rooms.

too high, it forms a steel which is too brittle and hard to forge. According to certain manufacturers' classifications,[1] steels containing about 12 to 17 per cent chromium and about 0.2 to 0.7 per cent carbon have been found most suitable for surgical instruments.

It is apparent that in the manufacture of instruments workmanship may vary considerably. It is good practice therefore to examine all new instruments. Observe if the points of scissors and forceps are equally long on each instrument; that the jaws of forceps are equally thick; that curved jaws are bent to a smooth, even curve; that serrations mesh properly and are beveled at the edges of the jaws; and that the jaws close evenly, starting at the point and being fully closed when the last ratchet has been reached. It is also important to note if the teeth of all forceps are even, of proper shape and sharpness, and mesh uniformly. There should be no sharp points or edges which may scratch or tear the surgeon's gloves. Scissors should close smoothly and cut well at the points, also along the entire edges. The box lock of forceps should work smoothly, yet show no evidence of looseness. The shanks should be springy and soft enough to permit closing to the last ratchet without undue effort. The ratchets should glide smoothly over each other, hold firmly, open easily, even from the last ratchet. All thumb and tissue forceps should be tested for the proper tension.

HAND WASHING OF INSTRUMENTS

Instruments must be cleaned as soon as possible after use, to avoid rusting and to remove soil before it can dry and harden in the serrations, crevices, etc. If stainless steel instruments are permitted to lie around for several hours before cleaning they may acquire a tarnish which is difficult to remove. Likewise, plated instruments may show evidence of rusting at points where the plating has been damaged or worn through by previous cleansing processes. Therefore, immediately after use the instruments should be rinsed in cold water to assist in the removal of blood. Then, if the instruments must be exposed for any period of time before washing, they should be covered with water containing some effective blood solvent or detergent.

The final washing process should be conducted with care and each step should be thoroughly understood by the person performing the duty. It is essential to remove all particles of adhering tissue, dried blood, scale and accumulations of lime salts in the serrations, ratchets and box locks of the instruments. In the scrubbing process, a hand brush with fairly stiff bristles may be used to advantage. The use of abrasives or other sharp cleaners should be avoided because continued use of an abrasive compound may roughen the surface, thereby minimizing the "stainless" properties. To assist in the removal of inaccessible soil, it is necessary to establish a routine consisting of preliminary soaking of the instruments in warm water at a temperature of about 125° F. (52° C.), to which has been added an effective detergent such as Haemosol, Pyrem or Edisonite. Thorough cleaning is extremely important because organisms concealed and protected by dried blood and scale in inaccessible parts of the instruments render sterilization more difficult.

Immediately after washing, the instruments should be rinsed with boiling water for a brief interval and then dried thoroughly, while still hot.

Rinsing with boiling water is important in the hand washing of instruments because the residual heat assists greatly in drying. If any moisture remains on the instruments, they may rust in storage. At best, the manual cleaning of instruments is a difficult and time-consuming process. It is almost impossible to remove all traces of soil from the inaccessible areas of box locks, serrations, ratchets, etc. The mechanical cleaning process, described below, utilizing the pressure instrument washer-sterilizer makes it possible to employ a superior technique in a fraction of the time normally required for the hand washing of instruments.

INSTRUMENT WASHER-STERILIZER

I) *Development:* The need for a safe and rapid mechanical process for the routine cleansing and sterilization of instruments in the operating room has been recognized for many years. It was not until 1938 that Walter[2, 3] described such a process together with appropriate illustrations of an instrument washer-sterilizer. The first apparatus, as shown in Figure 71, was designed along the lines of a vertical autoclave, constructed to withstand an operating pressure of 27 pounds. It utilized a stainless steel bucket as a receptacle for the soiled instruments. The bucket was placed in the washer-sterilizer directly over a baffle which forced the water to circulate through perforations in the bottom of the bucket. A steam coil in the bottom of the chamber supplied heat for sterilization and produced convection currents in the water to carry oil and grease released from the instruments to the surface and then to an overflow at the rear of the washer-sterilizer. The addition of a suitable detergent to peptonize proteins and saponify greases was necessary for proper cleansing. After the water reached a temperature of 273° F. (133° C.), requiring seven minutes' time, the steam was shut off and the water drained into a flash tank equipped with atmospheric vent. The instruments could then be removed from the washer-sterilizer in a clean, dry and sterile condition, ready for immediate use if so desired.

The latest development in the design of an instrument washer-sterilizer is shown in Figure 72. This unit was introduced to hospitals in 1947.[4] The horizontal (cabinet type) design, in contrast to the vertical type, makes it possible to utilize standard instrument trays which, in turn, permit easier and more efficient loading and unloading of instruments. The trays of instruments are automatically lowered into the chamber or raised by means of a hydraulic lift, powered by the water supply line pressure. The complete cycle of washing and sterilizing is governed solely by the moving of a single control handle to progressive positions shown on the front panel of the cabinet. The washing process is accomplished by means of a vigorously agitated detergent bath, heated directly by a muffled steam jet. During the washing phase the agitated detergent solution disengages blood, grease and tissue debris from the instruments, carries the soil to the surface and then to an overflow at the front end of the chamber. As the heated water expands in the chamber, the level rises and the released soil and scum overflow into a reservoir from which it is discharged through a thermostatic trap into the waste.

In the normal process of operation the temperature of the bath is raised to 270° F. (132° C.) in about 12 minutes. At this temperature sterilization is practically instantaneous and no holding period is required. The water

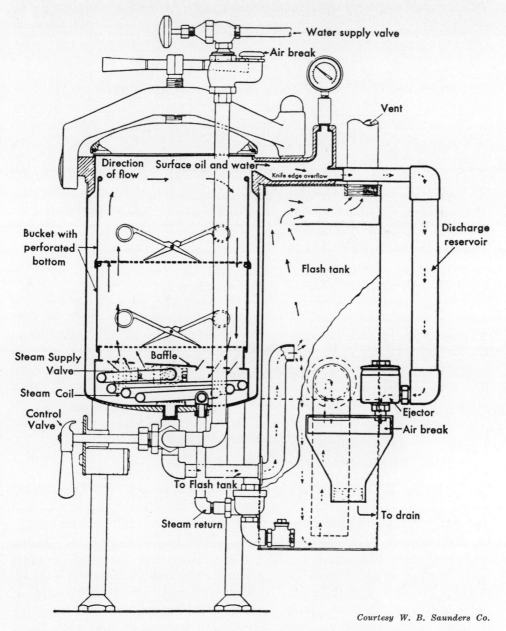

Courtesy W. B. Saunders Co.

Fig. 71. An early model of the instrument washer and sterilizer as illustrated by Walter.[3]

and steam are then rapidly exhausted and the high residual heat in the instruments is sufficient to flash any adherent moisture. The clean, dry, sterile instruments are then ready for immediate use upon removal from the washer-sterilizer or they may be placed in the instrument storage cabi-

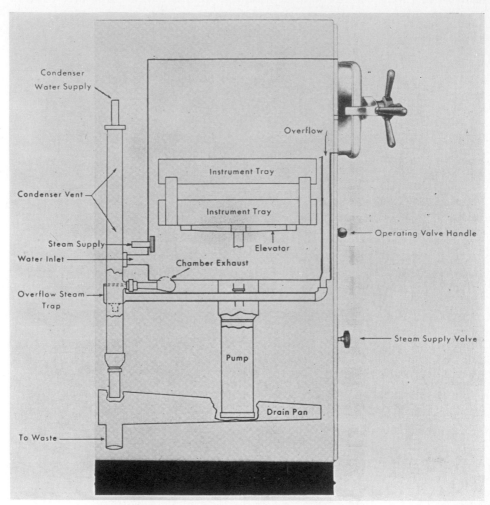

Fig. 72. Longitudinal diagram of pressure instrument washer-sterilizer, horizontal type.

net until needed. A typical process chart showing time required and resulting temperature of instruments for each phase of the washing-sterilizing cycle is given in Fig. 73.

II) *Technic of Operation:* The pressure instrument washer-sterilizer of the type shown in Figure 74 may be used with equal efficiency for routine preoperative sterilization, post-operative washing or for washing and terminal sterilization from septic cases. The technic of operation is as follows:

Routine practice demands that immediately upon completion of surgical procedure in operating room the instruments be placed in a basin of water to prevent excessive drying of blood in serrations, depressions, etc.

1) To LOAD. Promptly after use, collect soiled instruments and place in trays furnished with washer-sterilizer, making sure jointed instruments

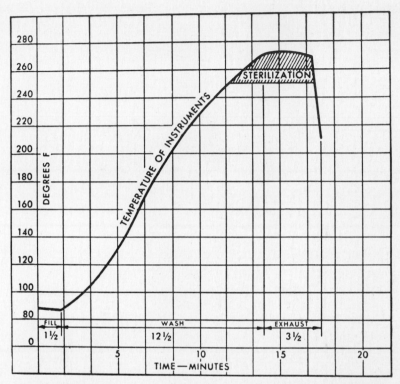

Fig. 73. Process chart showing time required and the resulting temperature of the instruments during each phase of the washing-sterilizing cycle.

are unlocked and fully opened. Place trays on sliding supports and push fully into chamber. Turn "Operating Valve" to "Lower." Trays will descend into chamber by means of hydraulic elevator.

2) To WASH AND STERILIZE. Turn "Operating Valve" to "Fill," add one ounce of liquid detergent directly on top of lowered trays. Operator should remain at close attention until water begins to overflow into the reservoir at front of chamber. Immediately turn "Operating Valve" to "Ster." Then close and lock door. Open "Steam Supply Valve." In about 12 minutes, temperature will reach 270° F. (132° C.) (27-28 pounds pressure). At this temperature the red "Signal Light" will come on indicating completion of sterilization.

3) To EXHAUST WATER AND STEAM FROM CHAMBER. At close of exposure period (Step 2), close "Steam Supply Valve," turn "Operating Valve"

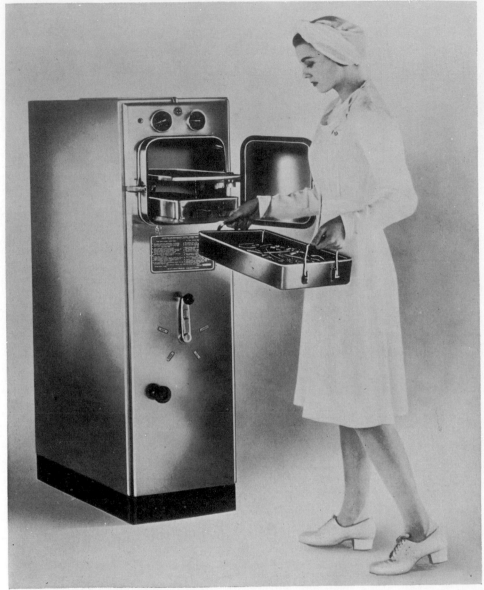

Fig. 74. An open-mounted installation of the washer-sterilizer. This utilizes standard instrument trays which permit efficient loading and unloading of the instruments. The single rotary operating valve controls each phase of the washing-sterilizing cycle.

to "Exhaust." When "Chamber Gauge" shows zero pressure turn "Operating Valve" to "Raise." Unlock door and remove load.

4) To Sterilize Instruments Only Without Washing.
   A) With a layer of muslin in bottom of tray, place clean instruments in tray and cover with layer of muslin for protection and to facilitate drying.

B) With load in chamber, trays in normal "Raise" position (do not "Lower" trays when machine is to be used as sterilizer only), door locked, open "Steam Supply Valve." Then turn "Operating Valve" to left (counterclockwise) to "Ster." Note time when thermometer shows 270° F. as beginning of exposure period. The "Signal Light" will come on at this temperature. Allow exposure period to continue for 7 minutes. For emergency sterilization of one or two instruments only, uncovered, the exposure period may be reduced to 3 minutes at 270° F.

C) At the end of exposure period, close "Steam Supply Valve" and turn "Operating Valve" to right (clockwise) to "Exhaust." When "Chamber Gauge" shows zero pressure, turn "Operating Valve" (clockwise) to "Raise." Open door slightly so that vapor can escape for about 3 minutes, before fully opening door and removing trays.

5) Chamber drain screen should be removed and cleaned at least once a week.

III) *Factors that Influence Removal of Soil from Instruments*: In the washing of surgical instruments there are certain basic factors which must be considered in order to evaluate the functional efficiency of the process. As a practical approach to the problem the functions of all the components in the washing system should be studied. In the case of the instrument washer-sterilizer these components are:

a) Kind of soil.
b) Quality of water.
c) Type of detergent.
d) Types of instruments.
e) Efficiency of washer.

Certainly one of the most important factors is the kind and amount of soil present on the instruments. Blood, feces, tissue fats and extraneous debris constitute the common types of soil encountered on surgical instruments. The amount of blood and organic matter present, as well as the total number of instruments soiled, is greater in certain operations than others. Consequently the efficiency of the washing process is influenced by the total number of soiled instruments in the load. If the blood has been permitted to dry on the instruments for a period of hours it will be difficult to properly clean them in any mechanical washer. As the result of this limitation, routine practice requires that immediately upon completion of the surgical procedure in the operating room the instruments be placed in a basin of water to prevent excessive drying of blood in serrations, depressions and other inaccessible surfaces.

Water is perhaps the most important single component of the washing process. In many cases it can be demonstrated that the solvent action of water alone will remove a high percentage of soil from the instruments. This action is obviously enhanced by the factor of agitation when correctly applied in the washing machine. Water also serves as the medium for carrying the detergent to all surfaces of the instruments and for taking away the separated soil. Unfortunately the quality of tap water in many localities is not well suited for use in any mechanical washer. This statement is based upon the fact that the instrument washer-sterilizer does not utilize a rinse for the removal of inorganic or organic residue which may be present on the instruments following the washing process. When hard water or water of high mineral content is exhausted from the washer surface evaporation occurs, frequently leaving a deposit of mineral salts upon the surfaces of the instruments. As a rule, this condition can be prevented through the selection of a detergent best suited to the characteristics of the water supply in question. This eliminates the necessity for a rinse.

It is probably no exaggeration of fact to state that there is no one detergent best suited for use in the instrument washer-sterilizer under any and all conditions. The principal function of the detergent is to render non-wettable surfaces wettable. By virtue of its chemical and physical properties, the detergent lowers the surface tension of water, permitting more intimate contact of the water with the instrument. In addition, it assists in the solubilization of albuminous soil, emulsifies grease and suspends soil particles in the solution. Most detergents are chemical mixtures of crystalline substances comprising a surface-active or wetting agent in combination with one or more builders, such as the sodium phosphates, carbonates, or silicates. Representative of this group are the detergents known as "Haemosol," "Edisonite," "Calgonite," "Alconox" and many others. All of these products have been evaluated for use in the washer-sterilizer. They have been found relatively unsatisfactory in that they leave a residue or film of powder upon the instruments after the washing and sterilizing cycle has been completed. Some workers have attempted to overcome this condition by first dissolving the detergent in a small amount of water and then adding this solution to the washer. Such a procedure is of little benefit because the powder will still be found on the instruments, due to surface evaporation during the phase of exhausting the water from the washer. Of the various powdered or crystalline detergents tested, the product known as "Finish" has given the best results.

Some of the common phosphate detergents recommended for use in mechanical dishwashers have been tried in the instrument washer-sterilizer. Not only were the results disappointing from the standpoint of cleaning but the instruments underwent a severe metallic staining. The brassy tarnishing of the instruments was due to the copper solubilizing action of the polyphosphated detergent upon internal parts of the washer-sterilizer. The dissolved copper was then deposited upon the instruments by electrolytic action. Bacon and Nutting[5] have described a similar condition which occurred from the use of polyphosphate detergents in mechanical dish-washers.

A special detergent* has been developed for use in the washer-sterilizer. It is all-liquid in composition and is made from a coconut oil base. It has remarkably good surface-active properties with a special affinity for metallic

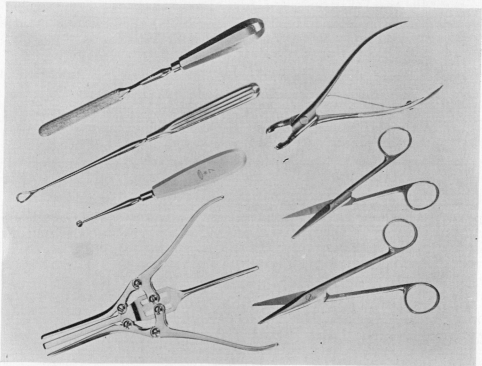

Fig. 75. These instruments are usually found to be the most difficult to clean by the mechanical process. Careful attention to prevent excessive drying of blood upon their surfaces will enhance considerably the mechanical cleansing process.

surfaces. When used in a concentration of one to two ounces in the washer, it leaves an invisible protective film on the instruments which resists corrosion.

Under the most careful operating conditions there are certain instruments difficult to clean by the mechanical process. Of primary importance are those shown in Fig. 75. The flat ground surfaces of scissors may occasionally present a problem if blood has been permitted to dry on them. Instruments used in bone surgery such as curettes and files may contain extremely adherent particles of tissue in the depressions and teeth which resist removal and cleansing in the washer-sterilizer. Likewise, multiple action bone cutting forceps and Rongeurs may offer difficulty in cleansing

---

* A product of American Sterilizer Co., Erie, Pa.

because of the multiple joints, inaccessible and tightly apposing surfaces. For these instruments a special treatment is recommended consisting of a preliminary soaking period in warm water containing one ounce per gallon of an effective detergent. Following this procedure the instruments may be subjected to the normal washing and sterilizing process given above.

IV) *Economics of Instrument Washer-Sterilizer:* The economic advantages of the instrument washer-sterilizer have for long been a popular subject of discussion among hospital administrators, professional personnel and the manufacturers. No one cares to argue the point that most hospitals maintain a heavy investment in surgical instruments. It is also agreed that the life of these instruments is influenced considerably by the care they receive. Furthermore, the processing of used surgical instruments is one of the highly repetitive jobs in every operating room. It frequently causes confusion in the flow of work, especially at the close of a busy operating day. A thorough and well-planned investigation of this subject was recently conducted by Prickett,[6] in cooperation with the Methods Engineering Council, University of Pittsburgh. In this study a flow process analysis was made of both the manual and the mechanical methods for processing surgical instruments. The unit used for analysis purposes was two trays of 150 instruments each. All steps in the process were charted, including washing, drying and inspection. The results of this study are summarized below:

Manual	*Time*	Mechanical
109 min.	TOTAL	35.4 min.
30 min.	PROFESSIONAL WORKER	30.0 min.
79 min.	NON-PROFESSIONAL WORKER	5.4 min.

Manual	*Labor Cost*	Mechanical
$2.09	TOTAL	$0.84
.75	PROFESSIONAL (@ $1.50/hr.)	.75
1.34	NON-PROFESSIONAL (@ $1.00/hr.)	.09

Savings Using Washer-sterilizer
TIME: 73.6 minutes/2 trays
LABOR COST: $1.25/2 trays
ANNUAL LABOR SAVING WITH AN AVERAGE WORK LOAD
OF 10 TRAYS/DAY AND A WORK WEEK OF 5½ DAYS = $1,787.50

Amortization of Equipment Cost
Cost of washer-sterilizer = $1,665.00
Savings less cost = $1,787.50 − $1,665.00 = $122.50

Thus the initial cost of the mechanical washer-sterilizer is paid for by direct labor savings in less than one year.

OILING OF INSTRUMENTS

The inconsistency of oiling instruments, prior to sterilization, as practiced in some hospitals is a hazardous procedure and it should not be permitted. The presence of a film of oil on an instrument simply serves as a protective barrier for any organism that may reside under the film.[7] It should be understood that sterilization is dependent upon moisture and that even a thin coating of oil will prevent moisture contact with instrument surfaces. The apparent need for oiling is indicative of the presence of soil or foreign matter which has accumulated in the joints of instruments. To relieve this stiffness so they will operate smoothly, it is recommended that a small amount of water-soluble grinding and lapping compound* (Grit No. 180) be placed in the box locks or joints, and worked in by opening and closing the instrument several times. This will remove the rough spots from the joints and, after cleaning, the instruments should operate satisfactorily.

SHARPENING INSTRUMENTS

In most cases, sharpening of instruments in the hospital is not recommended because to do the job well demands experience and skill which the average individual lacks. The instruments should be checked daily and at intervals of about three months or more frequently all instruments requiring attention for sharpening, plating or other repair should be sent outside to an expert. It is sound economy to take advantage of the specialized experience and equipment offered by a competent repair man. Even though the initial charges are a little higher the difference is definitely a good investment. Good repair work if done in time will usually make the instruments as good as new, whereas poor work will have to be repeated frequently, and damage may be done to the instruments, materially shortening their life.

ROUTINE STERILIZATION OF INSTRUMENTS

In the sterilization of instruments, care must be taken to insure that all instruments have been thoroughly cleaned beforehand and free from oil or grease. In no sense can the sterilizing process be considered as a substitute for adequate preliminary cleaning or to partially compensate for inadequate cleaning of instruments. The technic selected for sterilization must be adequate for the destruction of heat resistant spores. This requires the use of saturated steam under pressure at a temperature of 250° F. (121° C.) for a minimum of 15 minutes or 270° F. (132° C.) for a minimum of 7 minutes.

In arranging instruments for sterilization a serious attempt should be made to standardize on a basic set. Investigations[8] have shown that there is practically no standardization in operating rooms today and very little agreement as to the content of the basic set. In fact, the so-called basic sets have had a tendency to grow to such an extent that personnel complain about the large number and kinds of instruments which are being handled but not used.

For the routine sterilization of instruments the method shown in Figures

---

* A product of Clover Mfg. Co., Norwalk, Conn.

76 and 77 has proved highly satisfactory. The first step in the procedure is to place a layer of muslin in the bottom of the tray, making sure to always use a tray with a wire mesh or perforated bottom. Never use a solid bottom, water-tight tray or basin because it will trap air. The instruments are then arranged in the tray in a definite and fixed pattern. (This is important if the tray is to be located later as a unit on the nurse's table from which the instruments are removed as needed.) *All jointed instruments must be open or unlocked to permit prompt contact of steam to all surfaces.* Finally a towel or layer of muslin is placed on top of the instruments. The muslin cover is not considered essential if the instruments are sterilized in the conventional sub-sterilizing room. However, in many operating

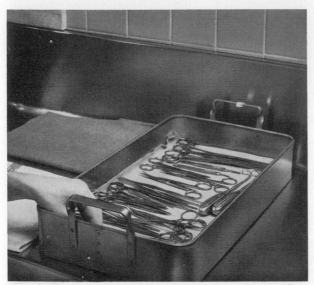

Fig. 76. In preparing instruments for sterilization it is good practice to place a layer of soft fabric in the bottom of the tray, then lay the instruments on this cloth. A wire-mesh or perforated bottom tray is necessary for effective sterilizaton. All jointed instruments must be open.

suites the instruments are sterilized in a central instrument room located some distance from the operating rooms. Where this condition exists the muslin cover offers protection against contamination in transit. The minimum exposure period is 15 minutes at 250° F. (121° C.) or 7 minutes at 270° F. (132° C.). Following completion of the exposure period the instruments should be allowed to remain in the sterilizer for 15 minutes with the door slightly open, about ¼ inch, to insure thorough drying. If the sterilizer is equipped with automatic control the drying phase will become a part of the normal cycle of operation.

When it is desired to hold sterilized instruments in temporary storage they should be arranged as suggested above and the entire tray wrapped with double thickness muslin. The exposure period should be no less than 20 minutes at 250° F. (121° C.). If completely wrapped trays of instruments are to be sterilized in the high-speed pressure instrument sterilizer, adjusted for 27 pounds pressure, the minimum exposure period should be 10 minutes at 270° F. (132° C.). The time required for killing of heat resistant spores in direct contact with steam at this temperature is two minutes. The additional eight minutes allow for penetration of steam through the muslin wrapper plus a reasonable factor of safety.

Occasionally it is found that instruments are wet following routine sterilization and drying. The condition occurs more frequently in the elec-

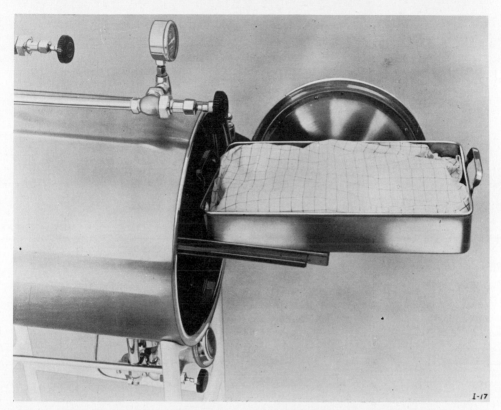

I-17

Fig. 77. This method of covering the tray of instruments affords protection against contamination in transit from the sterilizer to the operating room.

trically heated instrument sterilizer equipped with steam generator. Many times the cause is the same as that responsible for wet dressings, discussed on page 113. If the sterilizer is operating properly and the principles of good technique have not been violated, the difficulty of wet instruments may be overcome by preheating prior to sterilization. This can be accomplished by simply placing the trays of instruments in the sterilizer, closing the door, and maintaining steam in jacket only for 15 minutes. At the end of the preheating period steam may be admitted to the chamber and the instruments sterilized in the usual manner. The process of preheating reduces to a minimum the amount of condensate formed on the instruments during sterilization, thereby making drying less troublesome.

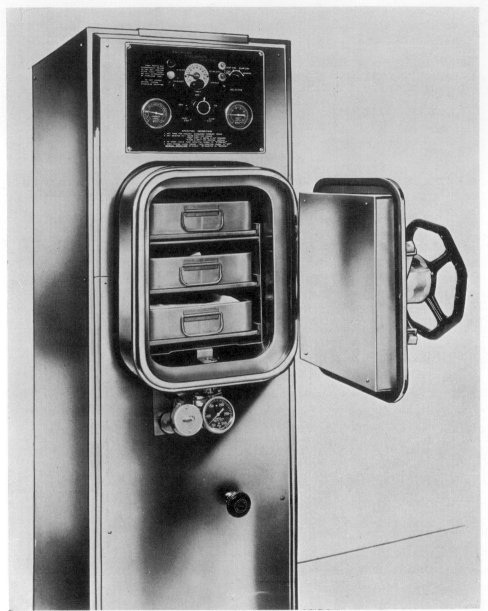

Fig. 78. The high-speed pressure instrument sterilizer, adjusted for operation at 270° F., meets the requirements for either emergency or routine sterilization.

EMERGENCY STERILIZATION OF INSTRUMENTS

In the emergency sterilization of instruments no compromise with safety can be tolerated. The method selected must be adequate for the destruction of resistant spores and it should be sufficiently rapid so as not to greatly inconvenience the surgeon. These requirements can be met through the use of a high-speed pressure instrument sterilizer, adjusted for operation at 270° F. (132° C.) and 27-28 pounds pressure, shown in Figure 78. When an instrument is urgently needed, as for one that has been accidentally dropped or inadvertently left out of a kit, it is possible for the nurse to wash, degrease, sterilize the instrument and return it to the operating table in 5 to 6 minutes with no compromise in safety.[3] The detailed steps of the technic are as follows:

STEAM SHOULD BE MAINTAINED IN THE JACKET OF THE HIGH-SPEED PRESSURE INSTRUMENT STERILIZER PRIOR TO AND DURING THE ENTIRE SURGICAL PROCEDURE.

1) Scrub the instrument with warm water containing detergent for about 15 seconds, followed by another 15 second wash in fat solvent, such as Soltrol 130* or Stoddard Solvent.

2) Place the opened instrument in a tray with wire mesh or perforated bottom, insert tray in sterilizer, close and lock door.

3) Open "Steam to Chamber" valve and note time when thermometer shows 270° F. The exposure period should be 3 minutes at this temperature.

If the sterilizer is equipped with "Cyclomatic Control," set "Timer" for 3-minute exposure period, turn "Selector" switch to "Fast Exhaust," and then turn "Operating Valve" (clockwise) to "Ster."

4) At end of exposure period, close "Steam to Chamber" valve and open "Exhaust" valve. After pressure has exhausted to zero, open door, remove instrument and deliver to operating table.

STERILIZATION OF UTENSILS

The most reliable method for the sterilization of utensils, basin sets and other containers is by means of steam under pressure. In most hospitals the procedure is fairly well standardized. The utensils are wrapped in muslin, sterilized in Central Supply, and stored for use, just the same as for dressings (fabrics) and other dry goods. It is important to observe certain details with respect to wrapping and loading in the sterilizer. If several utensils are nested, snugly fitting into each other, they should be separated by a layer of muslin to prevent tight contact of the metal surfaces and to allow some space for direct steam contact to all surfaces.

Utensils should be wrapped in double thickness muslin. In the case of the standard basin set the wrapper may then serve as the sterile drape for the basin stand. Always place the wrapped kits of utensils in the sterilizer on edge so that any water contained in them would drain out completely. This facilitates both sterilization and drying. The utensils can be sterilized separate from other supplies in a minimum exposure of 15 minutes at 250° F. (121° C.). If desired, they may also be sterilized as a part of the

---

* A product of Phillips Petroleum Co., Bartlesville, Okla.

bulk load of dry supplies, provided the utensils are not placed above or below other packs. In close contact with packs of dry goods, the basins may interfere with sterilization of the other materials, and they are almost certain to cause some wetting of the packs in contact with them. It is good practice to arrange the utensils at one end of the sterilizer, when included as a part of the bulk load of fabrics.

STERILIZATION OF SUTURES

Catgut: The catgut sutures produced today by reliable manufacturers can be depended upon for sterility. The suture material is available in two types: the anhydrous or boilable gut and the hydrated or non-boilable gut. The advantage of the boilable type is that the exterior of the tube can be sterilized by steam under pressure, in the same manner as surgical instruments. Non-boilable catgut, on the other hand, cannot be heated and the exterior of the tube must be disinfected by chemical means.

Silk Sutures, Untreated: Silk sutures should be sterilized by steam under pressure, not by boiling. For immediate use it is good practice to loosely wind the small amount of suture material needed for an operation on a gauze pad and subject it to sterilization with the instruments at 250° F. (121° C.) for 15 minutes. Repeated sterilization decreases strength somewhat, and procedures should be arranged to avoid more than three sterilizations of silk. If it is desired to prepare sutures for emergency use, they may be wound loosely on gauze as suggested above, covered with muslin wrappers and sterilized in the pressure sterilizer for 30 minutes at 250°-254° F. (121°-123° C.) along with other dry supplies.

Silk Sutures, Treated: Most silk sutures now in use are black, braided strands which have been waxed by the manufacturer. Tubed strands are sterilized by the manufacturer generally by a process equivalent to dry heat sterilization and therefore require sterilization of the outside of the tube only. This may be accomplished in the autoclave or by prolonged storage in germicidal solutions. Waxed braided silk supplied on spools should be sterilized by autoclaving at 250° F. (121° C.) for 30 minutes. The silk should be removed from the wooden spools to avoid possible contamination with resins extracted from the wood during the heating process, and loosely wound on reels designed to permit cutting all strands to 9-, 15- or 18-inch lengths as required.

Cotton Sutures: These should not be sterilized on the original spools because of the possibility of contamination from the wood, and of serious loss in strength due to normal shrinkage being prevented by the tight winding.[9] It is advisable to wind cotton suture material loosely in coils or on reels that will provide the desired lengths for use, and then sterilize by autoclaving. Cotton is not greatly affected by repeated sterilizations, but a maximum of three times is suggested for maintaining high quality of the sutures. Some surgeons prefer that sutures be boiled, and kept wet until used, as the tensile strength is greater after boiling than after autoclaving. In this case, Harms[10] has recommended that the approximate amount

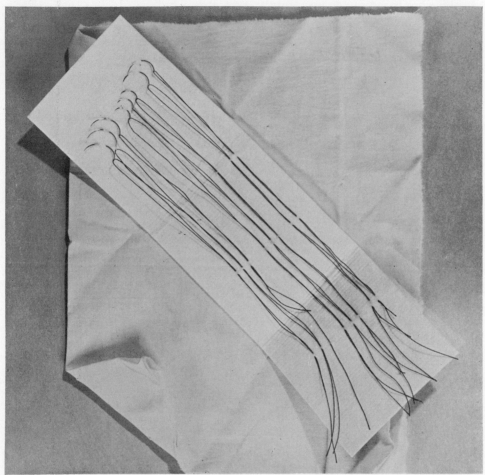

Fig. 79. Fine sutures of silk, cotton or nylon may be threaded on to needles, basted through gauze, wrapped in muslin and sterilized with other dry supplies for 30 minutes at 250° F.

needed for an operation be boiled 20 minutes and placed immediately in a bowl of water on the sterile table.

Nylon Sutures: Monofilament nylon is a relatively coarse strand used for cosmetic surgery and as a stay or tension suture. Multifilament nylon is in form and appearance quite similar to black braided silk. The suggestions given under silk apply completely to either form of nylon, whether distributed in sterile tubes with or without needles or on non-sterile coils or spools.

Fine sutures of silk, cotton or nylon may be threaded on to needles, basted through gauze, wrapped with muslin and sterilized with other dry supplies for 30 minutes at 250° F. (121° C.), as in Figure 79. It is well to remember that these suture materials are also subject to the condition of superheating as are all fabrics and textiles. To avoid superheating, the strands should be moistened lightly with water before placing them in the sterilizer.

REFERENCES

1. "How to Double the Life of Your Instruments." Master Surgical Instrument Corp., Irvington, New Jersey, p. 6, 1947.
2. WALTER, C. W.: Technique for the Rapid and Absolute Sterilization of Instruments. *Surg., Gynec. & Obst.,* 67:244, 1938.
3. WALTER, C. W.: *Sterilization.* Surgical Clinics of North America, New York Number, April 1942, p. 350, W. B. Saunders Co., Philadelphia, Pa.
4. PERKINS, J. J.: Preparation and Sterilization of Surgical Instruments. *The Surgical Supervisor,* 8:15-22, Sept. 1948.
5. BACON, L. R. AND NUTTING, E. G., JR.: Polyphosphate Detergents in Mechanical Dishwashing. *Ind. and Eng. Chem.,* 44:146-150, 1952.
   Ibid.: Metallic Staining of Silverware, p. 150-155.
6. PRICKETT, E.: *Processing of Surgical Instruments.* From a Study of the Operating Room, School of Nursing, Univ. of Pittsburgh and Methods Engineering Council, May 7, 1953.
7. ECKER, E. E. AND SMITH, R.: Sterilizing Surgical Instruments and Utensils. *Mod. Hosp.,* 48:92-98, 1937.
8. PRICKETT, E.: *A Study of the Operating Room.* Sect. III, p. 22-39, School of Nursing, Univ. of Pittsburgh, 1954.
9. MEADE, W. H. AND LONG, C. H.: The Use of Cotton as a Suture Material. *J.A.M.A., 117:*2140-2143, (Dec. 20) 1941.
10. HARMS, M. T.: Preparation and Use of Cotton Sutures. *Amer. J. Nursing, 48:*651-652, (Oct.) 1948.

Chapter 9

Water Sterilizers

IN THE HOSPITAL sterile water is as essential to clean surgery and aseptic technic as sterile instruments and dressings. It obviously should be protected from recontamination with the same care. Through the aid of modern methods it is not a difficult procedure to render water sterile. To maintain water in the sterile state is not, however, easily accomplished except through the use of equipment designed specifically for this purpose.

Since water as normally supplied to hospitals and institutions contains but few bacterial spores, and because the organisms present are wet, they are easily destroyed upon heating the water to 250° F. (121° C.) for a brief period of exposure. The real difficulty encountered is in effectively guarding the sterility of the water against air-borne, insect and contact contamination following the sterilization process, especially at the point of draw-off from the storage reservoir or tank.

THE MEANING OF "STERILE WATER"

General use of the term "sterile water" should be discouraged chiefly because it does not denote any particular quality of water from the standpoint of mineral impurities, freedom from pyrogens, chemical or physiological compatibility. In order to avoid possible misunderstanding or confusion as to the acceptability of the water for a particular surgical requirement it is desirable to designate the product as "sterile tap water," "sterile water for external use" or "sterile distilled water," whichever the case may be. Ordinary water as supplied for drinking purposes is usually designated "tap water," meaning that it has undergone only the common purification process of chlorination required of a public water supply so as to make it safe for human consumption. While tap water is generally recognized as being free of pathogenic organisms it is definitely not sterile. After sterilization it will still contain most of the original chemical impurities, including dead bacteria and pyrogens which render it unsafe for use in the preparation of parenteral solutions, isotonic fluids, or for other surgical application where a physiological environment for wound healing must be maintained.

Sterilized tap water produced in water sterilizers of the pressure type is widely employed in hospital operating rooms and delivery rooms for routine use in hand basins, irrigations, hot packs, etc. Many surgeons feel that sterile tap water is satisfactory for such applications. However, other surgeons, increasing in number within the last few years, recognize that sterile tap water does not fulfill the requirement for an ideal irrigating fluid and this group advocates the use of strictly isotonic solutions in the operating room.

The use of nonpressure reservoirs for water sterilization is no longer recognized as a reliable method. Long experience has proved that water in this type of container may not always be rendered sterile because the highest temperature attainable is 212° F. (100° C.); and it is almost immediately exposed to contamination occurring through unfiltered air contact and through unsterile gauge glasses or draw-off faucets. Loose fitting reservoir covers make it impossible to provide for air filtration and, lacking steam under pressure, there is no means for flushing out gauge glasses or draw-off faucets. If a water filter is provided it is impossible to sterilize it or the pipe connections leading to the filter. These factors constitute the principal objections to the nonpressure method for water sterilization.

Because of more dependable operation, the pressure method for the sterilization of water has become the commonly accepted standard of hospital practice. Recent trends would indicate that the pressure method will likewise give way in the not too distant future to an even more reliable process, namely, the individual flask method for the preparation, sterilization and dispensing of sterile water and other solutions in the hospital (see Chapter 18).

WATER STERILIZERS SHOULD PROVIDE FOR EFFECTIVE WATER AND AIR FILTRATION

The essential features of construction and operation of a pair of modern water sterilizers are shown in Figures 80 and 81. Other units, whether heated by gas or electricity, are similar in design and operation. Steam is the preferred source of heat because it is fast, economical and safe. The steam supply for each reservoir is controlled by a single valve and the return line from each heating coil is equipped with a thermostatic trap and check valve. Automatic pressure regulators, one for each reservoir, maintain the correct steam pressure and temperature of 15-17 pounds and 250°-254° F. (121°-123° C.) throughout the sterilizing period. The left-hand (cold) reservoir contains a cooling coil and the flow of cooling water is controlled by a dialed regulator adjustable for varying water pressures.

Each reservoir is also equipped with an individual, self-sterilizing, combination water and air filter—controlled by a single valve. In filling the tanks, the flow of water is visible through the glass front of the filter case. A percolating system is also provided for each water level gauge which automatically circulates water through the gauge while the reservoir is undergoing sterilization. Each gauge connection to the reservoir includes a

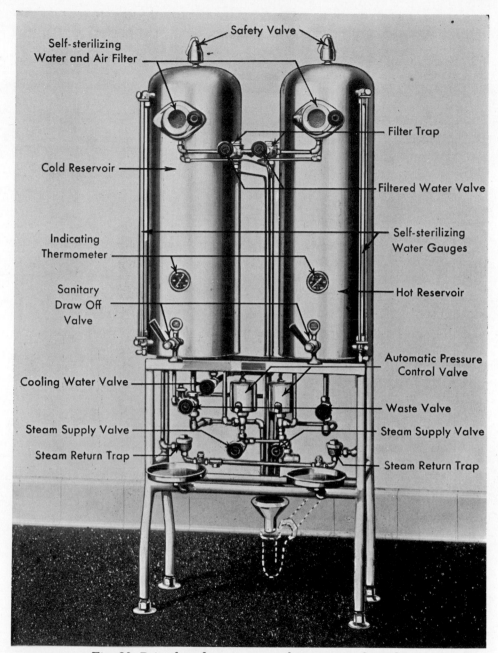

Fig. 80. Pair of modern water sterilizers—steam heated.

valve which closes automatically if the gauge glass is broken when the reservoir is under pressure.

When water is sterilized in any vessel opportunity for recontamination immediately begins when the water cools and continues until the reservoir has been emptied. Hot water, upon cooling, absorbs air until it is in equilibrium with the atmospheric (room) temperature and with every withdrawal

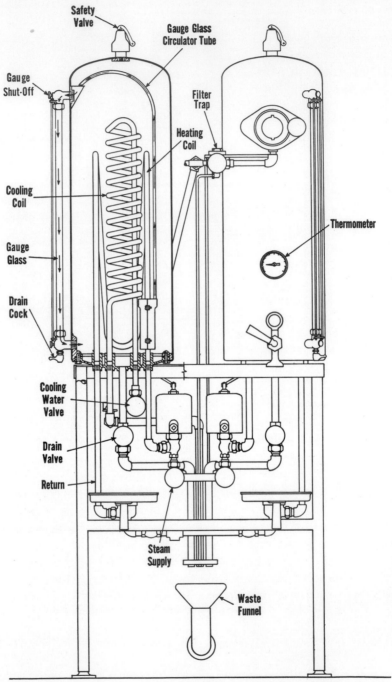

Fig. 81. This diagram shows essential features of construction and operation of the steam heated water sterilizers.

of water from the reservoir, an equal amount of air is drawn in to replace it. To illustrate, a 25-gallon reservoir of water was heated to 250° F. (121° C.) and then allowed to cool to atmospheric temperature. The reservoir was so arranged that all air was taken in through a glass water trap. Twenty-four hours after the heat was turned off, air bubbles were still being drawn in visibly through the water trap in appreciable quantity. This air absorption and air contact definitely permits contamination, unless the air is passed through an effective bacteria-retentive filter. All room air carries a certain amount of dust, a considerable portion of which is laden with microorganisms which may or may not be pathogenic.

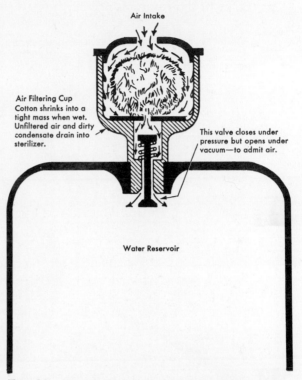

Fig. 82. A common type of vacuum release valve and air filtering cup found on older water sterilizers. It is worthless as an air filter.

Some of the older water sterilizers, still in use today, are equipped with air filters similar to that shown in Figure 82. This device consists of a small metal cup containing cotton wool as the filter medium, mounted above an automatic valve on the dome of the reservoir. The valve closes approximately tight but rarely completely tight, when the reservoir is subjected to internal pressure during sterilization. It opens freely to relieve vacuum when the water cools and when water is withdrawn, for the intake of air. The cotton in the cup serves poorly as a filter because it becomes moistened by steam escaping through the valve during sterilization. This causes the cotton to shrink away from the walls of the cup. When moist, the cotton becomes so dense that air can be forced through it only with difficulty. As the result, there is little filtration of air but a definite intake of dust particles and condensate from the cup back into the reservoir. This type of filter on a water sterilizer is worthless.

The combined water and air filter used on sterilizers shown in Figures 80 and 81 is so constructed that it can be automatically sterilized by steam each time the water is sterilized. The water filtering element (Fig. 83) consists of three removable filter discs made from a specially prepared fibrous material which will withstand the action of steam without serious loss of efficiency. The water filter is mounted in the filter case behind a glass cover through which the operator can see the passage of water as the reservoir is being filled.

Air intake to the reservoir occurs through the same filter case and might

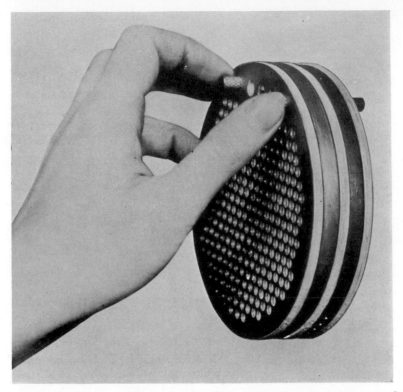

Fig. 83. This is typical of one type of water filter used on modern water sterilizers. It consists of three removable filter discs made from a compressed fibrous material.

be drawn back through the water filtering element except that it is so dense that air will pass through it only by considerable pressure. For the filtration of air a secondary element is provided consisting of tightly compressed noncorrosive metal wool, maintained in a moist condition. The air filtering element is backwashed by steam every time water is sterilized. It possesses a fair degree of efficiency in the removal of bacteria and dust particles. No air filter will assure complete protection. In fact, the sterilization of air by filtration through a fibrous medium means nothing more than the establishment of a permissible probability for passage of a contaminant.

The valve controlling raw water supply to the filter is a double action valve which when opened admits water to the filter and automatically closes the rear connection on the valve leading to the drain. When the valve is closed, water flow is shut off and the rear connection to the drain is opened. Then, should the valve leak slightly, leakage is conducted directly to the drain instead of the water reservoir. During sterilization steam from the reservoir passes through the filter to the drain and this flow continues until the filter (thermostatic) trap is heated and closes, holding the entire filtering system under pure steam pressure as long as sterilization continues.

An air intake tube connects the air filtering compartment directly to the air-vented waste. A ball check in the filter case prevents flow from the filter to the waste but admits air freely under slight back pressure as when water is withdrawn from the reservoir or when the sterilized reservoir cools down. In this manner modern water sterilizers give fairly reliable protection against the hazards of recontamination.

STERILIZATION OF GAUGE GLASSES

Of the water sterilizers in use today there are many with no provisions for the automatic sterilization of gauge glasses. These units present special problems because the water contained in the gauge glasses is not subjected to the sterilizing influence of the heat applied to the reservoir. If the gauge glasses are not flushed out during sterilization the unsterile water will later contaminate the reservoirs. Fortunately many of these older sterilizers have valves on the gauge fittings permitting the gauge to be closed off from the reservoir and the unsterile water then drained from the pet cock in the bottom fitting. Following this, steam is permitted to blow through the gauge glass for about 15 seconds in order to provide for sterilization. Then when the pet cock is closed and the valve to the reservoir opened, the gauge will refill with sterile water to the level in the reservoir.

The system employed for the automatic sterilization of gauge glasses operates on the principle of a coffee percolator, as shown in Figure 81. A metal tube is attached to the source of heat so that a small volume of water is heated sufficiently in advance of the main body of water to force it through the tube, the other end of which leads to the top of the water gauge. This circulation, indicated by a film of water flowing into the top of the gauge, continues, vigorously at first, but slowing down as the water in the gauge and the water in the reservoir approach the maximum temperature. This circulation eliminates accumulation of sediment in the bottom of the gauge glass and subjects the water in the gauge to the same sterilizing effect as the water in the reservoir.

DRAW-OFF FAUCETS

One of the most serious criticisms in the use of water sterilizers is that no positive method has ever been devised for the sterilization of the draw-off faucet. This is a most vulnerable location for the deposit of air-borne bacteria and it is extremely difficult to completely protect the draw-off faucet against insect or contact contamination. Present day faucets all have bell-shaped mouthpieces, designed to protect, insofar as possible, the water outlets from contact contamination. Probably the most effective method for the cleansing of faucets is as follows:

At the end of the sterilization period, before turning off the heat, place a wide-mouth pitcher or other large container under each draw-off faucet and permit the hot water and steam to flow through vigorously for at least 15 seconds. This will serve to sterilize the critical surfaces of the mouthpiece and to flush out the connection leading to the reservoir as effectively as can be done by any practical procedure. If care is taken to insure that this detail is carried out each time the reservoir undergoes sterilization the draw-off faucet will remain reasonably free of contamination.

Some hospitals require the mouthpieces of faucets to be flamed before use. This is a troublesome detail and the practice should be discouraged, especially if the sterilizers are located close to the operating room where explosive anaesthetic gases are used. It is also questionable if the flame as usually applied ever contacts the critical surfaces of the faucet with sufficient intensity to sterilize.

RESTERILIZATION OF WATER

The question frequently arises as to the maximum length of time water can be considered to remain sterile in water sterilizers. If the sterilizers are equipped with modern protective features and in good repair there is evidence to show that the water in the reservoirs will remain sterile for at least 24 hours. However, other factors justify the recommendation that the water should not stand more than 12 hours before resterilization. As must be acknowledged, the draw-off faucets can be contaminated easily and they may be covered with dust particles after standing many hours.

The degree of contamination within the reservoir, if it does occur, will likely increase with time. A slow leak in the cooling coil in the cold tank or a faulty air filter may contribute little, if any, contamination in a few hours, but the accumulated leakage or possible passage of contaminants during an entire day would definitely become a serious matter. The best procedure is to establish a routine for the sterilization of water on an 8 to 12 hour basis. This assures an added measure of protection in guarding against recontamination.

SAMPLING WATER FOR STERILITY TESTS

The collection of samples from water sterilizers for sterility testing should become a standard procedure in hospitals with properly equipped laboratories and trained personnel qualified to conduct this type of work. The first step in collecting the sample of water is to see that both reservoirs (hot and cold tanks) have been sterilized in the routine manner according to the operating instructions. This should be done in the afternoon preceding collection of the sample the following day in order that the sterilized water may stand for at least 12 hours. The purpose in permitting the sterilized water to cool overnight is to afford ample opportunity for contamination to enter the reservoir whether from a faulty air filter or a slow leak in the cooling coil in the cold tank.

The next step is to draw off approximately three-fourths of the volume of water in the reservoir and discard it. Then hold a previously sterilized bottle or flask of about 200 ml. capacity under the faucet and collect the sample from the remaining water. The flask should be immediately covered with a sterile stopper and delivered to the bacteriological laboratory. By following this procedure it is possible to collect a sample from the upper portion of water in the reservoir. This is desirable because a low order of contamination may not always be uniformly dispersed throughout the entire volume of water.

Another method which gives equally satisfactory results is to run the sample of water directly into a tube of sterile culture medium. However, this method requires extremely careful technique in order to collect no more and no less than the required aliquot of water for the volume of medium in the tube. When this method is used, the medium should be contained in large test tubes with dimensions of 30 x 200 mm., each containing 40 ml. of fluid thioglycollate or other approved sterility test medium. The sample of water undergoing test should then be limited to about 10 ml. All tests should be conducted in duplicate and the tubes incubated at a temperature of 32°-35° C.

OPERATING INSTRUCTIONS
(Refer to Fig. 80)

1) FILL RESERVOIR WITH WATER: Open filtered water valve and when water gauge indicates desired level in reservoir close valve tightly.

2) TO TURN ON HEAT: Open steam valve for the reservoir to be sterilized. During sterilization gauge glass is automatically sterilized, indicated by a film of water continuously flowing into top of gauge above the water level. Each water gauge fitting at top and bottom has a push button shut-off, for use only when gauge glass is broken. Normally these push buttons must be pushed all the way in. They are pulled out, with a twisting motion, only to close off the gauge.

3) TO STERILIZE: When thermometer indicates 250° F. (121° C.), note this time as beginning of exposure period. Exposure should continue for 15 minutes with the automatic pressure regulator adjusted to maintain temperature of 250°-254° F. (121°-123° C.)

4) STEAM FLUSH DRAW-OFF FAUCETS: At end of the exposure period, be-

fore turning off heat, hold a wide-mouth pitcher under the draw-off faucet and permit hot water and steam to flow vigorously for 15 seconds, to sterilize the valve and to flush out the connection into the reservoir.

5) CLOSE STEAM SUPPLY VALVE: Only after the draw-off faucet has been steam flushed, close the steam supply valve tightly.

6) TO COOL WATER: When sterilization is complete, open cooling water

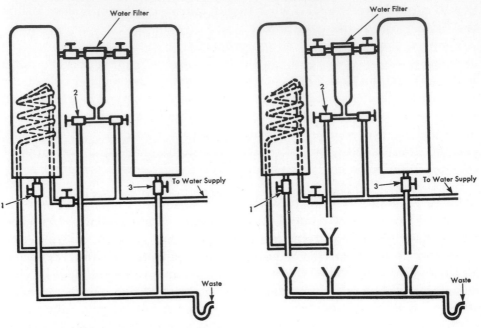

Fig. 84. Water sterilizers of all makes were formerly piped as shown here, with drainage connections leading direct to the sewage system with no intermediate air breaks. Leaky valves 1, 2 or 3 would permit the reservoirs, under negative pressure, to draw in sewage, or this might be occasioned by the backing up of sewage due to a clogged waste line. Present sanitary codes condemn this system of piping.

Fig. 85. This shows how air breaks can be applied to the piping (Figure 84) to guard against pollution from the waste. Air gaps in all such connections should be 1½ inches or more.

valve to left-hand reservoir and leave it open for about 30 minutes or until water has been cooled to desired temperature, indicated by thermometer. Then close tightly the cooling water valve.

7) RESTERILIZATION: Do not allow sterilized water to stand more than twelve hours before resterilization.

HAZARDS OF OBSOLETE TYPES OF WATER STERILIZERS

A dangerous source of sterile water contamination is found in obsolete equipment where the connections on the sterilizers are made direct to the waste, with no intermediate air breaks. This system, still occasionally encountered in hospitals, is shown in Figure 84. With such a system of piping there is no protection against the backflow of water from the waste to the sterile reservoirs. It is definitely hazardous and sanitary codes condemn the method of piping and require rearrangement to conform to the system shown in Figure 85. Here every drainage line is protected against back-flow from the waste by means of open funnel air breaks.

Any water sterilizers in use today lacking the latest protective features should be considered obsolete and prompt action should be taken to re-place or to modernize them. Whatever the circumstances may be, it is essential that the waste line piping conforms with modern plumbing codes. Each tank should be equipped with an individually controlled water and air filter, subject to automatic sterilization. Provision should also be made for automatic sterilization of gauge glasses. In addition, methods should be instituted for the routine inspection and control of water sterilizers, with special emphasis given to steam flushing of draw-off faucets each time the sterilizers are operated.

REMOVAL OF SCALE FROM WATER STERILIZERS

The water supply in many localities contains large amounts of lime, re-sponsible for hard water conditions. Application of heat to hard water causes the lime salts to deposit in the form of scale on the heating coils and on the bottom and side of the reservoir. Frequently this scale will accumu-late on the bottom of the reservoir, building up into a mass of considerable volume. As soon as any discoloration of water is noted, or if particles of scale appear when water is withdrawn, that is an indication that the tanks need to be cleaned.

The process of cleaning or removal of scale should not be attempted by nursing personnel, rather the work should be carried out by a trained mechanic or maintenance man after routine working hours. At weekly in-tervals or once each month, depending upon the quality of the raw water, the sterilizer should be filled to about one-third of its capacity and heated to sterilizing temperature. Cover the open funnel in the waste line with towels draped about it to prevent escape of steam and water into the room, then open the waste valve and permit the reservoir to blow down until it is empty. Then, while the coils are still hot, fill the reservoir completely and, without heating, permit the water to drain out. This will remove the loose scale quite effectively but will not remove the hard deposit on coils and other surfaces.

If the sterilizers are electrically heated, the accumulation of scale on the heaters will eventually cause burn out because the mass of scale becomes so dense that the heat builds up to a degree that will actually melt the metal sheath of the heaters. Usually it will be found necessary to dismantle the sterilizers for efficient cleaning, whether heated by direct steam or electricity. This is a major task and the following points should be kept in mind when performing the work: It is impractical to apply an acid or scale solvent to the interiors of tanks. Since comparatively little scale forms on these surfaces the use of a wire brush or coarse knife for scraping the scale loose will usually suffice. Before reassembling, the tanks should be thoroughly rinsed out with water. Coils or heating elements require soaking in warm muriatic acid (1 part acid to 9 parts water) until the scale has softened sufficiently for easy removal. The removal of scale from the interior of a coil can be accomplished by repeatedly filling the coil with the dilute acid while it is being subjected to moderate heating. Terminals on electric heaters must be protected from the acid and care should be exercised to prevent the acid fumes from contacting highly finished or plated surfaces. After soaking the coils or heaters in the acid solution for about an hour the residual can be removed by scraping with a coarse knife edge. The parts should be thoroughly rinsed in tap water before reassembling in order to remove all traces of acid.

LIMITATIONS OF WATER STERILIZERS

The continued use of water sterilizers in hospitals has been seriously attacked by several authorities in the field of sterilization. Walter,[1] for example, has stated that "there is no practicable way of guarding the sterilizers against contamination and that the water is likely to be contaminated when it is drawn off. . . . In summary, water sterilizers are decided luxuries that contribute little to aseptic technic." A more recent statement against the use of water sterilizers has been issued by the Advisory Committee on Sterilization Procedures for Queensland Public Hospitals.[2] This group is of the opinion that "sterility of the water can never be relied on—the only safe water is water that has been autoclaved."

Undoubtedly there is evidence to support the above statements when one considers the many elements of faulty design and the obvious neglect of protective sanitary features on water sterilizers installed in hospitals during the past fifty years. It is hardly fair, however, to direct such severe criticism against the modern types of water sterilizers—those installed in hospitals during the last two decades which for the most part have given satisfactory service. Many hospitals have instituted routine bacteriologic testing of water sterilizers and their results over a long period of time have shown that the sterilizers when maintained in good mechanical condition are capable of operating with a high degree of efficiency. Nevertheless, it must be acknowledged that water sterilizers have definite limitations and whenever such equipment is purchased by a hospital the facts should be honestly presented and clearly understood. Those features known to contribute to faulty operation and contamination of the water are:

a) Ineffective air filters.

b) Single water filter serving both reservoirs—always a potential source of contamination.

c) Cooling coil in cold tank. This may develop a slow leak.

d) No provision for automatic sterilization of side arm gauge glasses.

e) Leaky valves permitting raw water to enter sterile reservoirs. The most modern sterilizers are designed to prevent such an occurrence.

f) Drainage connections piped direct to the waste line, with no intermediate air breaks. This system of piping constitutes a violation of sanitary codes.

g) No practicable method for the positive sterilization of draw-off faucets.

REFERENCES

1. WALTER, C. W.: *Aseptic Treatment of Wounds.* New York, Macmillan. 1948, p. 302-307.
2. COMMITTEE ON STERILIZATION PROCEDURES: *Handbook of Sterilization Procedures,* Brisbane, Australia, A. H. Tucker, 1953, p. 70.

Chapter X

Dry Heat Sterilization

I T IS IMPORTANT for the student of sterilization to clearly understand the limitations of dry heat as a sterilizing agent. It should be used only where direct contact of the material or substance with saturated steam is impractical or unattainable. Dry heat in the form of hot air is difficult to control within narrow limits, except in a specially designed sterilizer. It penetrates materials slowly and unevenly and long exposure periods are required for sterilization. Because of the poor penetrability and the destructive effect of the high temperatures employed, dry heat or hot air is entirely unsuited for the sterilization of fabrics and rubber goods. On the other hand, it is well suited for the sterilization of keen, cutting edge instruments, needles and syringes. Dry heat does not exert a corrosive effect on sharp instruments as is commonly observed with steam, nor does it erode the ground glass surfaces of syringes.

The action of dry heat on objects is that of conduction. The heat is absorbed by the exterior surfaces of an article, eventually heating the interior, but the factor of moisture is lacking. It is a false assumption to believe that all substances normally in the liquid state, or those which become liquid upon heating, such as petroleum jelly ("Vaseline"), can be rendered sterile by the usual autoclaving process. Petrolatum, oils, oily suspensions, fats and powders have no appreciable water content and the moisture of the steam cannot be depended upon to permeate the substances. Heat resistant organisms concealed in these materials would, of course, be heated to the temperature of the surrounding steam, but lacking the moisture factor, the temperature would be inadequate for complete bacterial destruction in any practicable exposure period. Therefore, it is necessary for the sterilization of anhydrous oils, greases and powders to utilize a dry heat method, or its equivalent, with a safe time-temperature relationship, taking into account any appreciable time lag characteristic of heating a particular load.

RESISTANCE OF BACTERIA TO DRY HEAT

The phenomena responsible for the widely different temperatures required in dry and moist heat sterilization have been explained on the basis of the changes in the coagulability of proteins brought about by the abstraction of water. In the classic work of Lewith,[1] frequently cited, it was found that various proteins are coagulated by heat at lower temperatures when they contain an abundance of water than when water has been abstracted from them. The following data demonstrates this point:

Egg albumin + 50% water coagulates at 133° F. (56° C.)
Egg albumin + 25% water coagulates at 165°-176° F. (74°-80° C.)
Egg albumin + 18% water coagulates at 176°-194° F. (80°-90° C.)
Egg albumin + 6% water coagulates at 293° F. (145° C.)
Egg albumin + 0% water coagulates at 320°-338° F. (160°-170° C.)

If the heat coagulability of proteins as influenced by moisture is the determining factor, it is logical to state that a temperature of at least 320° F. (160° C.) should be used in dry heat methods of sterilization. It also follows that bacteria exposed to hot air may be dehydrated greatly before the temperature rises sufficiently to cause death by coagulation, complete dehydration necessitating their destruction by actual burning. For this reason, most authorities agree that death by dry heat is primarily an oxidation or a slow burning up process.

A review of the literature has shown that there is a lack of systematic study on death time temperatures of dry heat or hot air. The early findings of Robert Koch[2] and his coworkers demonstrated that the spores of *Bacillus anthracis* required a hot air temperature of 284° F. (140° C.) for 3 hours in order to insure their destruction. The resistance of both vegetative bacteria and spores varies considerably with different species, some being killed more readily than others. Mold spores appear to be intermediate in resistance between vegetative and sporulating bacteria in that they require a temperature of 230°-240° F. (110°-115° C.) for 90 minutes for their destruction.[3] In the author's laboratory it has been found that dry spores of *Bacillus stearothermophilus* which show maximum resistance to moist heat will survive dry heat at 250° F. (121° C.) for 2 hours, but they are destroyed at 320° F. (160° C.) for 1 hour. The data summarized in Table 9 are descriptive of the findings of various investigators in determining the time-temperature ratios required for the destruction of bacterial spores by means of dry heat. In dry heat sterilization an exposure time of 60 minutes at 320° F. is approximately the equivalent of 15 minutes at 250° F. in moist heat.

The microbicidal action of dry heat is markedly influenced by the nature of the fluid or substance surrounding the organism. In the presence of organic matter, such as a film of oil or grease, the organism is definitely protected or insulated against the action of dry heat. Walter[14] has emphasized the importance of this factor, particularly in the case of surgical instruments, which, if properly cleaned beforehand, may be sterilized in one hour at 320° F. If oil or grease is present on the instrument, safe sterilization calls for 4 hours exposure at 320° F. Rodenbeck[15] has studied the

TABLE 9

Destruction of Bacterial Spores by Dry Heat at Different Temperatures

(From Perkins[21])

TIME—MINUTES

Organism (Dry Spores)	248°F. (120°C.)	266°F. (130°C.)	284°F. (140°C.)	302°F. (150°C.)	320°F. (160°C.)	338°F. (170°C.)	356°F. (180°C.)	Investigator
B. anthracis	45	20						Murray[4]
B. anthracis			180					Koch et al[5]
B. anthracis				60				Stein and Rogers[6]
B. anthracis			180					Park and Williams[7]
B. anthracis	60				9			Oag[8]
B. subtilis				60				Perkins and Underwood[9]
Cl. botulinum	120	60	60	25	25	15	10	Tanner and Dack[10]
Cl septicum						7		Oag[8]
Cl. tetani		35	15					Murray and Headlee[11]
Cl. welchii	50	15	5					Headlee[12]
Cl. welchii						7		Oag[8]
Garden Soil					30	15		Ecker and Smith[13]

thermal death time temperatures of resistant dry spores in anhydrous oil. The findings of this investigator are deserving of serious consideration in the establishment of safe exposure periods for dry heat sterilization of oils, fats or other anhydrous fluids. For example, it has been determined that at a temperature of 320° F. (160° C.) a period of 160 minutes is required for the destruction of resistant spores in anhydrous oil or fat. If the oil is hydrated or contains a small amount of water, as little as 0.5 per cent, sterilization may be accomplished in approximately 20 minutes at this temperature. Rodenbeck also found that the addition of 1% water to fats, oils or paraffin made sterilization possible in the autoclave after 30 minutes at 120° C. or 10 minutes at 130° C. Fortunately most oils do contain a small amount of moisture, less than one per cent, unless subjected to a specific dehydration process.

REQUIREMENTS FOR DRY HEAT STERILIZATION

In setting up standards for dry heat sterilization, it is difficult and somewhat impractical to attempt to establish one time and temperature entirely suitable for all types of supplies. Several factors influence the time-temperature relationship required. The nature and properties of the article or material undergoing sterilization must be reckoned with, strict attention must also be given to the method of preparation, packaging or wrapping, as well as loading of the sterilizer. If these factors are ignored the exposure time selected may be inadequate for destruction of the most resistant and least accessible organisms. Instruments represent the ideal for dry heat sterilization because of the heat conducting properties of the metal, but the maximum temperature employed must be restricted to a safe range beyond which the temper of the metal may be drawn. For heat-stable articles such as glassware, it becomes possible to use a higher temperature for a shorter period of time, than when sterilizing certain powders which may undergo physical or chemical change unless the temperature is maintained below the critical point of the substance. In dry heat sterilization the basic point to keep in mind is that the time required to heat a quantity of one material to sterilizing temperature may differ markedly from that required to heat another material to the same temperature. Allowance must be made for any such differential in the exposure time.

For dry heat sterilization of hospital supplies the most widely used temperature is 320° F. (160° C.) for 1 hour, preferably 2 hours. This requirement refers to the actual temperature of the load. It does not make allowance for any appreciable time lag characteristic of a particular load after the sterilizer has reached this temperature. In establishing reliable methods for dry heat (hot air) sterilization, the following time-temperature ratios are considered adequate:

340° F. (170° C.)...........1 hour
320° F. (160° C.)...........2 hours
300° F. (150° C.)...........2½ hours
285° F. (140° C.)...........3 hours
250° F. (121° C.)...........6 hours, preferably overnight

HOT AIR STERILIZERS (GRAVITY CONVECTION TYPE)

There are two kinds of hot air sterilizers in common use, the gravity convection type, and the mechanical convection or forced air circulation type. For both units, the preferred method of heating is by electricity because it affords accurate and dependable temperature control within the desired range. For routine work the temperature range should be 320°-325° F. (160°-163° C.), but the automatic regulator should be readily adjustable

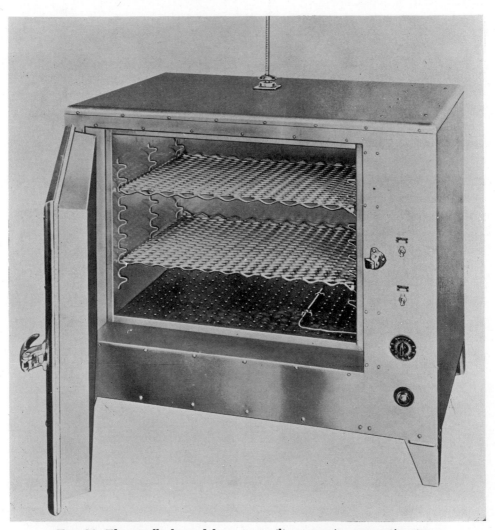

Fig. 86. Electrically heated hot air sterilizer, gravity convection type.

for lower temperature sterilization if the need occurs. When it is desired to sterilize glassware only, as in the laboratory, close temperature control is not so essential, and the temperature may advance to as much as 400° F. (204° C.) without harming the glassware. For this reason the laboratory hot air sterilizer is frequently just a plain, uninsulated, gas-fired oven, without accurate thermostatic control. To be sure, gas cannot be controlled with the same accuracy as electricity and the use of gas involves a definite fire hazard. Such equipment has no place in the modern laboratory or hospital and it should not be used for the sterilization of materials that require accurate temperature control or are known to be combustible in nature.

In the gravity convection hot air sterilizer shown in Figures 86 and 87, the air circulates in accord with existing temperature differences between various portions of the chamber. When air is heated, it expands with a corresponding decrease in density. The cooler air descends in the chamber and the

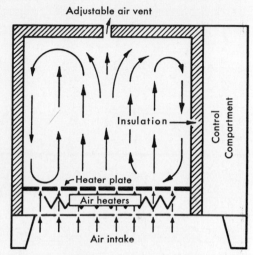

Fig. 87. Schematic diagram of air circulation in gravity convection hot air sterilizer.

heated air rises to displace it. The ascending warm air gives up some of its heat to the load in the chamber and also contracts in volume. At the same time the descending cool air is heated as it passes over the heating elements. In this manner the cycle is repeated, setting up "gravity convection" circulation in the chamber. The speed of circulation is dependent upon the ventilation provided through the adjustable air vent or exhaust located on top of the sterilizer, and also the temperature differential between the region of the heaters and the exhaust port.

The design characteristics of the gravity convection hot air sterilizer influence the functional efficiency. The design should not oppose the natural flow of air currents by directing the air stream around corners, through baffles, etc. The heater bank should be located beneath the chamber, separated from it by a perforated metal plate, which serves not only as the chamber floor, but as a diffusing surface to produce uniform heating effect over the full horizontal plane of the chamber. Pre-heated fresh air can then rise through the perforated plate, pass up through the chamber, flow through the perforated diffusing panel which forms the ceiling, and finally exhaust itself through the adjustable ventilating port on top of the cabinet. At best, the gravity convection type sterilizer is much slower in heating, requires longer time to reach sterilizing temperature, and less uniform in temperature control throughout the chamber than the mechanical convection type. It should be used only for applications where rapid and precise

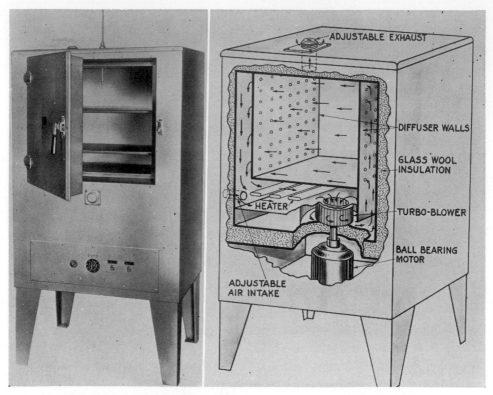

Fig. 88. Hot air sterilizer, electrically heated, mechanical convection type. Forced air circulation is accomplished by a motor-driven turbo-blower.

Fig. 89. Diagram of air circulation in mechanical convection hot air sterilizer.

heating, unrestricted loadability of chamber, and accelerated air circulation are not decisive factors.

THE MECHANICAL CONVECTION TYPE

For hospital use, particularly in the laboratory and the central supply department, the mechanical convection hot air sterilizer (Fig. 88) offers the maximum in functional efficiency at minimum cost. This type is usually equipped with a motor-driven turbo-blower which produces rapid movement of a large volume of heated air, to convey heat directly to the load under controlled temperature conditions. The heater bank (Fig. 89) is mounted in a compartment separated from the working chamber by a diffusing wall, directly in front of the turbo-blower. An adjustable air inlet opens into the heater compartment. As the incoming air is heated, it enters the turbo-blower where it is mixed and diffused with recirculating air. The heated air then passes through a duct, where a high static pressure is built up, forcing the air over to a compartment on the opposite side of the chamber. Here it passes through another perforated diffuser wall and the air is discharged uniformly over the entire vertical plane area of the chamber. This insures a positive airflow in the horizontal plane, thus maintaining uniform temperature and equal transfer of heat to all regions. As the heated air flows across the chamber and passes through the diffusing wall in front of the heaters, it is recirculated by the turbo-blower and the cycle repeated. Any portion of the circulating air can be exhausted to the outside through the adjustable vent on top of the sterilizer.

With the mechanical convection sterilizer, air velocity, direction of circulation and heat intensity are controlled to produce uniform temperature in the chamber regardless of the type of load. To meet the requirements of heavy usage in hospital work, an efficient hot air sterilizer should have performance characteristics as follows:

> Power consumption—approximately 520 watts per cu ft. of chamber capacity.
> Come up time to 320° F. in chamber (no load)—no longer than 30 minutes.
> Maximum temperature deviation throughout chamber (no load)—±2° F.
> Come up time to 320° F. with fully loaded chamber of glassware—no longer than 75 minutes.

In addition to the above characteristics, the sterilizer should have positive means for exhaust of gases or vapors liberated during the sterilizing process. Automatic controls are also a desirable feature, including a 5-hour timer and an alarm.

USE OF AUTOCLAVE AS HOT AIR STERILIZER

Supervisors frequently inquire as to the advisability of using the ordinary pressure steam sterilizer (autoclave) with steam in jacket only as a substitute for the hot air or dry heat sterilizer. Certainly this can be done, is being done in many hospitals, but the method is not deserving of recognition as a standard procedure, unless the sterilizer is equipped with proper controls. When operated with steam in jacket only at 15-17 pounds pressure, it is true that the chamber walls of the dressing sterilizer are uniformly heated to 250° F., and that conditions in the chamber are moderately suited to hot air sterilization. However, the thermometer located in the chamber discharge line does not function as an indicator of the chamber temperature when steam is applied to the jacket only. Moreover, it is just as important to record the true conditions of time and temperature for dry heat sterilization as it is for saturated steam under pressure. This constitutes the first serious objection to the method—there is no reliable means of checking temperature conditions in the chamber, without modification of the sterilizer.

Another disadvantage in the use of the autoclave as a dry heat sterilizer is that the standard steam pressure maintained in the jacket is 15-17 pounds, equivalent to 250°-254° F. (121°-123° C.). With this dry heat temperature in the chamber, safe sterilization calls for six hours exposure, preferably overnight. An exposure period of this order is indicative of a relatively inefficient process, especially when safe sterilization can be accomplished in a much shorter time at a higher temperature in a dry heat oven. In the interest of economy and for the hospital that does not have a dry heat sterilizer, there is some merit to loading the dressing sterilizer with syringes and needles for an overnight exposure at 250° F. During this period the dressing sterilizer would not normally be required for other purposes.

In the case of oils, greases and lubricated gauze, it is not uncommon to experience spillage or leakage of these materials in the sterilizer chamber. When this occurs in the autoclave, it necessitates careful cleaning to remove all traces of oil or grease from the chamber surfaces. Otherwise, supplies undergoing steam sterilization later may possibly become contaminated with a film of oil which serves as a protective barrier against moist heat sterilization. Oil or grease in the chamber eventually leads to partial clogging of the discharge line which then requires cleaning and service by an experienced mechanic to insure efficient operation of the sterilizer. The obvious answer to all of these shortcomings is not to use the autoclave as a substitute for the hot air sterilizer, except in an emergency or until such time as suitable equipment designed for dual-purpose sterilization can be procured.

PREPARATION OF SUPPLIES

The importance of thoughtful attention to details cannot be overemphasized in preparing supplies for dry heat sterilization. Instruments, syringes and needles must be free from traces of oil or grease. Wherever practicable the quantity of a liquid or a powder should be limited to that required for a single use application. An attempt should be made to standardize on types of containers, methods of packaging and loading to insure that when the sterilizer reaches the proper temperature the load also will be at this temperature or very close to it.

Cutting Edge Instruments: Selection of a satisfactory method for sterilization of cutting edge instruments frequently poses a problem for the operating room supervisor. Surgeons require both sharp and sterile instruments. Chemical disinfection is commonly resorted to, particularly for scalpel blades, but great care must be used to insure that the instruments are thoroughly cleaned before immersion in the germicide and that sufficient time be allowed for disinfection to take place. Then, if the germicide contains formaldehyde or any other irritating substance, it is necessary to rinse the instruments in sterile water and dry them under sterile conditions before use. In many cases it is apparent that chemical disinfection methods are employed for convenience rather than bacteriological efficiency or surgical safety.

Dry heat sterilization of sharp instruments can conveniently be carried out in the hot air sterilizer at 320° F. (160° C.) for one hour. The first requirement is that the instruments be clean, free from oil or grease, otherwise this exposure time may be inadequate. It is preferable to place the instruments on shallow aluminum trays in the sterilizer to enhance the rate of heating through the heat conducting properties of the metal. Caution must be exercised to guard against overheating. Exposure to temperature appreciably higher than 320° F. may destroy the keenness of the cutting edge. If the autoclave is used as the dry heat sterilizer with steam in jacket only at 250°-254° F., the exposure period should be no less than four hours for clean instruments prepared as above.

Walter[16] has described a dry heat sterilizer for cutting-edge instruments in which the instruments are heated by direct contact with a metal surface maintained at 320° F. This method provides rapid and uniform heating. Hawn and Walter[17] have also described a unique method of packaging scalpel blades for dry heat steriliza-

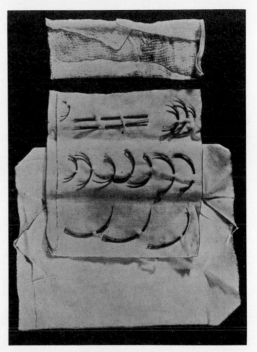

Fig. 90. Suture needles may be prepared in a gauze pad as shown here. They are then wrapped in muslin and sterilized by hot air at 320° F. for not less than 1 hour.

tion. The scalpel blade is hermetically sealed in an aluminum foil packet prior to sterilization. It is possible that blades packaged in this manner will become commercially available.

Suture Needles: When suture needles are sterilized by saturated steam serious rusting occurs which is difficult to overcome. Experience has shown that dry heat sterilization is the method of choice. The needles should first be cleaned by soaking in a detergent solution and then dried. If polishing is required they can be passed through a bag of fine emery powder. For packaging, it is desirable to insert the needles in a lightly folded gauze pack and wrap with muslin as in Figure 90. Sterilization may then be accomplished at a temperature of 320° F. for not less than one hour.

Powders: The slow rate of heat transfer through jars or canisters of powder makes it necessary to employ abnormally long periods of heating to insure sterilization. This point is illustrated graphically in Figure 91. A four ounce jar of powder of the type shown in Figure 92 requires 115 minutes to reach the sterilizing temperature of 320° F. in the hot air sterilizer.

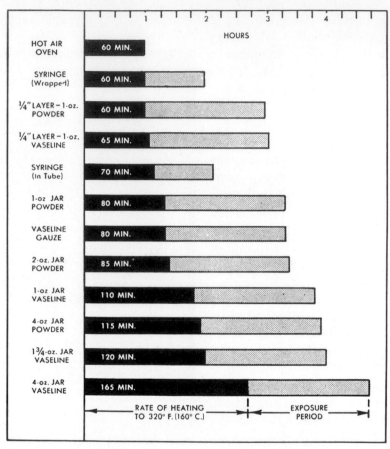

Fig. 91. Time required to heat specific quantities of materials from room temperature of 75° F. to 320° F. in hot air sterilizer. The lightly shaded section of each bar represents the exposure period after the material has reached a temperature of 320° F. The total time consumed in the heating process is equal to the entire length of each bar.

From the time that the sterilizer itself reaches this temperature, the powder still requires 55 minutes longer. Then, for safe sterilization it is necessary to add an exposure period of two hours which makes the total heating time about four hours. Similar conditions of slow heating prevail for the smaller 2-ounce and 1-ounce jars of powder. The poor heat conducting properties of the glass jar, the layer depth of powder and the surface area exposed are the chief factors which contribute to the slow rate of heating of powder. For example, 1-ounce of powder was placed in a Petri dish (Fig. 92),

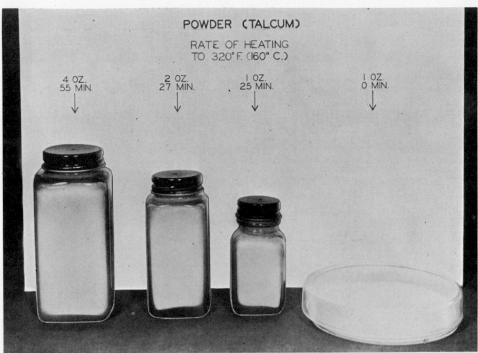

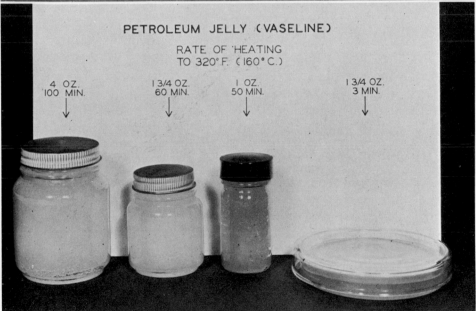

Fig. 92. Comparative rates of heating different quantities of powder to 320° F. in hot air sterilizer. The time recorded for each container is actually the additional time needed for the material to reach 320° F., after the sterilizer has attained this temperature.

Fig. 93. Comparative rates of heating different quantities of petroleum jelly to 320° F. in hot air sterilizer. The time recorded for each container is actually the additional time needed for the material to reach 320° F., after the sterilizer has attained this temperature.

forming a layer ¼ inch thick, and then heated in the hot air sterilizer. By means of a potentiometer and thermocouple it was determined that after 30 minutes heating, the temperature rise ran parallel to that of the sterilizer, and after 60 minutes both were at the same temperature of 320° F. This represents the ideal condition—uncommonly practiced in the hot air sterilization of powders. The use of containers for bulk powder involving quantities much greater than one ounce should be discouraged. Also, wherever possible, the quantity of powder should be restricted to a ¼ inch layer in a Petri dish or similar type of container. If these conditions are ignored the exposure period of 2 hours at 320° F. may be inadequate.

Sulfonamide Powders: The sulfonamides, including sulfanilamide, sulfadiazine, sulfathiazole and sulfamerazine are relatively heat-stable chemicals. In powder form they may be heated to a temperature of 311° F. (155° C.) for 1½ hours without decomposition. This temperature is, however, close to the melting point of sulfanilamide (165° C.), and for a greater margin of safety, it is recommended that the powders be sterilized at 285°-300° F. (140°-150° C.) for 3 hours. A convenient method of preparation is to place small amounts of the powder, not exceeding 4 or 5 grams, in double envelope paper containers. Test tubes with cotton plugs, individually wrapped, also serve as suitable containers.

Zinc peroxide is another substance which should be dry heat sterilized at 285° F. (140° C.) for four hours. This time and temperature is required to activate or mobilize the oxygen and at temperatures higher than 285° F. it begins to decompose. To be effective this material must conform to certain minimum standards which have been outlined in detail by Meleney.[18]

Other chemicals such as kaolin, zinc oxide, mercurous chloride and bismuth subnitrate can be dry heat sterilized at 340° F. (170° C.) for one hour or 320° F. (160° C.) for two hours.

Oils and Nonaqueous Vehicles: The slow rate of heating evidenced in the sterilization of powders is even more marked in the case of oils. For example, the time required to heat a 4-ounce jar of petroleum jelly ("Vaseline") from room temperature of 75° F. to 320° F. in the hot air sterilizer is 165 minutes, as shown in Figure 91. From the time the sterilizer reaches this temperature, the petroleum jelly requires 100 minutes longer heating to reach 320° F. If the exposure period of 2 hours is then added, the total heating time becomes 4¾ hours for sterilization of this quantity of petroleum jelly.

The time required to heat small quantities of petroleum jelly or petrolatum to sterilizing temperature is far greater than commonly observed in hospital practice. This statement is supported by the data given in Figure 91 which shows that a 1¾ ounce jar requires 120 minutes and a 1-ounce jar 110 minutes to heat to 320° F. This means that when the sterilizer reaches

320° F., an additional period of 60 minutes and 50 minutes respectively is required for the two smaller containers to reach sterilizing temperature. As in the case of powder explained above, the depth of the layer of oil and the surface area exposed greatly influence the rate of heating. To illustrate, a ¼ inch layer of petrolatum, 1¾ ounces, was placed in a Petri dish (Fig. 93) and then heated in the hot air sterilizer. With potentiometer and thermocouple it was determined that after 30 minutes heating the temperature rise

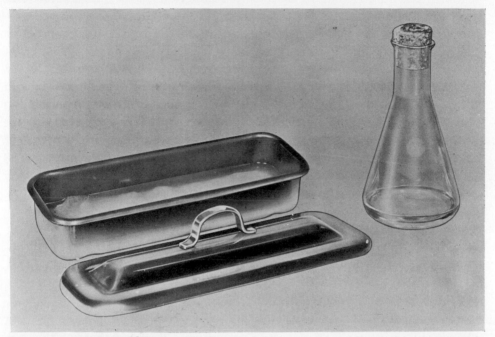

Fig. 94. A wide bottom flask is ideally suited as a container for petrolatum and other oils normally liquid at room temperature. The quantity of oil should be limited to a ¼ inch layer, about 1 oz., in order to provide some margin of safety in sterilization. Petrolatum gauze can be conveniently prepared in the catheter tray shown above. The gauze strips should be limited to about 20 and the petrolatum to no more than 4 oz., making a layer ½ inch deep in the tray.

in the petrolatum almost paralleled that of the sterilizer, and that at the end of 60 minutes the petrolatum required only 3 minutes longer heating to reach 320° F. Again, this condition approaches the ideal, and the results confirm the recommendation that for safe sterilization the quantity of oil should be limited to approximately one ounce.

Admittedly the Petri dish is not the most suitable container for oils because of its shallow depth and the possibility of spillage. It can serve as a convenient receptacle for petroleum jelly, ointments or other preparations not normally liquid at room temperature. A stainless steel needle jar, 3⅛ x 2½ inches, with cover, is a suitable container for oils; also the Erlenmeyer flask shown in Figure 94. Since the commonly used oils such as petrolatum, paraffin, olive oil and peanut oil are thermostable, they may also be sterilized at 340° F. (170° C.) for one hour. At this higher temperature small bottles with heat-resistant screw caps, containing no more than 1½ ounces of the material, are quite satisfactory. If larger quantities are required, then it becomes necessary to determine beforehand the additional time needed for the material to reach sterilizing temperature, after the sterilizer has attained that temperature. Failing this, it is useless to try and establish a minimum safe exposure period, especially where the operator must rely upon the chamber temperature indicated by the thermometer as the beginning of the exposure period.

Petrolatum ("Vaseline") Gauze: The preparation and sterilization of petrolatum gauze has long been a troublesome procedure. Observations in many hospitals have revealed the all too frequent error of preparing too much material, with large excess of petrolatum, inadequate exposure for sterilization or overheating at too high a temperature with consequent charring or partial destruction of the gauze strips. If proper attention is given to the details of preparation and heating the product easily can be controlled within safe limits. The procedure is as follows:

> Prepare about 20 strips of bandage gauze, each 6 to 8 inches long and 2 inches wide. Place the strips in a stainless steel catheter tray with dimensions of 2½ inches wide x 8 inches long x 1¼ inches deep. Cover the strips with 4 ounces of petrolatum, previously liquefied by heating. This should form a layer ½ inch deep in the tray with a thin layer of petrolatum over the topmost gauze strip (see Fig. 94). Sterilize in the hot air sterilizer at 320° F. for 2½ hours.

In the sterilization of petrolatum gauze prepared as above, a longer exposure period is required than in the case of oils, due to the greater depth of the layer in the tray. If the temperature is maintained within the range of 320°-330° F., there should be no evidence of charring or discoloration of the gauze. Repeated tests have shown that a temperature of 340° F. will produce some discoloration, while a temperature of 360° F. for a short period of time produces definite charring of the gauze.

Gershenfeld[19] recently made a thorough investigation of methods of preparation and sterilization of petrolatum gauze in hospitals. His findings showed no uniform satisfactory technique employed in the various institutions. He stated that "the homemade techniques vary widely as to details of preparations; and one cannot help but feel dubious of the efficiency of the procedures of preparation and sterilization, as to their yielding at all times a sterile product and one possessing pharmaceutical elegance." Yarlett, Gershenfeld and McClenahan[20] have also reported on methods for sterility testing and the preparation and sterilization of petrolatum gauze. Their findings indicate that steam processing of gauze impregnated with white petrolatum cannot be relied upon to produce a sterile product. In

TABLE 10

SUMMARY OF REQUIREMENTS FOR HOT AIR STERILIZATION OF SUPPLIES

Material	Exposure Period From Time Sterilizer Shows Temperature of—			Quantity and Preparation
	340°F. (170°C.)	320°F. (160°C.)	285°F. (140°C.)	
Glassware	60 minutes	60 minutes		Items must be clean and free from oil or grease.
Glycerine		120 minutes		Quantity should be limited to ¼" layer (approx. 1 oz.) in 200 ml. Erlenmeyer flask.
Instruments (Cutting Edge)		60 minutes		Instruments must be clean, free from oil or grease and placed on metal tray in sterilizer.
Needles (Hypodermic)		120 minutes		Needles may be placed in tubes having restricted sides, with cotton stoppers. Wire mesh baskets serve well as containers for tubes. Remove stylets.
Needles (Suture)	60 minutes	60 minutes		Sew needles into gauze pack, wrap in muslin.
Oils		120 minutes		Quantity should be limited to ¼" layer (approx. 1 oz.) in 200 ml. Erlenmeyer flask or similar container. Same as for Oils.
Petrolatum—Liquid	60 minutes	120 minutes		Quantity should be limited to ¼" layer (approx. 1 oz.) in Petri dish, ointment jar or other similar container.
Petroleum Jelly (Vaseline)	60 minutes	120 minutes		
Petroleum Jelly (Vaseline) Gauze		150 minutes		Quantity should be limited to 20 strips of 2" x 8" gauze and no more than 4-oz. Petroleum Jelly in catheter tray with dimensions of 2½" x 8" x 1¼".
Powders	60 minutes	120 minutes		Quantity should be limited to ¼" layer (approx. 1 oz.) in Petri dish or other container.
Sulfonamide Powders			3 hours	Quantity should be limited to 4-5 gm. in double envelopes or cotton-plugged test tube.
Syringes (in Test Tubes)		75 minutes		Place assembled syringe with needle attached in test tube of suitable size. Cover top of tube with muslin.
Syringes (Wrapped)		60 minutes		Remove plunger from barrel and wrap in muslin. The needle embedded in gauze may be included in pack.
Zinc Peroxide			4 hours	For clinical application, quantity should be limited to 15-20 gm. in suitable container.

fact steam treatment at 259° F. (126° C.) for 60 minutes failed in every instance to kill spores of an organism belonging to the *subtilis-pumilis* group of the genus *Bacillus,* even when the petrolatum gauze was processed in thin layers.

Operation of Hot Air Sterilizer: For efficient operation of any hot air sterilizer, the characteristics of the individual unit must be known. Close regulation of temperature is important to avoid over-exposure of the less heat-stable articles and to prevent under-exposure with the possibility of an unsterile load. Never load the chamber to the limit. Allow some space between each packaged article and between each basket or container of supplies. Keep all articles well away from chamber sidewalls, so that the free circulation of air is not cut off.

After placing load in sterilizer, check the thermometer to see that it is properly inserted in top of chamber. Adjust the air flow damper to "medium" position and partially open the air inlet and exhaust vents. The heat should then be turned on and the thermostat set to maintain the desired temperature range. Time the exposure only when the thermometer shows the correct temperature. Avoid opening the door during the exposure period because the chamber will cool rapidly. If the methods of preparation for the various supplies deviate greatly from those summarized in Table 10, then it is incumbent upon the operator to determine experimentally the time required for the material to reach sterilizing temperature.

REFERENCES

1. Lewith, S.: Ueber die Ursache der Widerstandsfahigkeit der Sporen gegen hohe Temperaturen. Ein Beitrag zur Theorie der Desinfection. *Arch. exper. Path. u. Pharmakol., 26:*341-354, 1890.
2. Koch, R., and Wolffhugel, G.: Untersuchungen uber die Desinfection mit heiser Luft. *Mitt. a.d.k. Gesundkeitsamt, 1:*1-21, 1881.
3. Wilson, G. S., and Miles, A. A.: Topley and Wilson: *Principles of Bacteriology and Immunity.* Baltimore: Williams & Wilkins, 1946, p. 113.
4. Murray, T. J.: Thermal Death Point. II. Spores of Bacillus anthracis. *J. Infect. Dis., 48:*457-467, 1931.
5. Koch, R., Gaffky, G., and Loeffler, F.: Versuche ueber die Verwerthbarkeit heisser Wasserdampfe zu Desinfectionszwecken. *Mitt. a. d. k. Gesundkeitsamt, 1:*322, 1881.
6. Stein, C. D., and Rogers, H.: Observations on the Resistance of Anthrax Spores to Heat. *Vet. Med., XL:*406-410, 1945.
7. Park, W. H. and Williams, A. W.: *Pathogenic Microorganisms,* 10th Ed., Philadelphia, Lea & Febiger, 1933, p. 555.
8. Oag, R. K.: Resistance of Bacterial Spores to Dry Heat. *J. Path. & Bact., 51:*137-141, 1940.
9. Perkins, J. J., and Underwood, W. B.: Unpublished Data. 1945.
10. Tanner, F. W., and Dack, G. M.: Clostridium botulinum. *J. Infect. Dis., 31:*92-100, 1922.
11. Murray, T. J., and Headlee, M. R.: Thermal Death Point, I. Spores of Clostridium tetani. *J. Infect. Dis., 48:*436-456, 1931.
12. Headlee, M. R.: Thermal Death Point, III. Spores of Clostridium welchii. *J. Infect. Dis., 48:*468-483, 1931.

13. ECKER, E. E., AND SMITH, R.: Sterilizing Surgical Instruments and Utensils. *Mod. Hosp.*, *48*:92-98, 1937.
14. WALTER, C. W.: *Aseptic Treatment of Wounds*. New York, Macmillan, 1948, p. 93.
15. RODENBECK, H.: Ueber die thermische Sterilisation wasserfreir Stoffe und die Resistenz einiger Bakterien bei Erhitzung in solchen Stoffen. *Arch. Hyg. u. Bakt.*, *109*:(2), 67-84, 1932.
16. WALTER, C. W.: Sterilization. *Surg. Clin. North America*, New York Number, Philadelphia, Saunders, April, 1942, p. 353.
17. HAWN, C. V. Z., AND WALTER, C. W.: The Sterile Scalpel, *Surg., Gynec. & Obst.*, *99*: 118-119, July, 1954.
18. MELENEY, F. L.: *Treatise on Surgical Infections*. New York, Oxford, 1948, p. 591.
19. GERSHENFELD, L.: Petrolatum Gauze. *Am. J. Pharm.*, *126*:112-130, April, 1954.
20. YARLETT, M. A., GERSHENFELD, L., AND McCLENAHAN, W. S.: Petrolatum Gauze I. Methods for Sterility Testing. II. Its Preparation and Sterilization. *Drug Standards*, *22*:205-215, Nov.-Dec., 1954.
21. PERKINS, J. J.: Dry Heat Sterilization. *Manual of Sterilization and Disinfection*, *11*:3-22, 1951.

Chapter XI

Sterilization and Care of Syringes and Needles

THE SUPPOSEDLY STERILE SYRINGE

DURING the past decade much has been written about the supposedly sterile syringe and its implications in a variety of conditions attributable to faulty injection technique. Mild inflammations and infections not uncommonly follow the inoculations and injections which play such an important part in modern treatment. Accidents following injections are especially serious when they occur in hospital practice or in the course of mass inoculations and, on more than one occasion, severe and even fatal results have occurred as the result of a contaminated syringe and needle—supposedly sterile. Viral hepatitis may readily be transmitted by contaminated syringes, needles and other equipment employed for taking venous blood or for capillary puncture.[1, 2] Multiple injections with a single syringe and venipuncture using inadequately sterilized syringes may spread the causative agent of serum hepatitis.[3, 4]

In a review of this subject by the Medical Research Council,[5] it was reported that alcohol is used more often than any other chemical disinfectant for sterilizing syringes, although the practice is not recommended. This widespread use of alcohol as a disinfectant is a perpetual cause of disquiet to those familiar with its germicidal properties. Alcohol is totally incapable of destroying bacterial spores. The literature records several cases of postoperative gas gangrene conclusively traced to instruments supposedly sterilized by alcohol.[6] Complete bacteriological sterility can be achieved only by sterilization in the autoclave with saturated steam under pressure or in the hot air sterilizer. Boiling in water will destroy pathogenic organisms but it cannot be relied upon to destroy resistant spores. A boiled syringe may, if thoroughly cleaned beforehand, be accepted as reasonably safe where sterilization in the hot air oven or autoclave is not possible, but a boiled syringe is not necessarily sterile and its safety cannot be guaranteed. Of the many recommendations made by the Research Council Committee, those deserving of special emphasis are:

A fresh sterile syringe and needle must be used for each injection or aspiration.

In clinics where many injections of the same fluid are given, the same syringe may be used for several subcutaneous or intramuscular injections, *but not intravenous*, provided a fresh sterile needle is used for each patient.

A syringe that has been used for aspiration, e.g., of blood from a vein, or pus from an abscess, or for intravenous injection, which always entails aspiration of blood, must be cleaned and sterilized before it is used again.

It is essential to keep syringes for injection separate from those used for aspiration.

Syringes and needles require thorough cleaning after use, before resterilization.

Contamination of syringes and needles may occur during assembly after sterilization as the result of contact with fingers, dust or droplets of saliva from either the doctor or the subject, or to contact of the needle with a non-sterile surface.

Handle needles with sterile forceps only, syringes with dry, washed hands, taking care to touch only the outside of the barrel and the handle of the piston.

Do not talk, cough or sneeze over a sterile syringe. Persons with known or suspected upper respiratory infections must wear masks while carrying out injections.

The practice of "dishing up" a sterile syringe and needle in an open bowl, especially one which contains any liquid, is condemned.

Sterile syringes and needles must be placed in sterile covered containers.

CLEANING OF SYRINGES

For the busy hospital a centralized syringe and needle service is considered essential. For maximum efficiency the service should be delegated to the central supply department, where the procedures of cleaning and sterilizing for all syringes are under one control. If syringes are not thoroughly cleaned after use, sterilization may be ineffective, particularly if the syringe contains traces of oil, grease or coagulable protein. The following procedure is recommended for the manual cleaning of syringes:

1) Immediately after use, separate barrel and plunger and rinse thoroughly with cold tap water. This is particularly necessary when the syringe has been used for aspiration of blood or body fluids.

2) Wash barrel and plunger in warm water to which has been added a safe and effective detergent (Fig. 95). Scrub outside surfaces with a good grade fibre brush and use a test-tube brush for cleaning inside of barrel. AVOID SCRATCHING. Be sure and force detergent solution through tip of syringe. (Care should be exercised in selecting a detergent for this application because alkalies, soaps and many detergents erode the ground glass surfaces, thereby causing the syringe to leak or bind.) A non-etching and low-sudsing detergent buffered to maintain neutral pH in use solution is best suited for cleaning of syringes.

3) Rinse in three changes of water. A brush should be used with the first rinse to make sure that all traces of detergent are removed from ground surfaces and graduation marks. The third or final rinse should be made with freshly distilled water.

4) After final rinsing, permit parts to air-dry and then assemble, taking care to match the serial numbers of barrel and plunger.

Failure to clean syringes immediately after use may result in the plunger sticking in the barrel or the needle sticking on the tip of the syringe. Various methods may be used to separate the "frozen" parts but probably the most

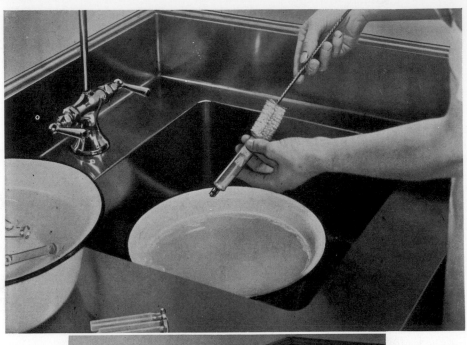

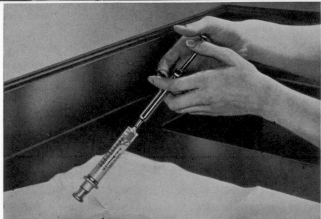

Courtesy Becton-Dickinson and Company.

Fig. 95. Syringes require thorough cleaning after use and before sterilization. If the manual procedure is followed, a test tube brush of appropriate size will facilitate cleaning inside of barrel. Avoid scratching of ground surfaces.

Fig. 96. Separating a frozen syringe with the B-D Syringe Opener. This all metal syringe provides a convenient means for loosening any frozen Luer-slip or Luer-lok syringe (Becton-Dickinson & Co.).

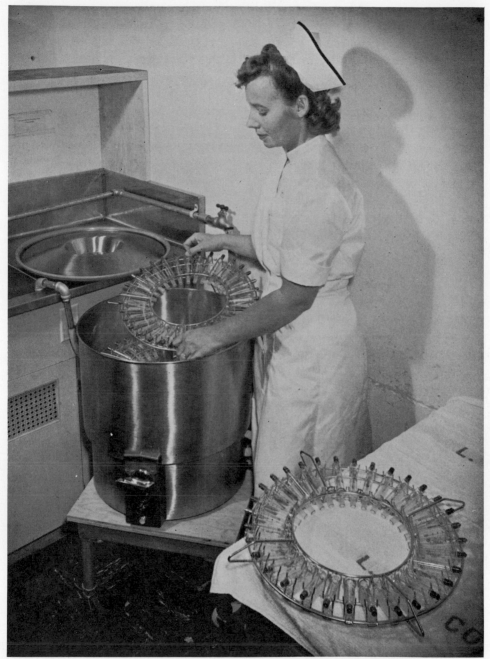

Courtesy Los Angeles County Health Dept., Los Angeles, Calif.

Fig. 97. Mechanical syringe cleaner. Washing action is accomplished by forced jets of detergent solution directed into and over barrel and plunger surfaces.

successful technic is to use the B-D Syringe Opener, as shown in Fig. 96. This is an all-metal syringe for loosening any frozen Luer slip or Luer-Lok syringe. The procedure is to first fill the syringe opener with warm water. Attach it firmly to the tip of the frozen syringe by holding at the base of the barrel. Then apply firm, steady pressure, gradually increasing the pressure until water infiltrates around the plunger and reaches the top of the barrel. Do not grasp the frozen syringe, but rather let it hang free. Keep the pressure steady, and the plunger will gradually be expelled from the barrel. A towel spread beneath the syringe will prevent breakage in the event that it separates with expulsive force. Other methods are sometimes used in an attempt to separate a frozen syringe but their success has not been altogether uniform. These include: Boiling the syringe in 25% aqueous glycerine for ten minutes, removing plunger while syringe is still hot. Placing syringe in ice water for five minutes and then immersing, up to the flange, in hot water for a few seconds, then quickly removing the contracted plunger from the expanded barrel.

MECHANICAL SYRINGE CLEANER

The ever-increasing use of syringes for immunization, antibiotic therapy and hematologic studies has created a major problem of supply for hospitals. The average general acute hospital of 200 beds may use anywhere from 200 to 300 syringes daily. To hand wash this number of syringes is unquestionably an arduous task which consumes a great amount of time and introduces the costly factor of breakage. The most feasible solution to this problem is the use of an efficient, automatic syringe cleaner or washer. Experience in many hospitals justifies the claim that the daily complement of syringes can be thoroughly cleaned, with less handling and less breakage, in approximately one-quarter of the time required by the manual cleaning process.

The mechanical syringe cleaner shown in Figure 97 is well suited to the needs of the average hospital. It employs five circular stainless steel racks to hold any combination of all standard makes of syringes. The capacity is 156 syringes, with barrels and plungers matched in their respective slots in each rack. Washing action is accomplished by forceful jets of detergent solution directed into and over barrel and plunger surfaces. The jets are fed by a centrifugal pump operated by an electric motor housed under the base of the drum. The total washing and rinsing cycle may be varied from 5 to 20 minutes by means of an automatic timer control.

STERILIZATION OF SYRINGES

Dry heat is considered the most satisfactory agent for the sterilization of syringes, principally because all moisture is eliminated, thereby minimizing erosion of the ground glass surfaces. A common method of preparation is to remove the plunger from the barrel and wrap the parts together in one muslin cover as shown in Figure 98. If desired, the needle can be embedded in gauze and included in the same package. With this method of preparation the exposure period should be not less than one hour, preferably two hours, from the time that the hot air sterilizer shows 320° F. (160° C.). Care must be taken to insure that the chamber is not overloaded and that some space is allowed between the wrapped syringes for free air circulation. In an efficient hot air sterilizer, moderately loaded, the rise of temperature in the load should closely follow that of the chamber (see Fig. 91).

Another method which has certain advantages, especially for the larger syringes, is to place the plunger in the barrel with the needle attached. The assembled syringe is then placed in a Pyrex test tube of such diameter that the barrel of the syringe fits loosely in the tube with the flange resting on the top rim as illustrated in Figure 99. The tube should be of sufficient length to accommodate the syringe with needle attached, without the point of the needle touching the bottom of the tube. (A 10 ml. syringe requires a test tube 200 mm. in length

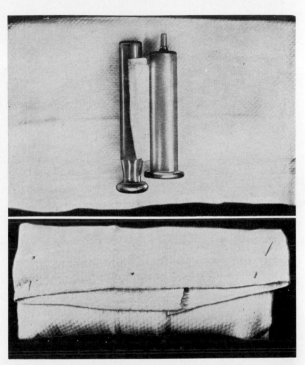

Fig. 98. This method of packaging syringes is suitable for either hot air or pressure steam sterilization. The plunger is removed from the barrel and the parts are wrapped in muslin.

and 25 mm. outside diameter; whereas a 5 ml. syringe requires a tube 150 mm. in length and 20 mm. outside diameter). With this method the cotton stopper is eliminated because a portion of the syringe extends above the rim of the tube. The upper portion of the tube should, however, be covered with a muslin wrapper.

A recent technic described by Walter[7] for preparing syringes for dry heat sterilization is worthy of note. After washing the syringes in a mechanical cleaner, they are dried, assembled, and a plastic shield* placed over the syringe tip, as in Figure 100. The syringes are then sorted into baskets

---

* Plastic tips for syringes are available from Fenwal Laboratories, Inc., 47 Mellen, Framingham, Mass.

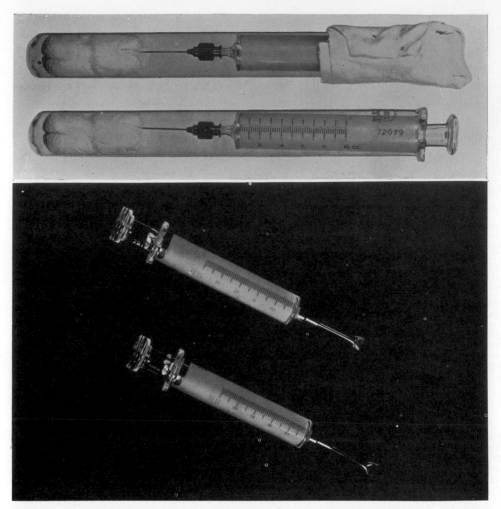

Fig. 99. This method of preparing the syringe for hot air sterilization is advantageous for certain types of work, the syringe being completely assembled with the needle attached. The test tube should be of such diameter that the syringe fits loosely in the tube, with the flange resting on the rim of the tube.

Fig. 100. This method of preparing syringes (assembled) for dry heat sterilization is rapid, efficient and economical. A plastic shield is placed over the syringe tip as shown. The plunger cannot be removed until the seal is broken between the shield and syringe.

by size, loaded into the autoclave (at the end of the day's schedule), and with steam admitted to the jacket only they are dry heat sterilized in an overnight exposure. Upon removal from the sterilizer the syringes are available for immediate use. "The plastic shield seals off the tip of the syringe so that the plunger cannot be removed until the seal is broken between the shield and syringe. This is accomplished by gently twisting the shield and pushing it against the tip. Added advantages of this technic are quick identification of syringe size and storage requiring less space."

The principal disadvantage in the use of dry heat for the sterilization of syringes is the time required to do the job. Even with the most efficient of hot air sterilizers the time required to process a heavy load of syringes averages 3 to 4 hours. The autoclave with steam to jacket only, serving as a hot air sterilizer, requires a minimum of 4 hours exposure. It cannot conveniently be used for this purpose during the day because of the demands placed on it for steam sterilization of other supplies. This leaves the hospital with the alternative of either using the autoclave as a hot air sterilizer with an overnight exposure or, during the day, use the more rapid process of sterilizing the syringes with saturated steam under pressure. In the interest of expediency many institutions favor the steam sterilization process.

When preparing syringes for steam sterilization they should always be disassembled—the plunger separated from the barrel. If this is not done direct steam contact to all surfaces cannot be assured and the sterilizing process may be ineffective. The attempted steam sterilization of a dry assembled syringe is contrary to established principles. If assembled syringes are to be sterilized by steam, it is necessary to rinse the parts with distilled water, leaving them distinctly moist, just before assembling, packaging and placing in the sterilizer. The residual film of moisture will then

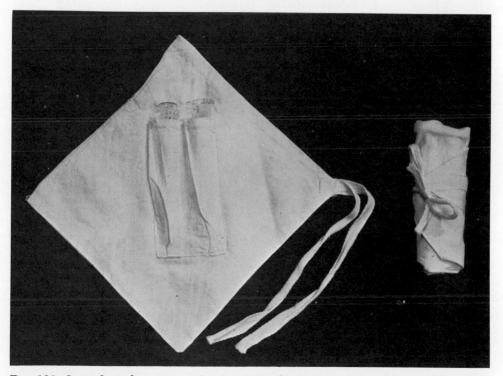

Fig. 101. Special muslin wrapper for steam sterilization of disassembled syringe. Two pockets are provided for the barrel and plunger. The size of the wrapper is sufficient to allow for complete coverage and the tie strings facilitate rapid preparation.

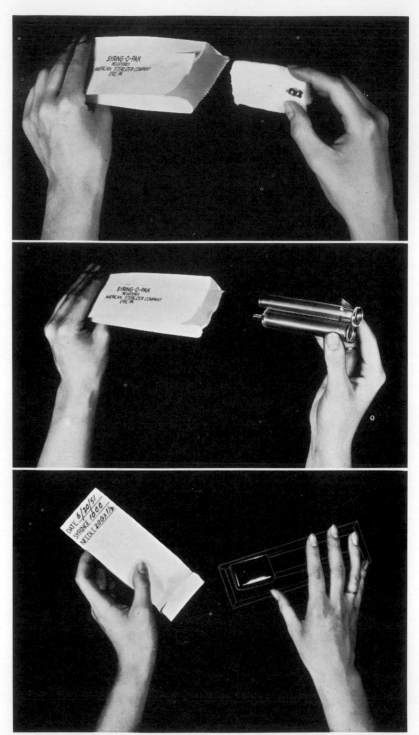

Fig. 102. Place folded gauze square, 3″ x 3″, containing needle in Pak, with hub of needle pointing up.

Fig. 103. Place disassembled syringe in Pak.

Fig. 104. Fold over top portion of Pak twice and staple or seal for tight closure.

186

provide steam contact to the inside surfaces. Unfortunately this method is also objectionable, because the residual water in the assembled syringe during sterilization will attack the ground glass and leach out alkali, which later will destroy certain drugs admitted into the syringe.

Special muslin wrappers facilitate preparation of syringes for steam sterilization (Fig. 101). There are two pockets in the wrapper, one for the barrel and one for the plunger. The tie strings sewed to the outside of the wrapper assist in rapid packaging. Syringes packaged in this manner can conveniently be sterilized with bulk loads of dry supplies at 250° F. for 30 minutes.

The use of specially fabricated paper bags for packaging of syringes has become very popular in the past few years. When properly carried out, the method is safe, efficient and economical, especially for the hospital where large numbers of syringes must be processed daily. To realize the maximum from this technique the first requirement is to select a paper bag of the right characteristics. It should be made preferably from a white sulfite bond paper of high bursting strength, with con-

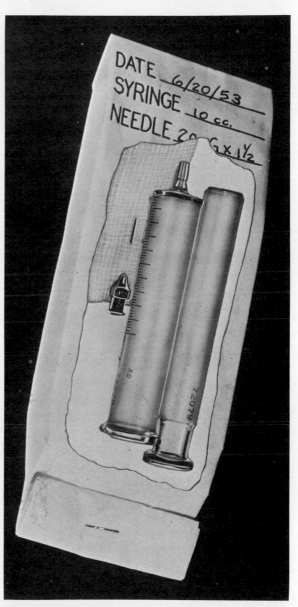

Fig. 105. When properly packaged, the syringe and needle will rest in bag as shown. Sterilize in the autoclave at 250° F. for 30 minutes, followed by 15 minutes drying.

trolled porosity to permit adequate steam permeability during sterilization and limited air permeability following sterilization. In addition, all seams and folds of the bag should be uniformly sealed with heat-resistant adhesive

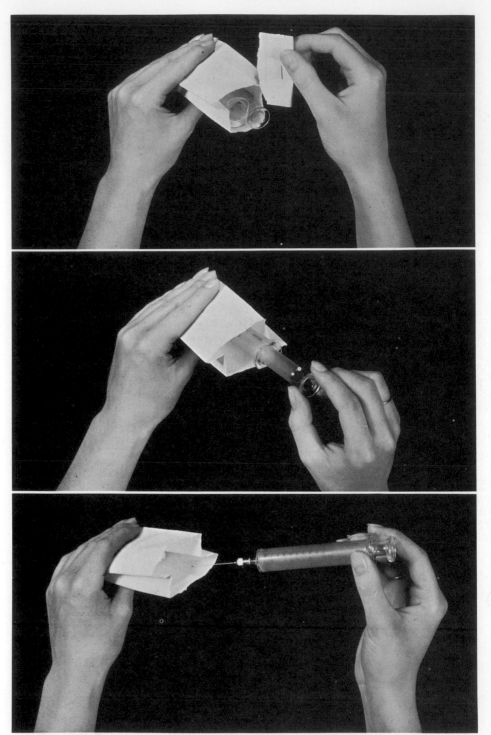

Fig. 106. To use, tear off top portion of Pak, exposing contents as shown.

Fig. 107. By holding Pak firmly, insert plunger in barrel. Then, by holding hub of needle from outside of Pak, force lightly tip of syringe into needle.

Fig. 108. Finally withdraw assembled syringe with needle attached from Pak, ready for immediate use. The gauze square remaining in Pak may be used as a scrub or compress for the inoculation site.

to prevent opening up during sterilization. The technique of packaging, sterilization and use is described under Figures 102 to 109B, inclusive.

CLEANING OF NEEDLES

Like syringes, needles require thorough cleaning as soon as possible after use. Particular attention must be given to the inside of the hub where blood or dirt may have accumulated. The following procedure should be observed in the manual cleaning of needles:

1) Immediately after use flush thoroughly with cold water.

2) Insert stylet or needle wire through needle to make sure there is no

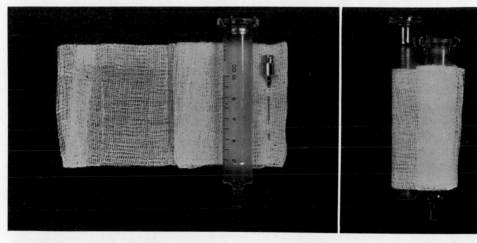

Fig. 109A. Alternate method of packaging syringe and needle in paper bag. Open gauze square (3″ x 3″) one fold. Thread needle into gauze and place barrel beside needle as shown.

Fig. 109B. Roll barrel and needle one turn in gauze, place plunger beside barrel and finish roll as shown. Insert in Pak and sterilize as in Figure 105. For removal follow the procedure shown in Figures 106, 107 and 108.

clogging or obstruction in the cannula. (Always insert stylet through the hub—not from the point.)

3) Place needles in basin of hot water to which an alkaline detergent capable of dissolving blood has been added. Wash thoroughly inside and out. Use syringe to flush the cannula. Carefully clean inside of hub with a tightly wound cotton applicator.

4) Rinse well with freshly distilled water and inspect for cleanliness and sharpness. The use of ether, acetone or alcohol as a final rinse contributes little to the cleaning process. To hasten drying the needles may be placed over a warm radiator or on top of the sterilizer. *If the needles are to be sterilized by steam some moisture must be present in the cannula at the time of placing in the sterilizer.*

As with syringes, the manual cleaning of large numbers of hollow needles is a difficult and time-consuming task. Human fatigue must eventually take its toll and when this occurs a percentage of the needles will be poorly cleaned, especially on the inside of the hub and some, perhaps, not at all. The mechanical needle cleaner, now employed in many hospitals, will do much to safeguard cleaning efficiency and to standardize technique. Time

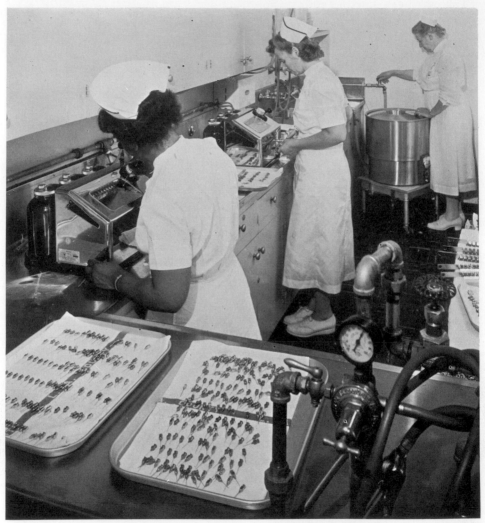

Courtesy Los Angeles County Health Dept., Los Angeles, Calif.

Fig. 110. The two mechanical needle cleaners shown here are typical of those commonly used in hospitals.

study measurement figures show that 2 minutes (average) is required to properly clean one needle.[8] At the top rate of 30 per hour, only 240 needles can be cleaned per day per person by the manual process. In this same period of time, one person operating the mechanical needle cleaner can wash 100 needles every 10 minutes or 600 per hour. Obviously the mechanical cleaner effects a tremendous savings in personnel time, insofar as the actual process of washing is concerned. The needle cleaners shown in Figure 110 are typical of those in common use. The sequence of operation

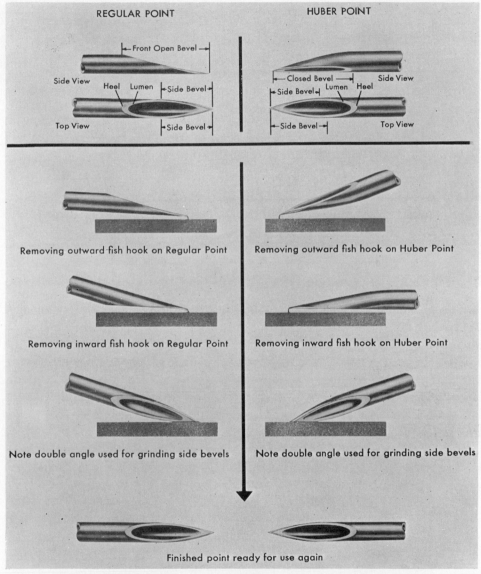

REGULAR POINT   HUBER POINT

Front Open Bevel

Side View   Heel   Lumen   Side Bevel

Top View   Side Bevel

Closed Bevel   Side View
Side Bevel   Lumen   Heel

Side Bevel   Top View

Removing outward fish hook on Regular Point   Removing outward fish hook on Huber Point

Removing inward fish hook on Regular Point   Removing inward fish hook on Huber Point

Note double angle used for grinding side bevels   Note double angle used for grinding side bevels

Finished point ready for use again

Fig. 111. Needle sharpening technique (Becton-Dickinson & Co.).

comprises: 1) cleaning out the hub of the needle with a power-driven swab; 2) forcing under pressure three separate cleaning liquids through the cannula, and 3) forcing compressed air through the cannula, leaving it dry and ready for sterilization. The needles are placed in the machine in units of 12 by means of specially designed holders or racks which accommodate all lengths and sizes.

SHARPENING OF NEEDLES

Before sterilization, the point of each needle should be carefully inspected with the aid of a hand lens or magnifying glass to determine if it is damaged and in need of sharpening. Particular attention must be given to the detection and removal of burrs, "fish-hooks," and dull, broken, or misshaped points. The use of a fine Arkansas oil stone is essential for sharpening, also a needle adapter fitted with a handle to hold the needle. A light mineral oil on the stone hastens sharpening, prevents clogging of the grinding surface, and gives a smoother finish. The first step is to grind off any hook on the tip of the needle (see Fig. 111). Then the bevel must be restored and sharpened. This may be accomplished by placing the bevel flush on the stone at the proper angle, followed by movement of the needle in an elliptical pattern, until it is smooth and shiny. The sides of the bevelled point should then be lightly rubbed on the stone so that it will penetrate skin easily and smoothly. In sharpening a needle with a fitted stylet care must be taken to keep the stylet in place so that perfectly matched bevels are maintained.

STERILIZATION OF NEEDLES

The preferred method for the sterilization of hollow needles is dry heat in the hot air sterilizer. They may also be sterilized in the autoclave with steam in jacket only at 250°-254° F. (15-17 pounds pressure) and an overnight exposure period. The dry heat process leaves the needles absolutely dry and assures sterility of the cannula, even when the stylet is left in place. Routinely needles should not be sterilized with stylets in place because of the possibility of corrosion due to electrolytic action between stylet and needle.

Special tubes of the hour-glass type serve ideally as containers for needles. The restricted sides suspend the needle in the tube and thereby protect the point (Fig. 112). The open end of the tube is stoppered with a cotton plug. Needles prepared in this manner may then be placed in wire-mesh metal baskets for loading in the sterilizer. It is important to note that the tubes and needles in the middle of the basket will not attain sterilizing temperature as rapidly as those near the sides. In fact, when the sterilizer shows 320° F. (160° C.), the temperature of the needle in the most centrally located tube is only 277° F. (136° C.). This needle requires 55 minutes longer heating time to reach 320° F. Therefore, when needles are prepared as in Figure 112 the absolute minimum exposure time is two hours after the sterilizer shows 320° F.

Needles prepared as in Figure 112 can also be sterilized with steam under pressure in the autoclave. If this procedure is followed, each needle should be flushed with freshly distilled water and left distinctly moist, just before placing in the sterilizer. Also the tubes containing the needles should rest on their sides in the sterilizer to facilitate air removal and steam intake to each tube and needle. Under these conditions the exposure period is 30 minutes at 250° F., followed by drying for not less than 15 minutes.

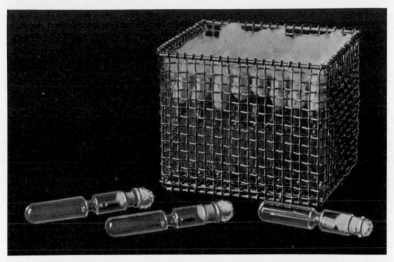

Fig. 112. Needles in special tubes of the hour-glass type with restricted sides, stoppered with cotton plugs, may be sterilized by dry heat or by steam under pressure. The metal baskets facilitate loading in the sterilizer and later handling in storage.

UNIT CONTAINERS FOR ISSUE AND RETURN OF SYRINGES AND NEEDLES

Methods in force for the preparation, sterilization, issue and return of syringes and needles in hospitals show a serious lack of standardization. It is fair to state that of the variety of technics in use relatively few meet the requirements for a comprehensive syringe and needle service. To be sure, there are perfectly acceptable methods for cleaning these items, the rules for packaging are well defined, and the methods of sterilization are reliable when properly conducted. Still, in most instances, there is an important element lacking—a convenient system for the daily issue and return of syringes and needles to and from the various floors or stations throughout the hospital. As a practical approach to this problem, the first step is to establish a centralized syringe and needle service. This is one of the specific functions of the central (supply) service department in the hospital. An area should be set aside within the department for the daily care and preparation of syringes and needles as in Figure 110. Secondly, a standardized unit container should be developed for the daily issue of sterile syringes

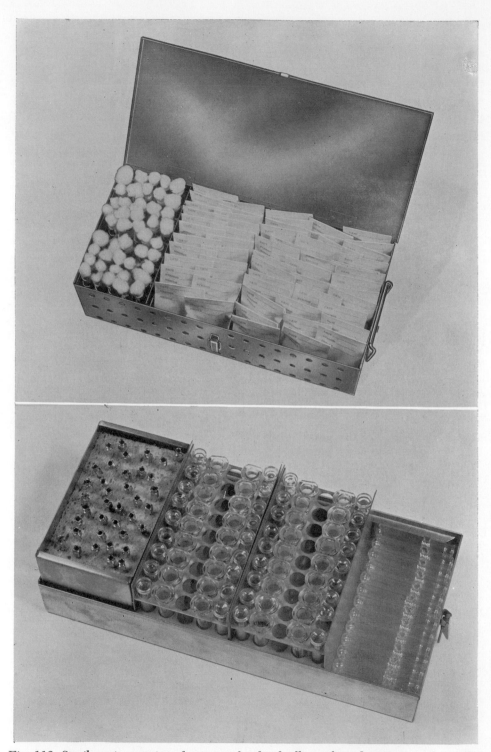

Fig. 113. Sterile unit container for issue of individually packaged syringes and needles.

Fig. 114. Soiled unit container for return of used syringes and needles to central service department.

and needles to the various floors throughout the hospital. A similar, companion-type, unit container should likewise be employed for the return of the soiled items to the central service department.

The assembled unit containers shown in Figures 113 and 114 demonstrate the principle of the proposed system. The sterile unit (Fig. 113) contains a sufficient number of 2, 5, and 10 ml. syringes and needles of appropriate sizes to satisfy the normal daily complement of a 25-bed nursing unit. Both syringes and needles are individually packaged for effective protection against contamination. The unit container may be sterilized either by steam under pressure at 250° F. for 30 minutes or by hot air at 320° F. for 1 hour or 250° F. for 6 hours.

The soiled unit container shown in Figure 114 is for the return of the used syringes and needles to the central service department. It contains one water-tight tray in which is placed a thick cellulose sponge. The sponge is saturated with an effective detergent-germicide. Immediately after use, the needles are flushed out with water and stuck in the sponge as shown. This treatment keeps the needles moist, prevents residual soil from drying, and facilitates safe handling upon their return to central supply. The used syringes are likewise rinsed with water immediately after use, disassembled, and placed in the special rack as shown. The empty needle tubes are placed in one end of the container. If terminal sterilization of the needles and syringes is necessary, the entire unit container can be subjected to autoclaving. The unit container system helps to standardize methods and promote safety in the routine handling of syringes and needles.

REFERENCES

1. Capps, R. B., Sborov, V., and Scheifley, C. H.: A Syringe Transmitted Epidemic of Infectious Hepatitis. *J.A.M.A.*, *136*:819, 1948.
2. Capps, R. B.: Viral Hepatitis. *Mod. Hosp.*, 78:65-67, Jan., 1952.
3. Morton, R. S.: Syringe-Transmitted Jaundice. *Brit. M.J.*, 2:938, 1948.
4. Malmros, H., Wilander, O., and Herner, B.: Inoculation Hepatitis. *Brit. M.J.*, 2:936, 1948.
5. *The Sterilization, Use and Care of Syringes.* By Committee of Medical Research Council, His Majesty's Stat. Off., York House, Kingsway, London, W.C. 2.
6. Nye, R. N., and Mallory, T. B.: Fallacy of Using Alcohol for Sterilization of Surgical Instruments. *Boston Med. & Surg. J.*, 189:561-563, 1923.
7. Walter, C. W.: Severe Dermatitis Is Eliminated by Complete Removal of Residual Drugs from Syringes, Hospital Topics (Central Supply Room Section) Feb., 1954, p. 81-82.
8. Personal Communication, C. J. Curran, Nov. 24, 1952.

CHAPTER XII

Disinfection of Instruments and Utensils by Boiling Water

THE USE of the word "sterilization" is incorrect when applied to boiling water as an agent for rendering instruments and utensils free from all microbial life. Several investigators have shown that boiling water or moist heat at a temperature of 212° F. (100° C.) is inadequate for the destruction of resistant bacterial spores. (See Table 5, p. 42.) There is also some question as to the efficacy of boiling water for the inactivation of certain viruses[2, 3] under ordinary methods of use. It is considered more appropriate to designate the process as one of disinfection or sanitization. The official definition of the word "disinfection" adopted by the American Public Health Association is "killing of pathogenic agents by chemical or physical means directly applied."[1] Sanitization implies a process whereby the number of organisms present on utensils is reduced to a safe level as judged by public health requirements. It does not imply complete freedom from bacteria. Sanitization is a less precise term than disinfection and is more appropriately applied to a cleaning process.

THE STATE OF BOILING

The highest temperature that can be attained in boiling water in any open or non-pressure vessel is 212° F. (100° C.) at sea level. At higher altitudes, the atmospheric pressure is reduced and water will boil at lower temperatures, for example, in Denver boiling occurs at 202° F. (94.4° C.), and in La Paz, Bolivia at 188° F. (86.6° C.). It makes no difference how much heat is applied to the vessel—when ebullition occurs, the temperature will have reached the maximum. The application of more heat will simply increase the rate of evaporation and produce more violent boiling. When water boils slowly with the formation of only a few bubbles, liberating very little steam, the condition may be described as "mild boiling." When water boils so rapidly that bubbles form all over the surface, continuously but not violently, the condition may be described as "vigorous boiling." There is no advantage gained in applying so much heat that the water boils violently, giving off clouds of steam. Also, too vigorous boiling will rapidly deplete the water in the vessel and require frequent refilling which is objectionable. The heat should be regulated to maintain a moderate boiling condition.

Instrument and utensil boilers may be vented to the atmosphere to dispose of excess steam, or they may be equipped with condenser vents in which cold water is permitted to flow through a condensing device at the rear of the chamber in such manner as to condense excess steam as fast as it forms. Neither of these methods makes any attempt to conserve heat, they merely dispose of the excess steam created by too vigorous boiling. Regardless of the venting system employed on the boiler, some steam should escape from under the cover to inform the operator that the chamber is filled with free flowing steam. Not infrequently, in the attempt to keep all steam out of the room or perhaps to conserve heat, the apparatus is regulated for the production of steam at so slow a rate that the temperature above the water may drop below the range at which disinfection should be conducted. Under this condition the water just simmers, very little steam is formed, and the temperature above the water may never get higher than 170° F. (76° C.). This is hazardous for any article that may extend above the surface of the water or when the apparatus is being used as a steamer only for disinfection.

With the usual simple boiler, the rate of heating can be controlled only by manual regulation of the valve or switch. The operator will turn on the heat to the highest range until the water boils, then the heat is turned down until the desired range is maintained. This requires close attention and some acquired skill. Within recent years automatic devices have been made available for all hospital types of boilers which control the rate of heating. They are known as "excess vapor regulators." In service, they utilize the full amount of heat to bring the water to a boil quickly, then automatically reduce the heat to maintain the proper rate of boiling without creating an excess of steam. Figure 115 shows application of this type of control to a steam heated instrument boiler.

BOILING OF INSTRUMENTS FOR DISINFECTION

The preoperative boiling of surgical instruments for disinfection is not recommended except where steam under pressure is unavailable. This statement is made with full knowledge that in certain hospitals and clinics, where comparatively high standards prevail, instruments are boiled for 20 minutes in ordinary tap water—with apparently good results. Nevertheless, in comparison with established standards for surgical sterilization the technic is open to question, and its use should be discouraged wherever steam under pressure is available. If the boiling process must be used, it is imperative that the instruments be thoroughly cleaned beforehand to remove traces of dried blood, oil and grease. Jointed instruments must be opened or unlocked before placing in the boiler. With water boiling at 212° F. (100° C.) the minimum exposure period should be 30 minutes. At high altitudes the exposure period should be increased about 5 minutes for each

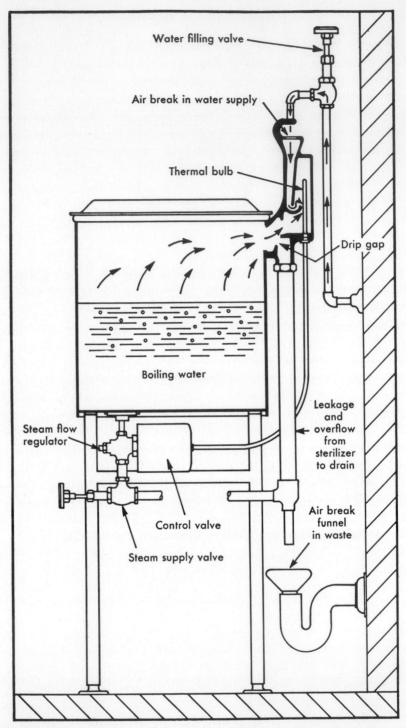

Fig. 115. Excess vapor regulator and heat control as applied to a steam heated instrument boiler. This device is neither vent nor temperature regulator. Instead, it automatically controls the rate of heating, to keep water boiling without creating excess vapor or needless waste of fuel.

1000 feet elevation above sea level. It is necessary that the boiler contain sufficient water so that all parts of the instruments are well covered. The water level should be adjusted before boiling with at least an inch of water above the instruments.

The bactericidal efficiency of boiling water may be increased by the addition of sufficient sodium carbonate (sal soda) to make a 2 per cent solution or by the addition of sodium hydroxide (caustic soda) so as to make a 0.1 per cent solution in the boiler. Mundel[4] reported that the addition of this amount of washing soda markedly increases the disinfecting power of boiling water and also decreases its corrosive action on metal instruments. Bacterial spores in water resisted boiling for about 10 hours, but they were destroyed in a 2 per cent soda solution at 208° F. (98° C.) in 10 to 30 minutes. Other workers[5] employing a similar technic demonstrated that when contaminated and oiled instruments were boiled in a 2 per cent soda solution, a period of 10 minutes' boiling was necessary to produce sterilization. Boiling water to which alkali has been added in the above-mentioned concentrations is adequate for the destruction of most spores in an exposure period of 15 minutes.

Scale formation resulting from deposition of lime salts on instruments and utensils routinely boiled is difficult to control, especially in hard water areas. The scale formation can be reduced appreciably by boiling the water for ten minutes before placing the instruments in it. During this interval, a part of the lime salts in the water will deposit on the heating coils, leaving less to accumulate on the instruments. Frequent draining of the boiler as well as too vigorous boiling contribute to scale formation. The addition of fresh water means the presence of more lime salts. The desirable procedure is to use the water in the boiler throughout the day, then drain and carefully clean the boiler at the close of the day. Water softeners are also of some advantage, but they do not entirely overcome the difficulty. Oil or grease should never be permitted in any instrument boiler. These substances provide a protective barrier for bacteria through which the moist heat cannot penetrate. The use of boiling type "sterilizers" for surgical sterilization of instruments and utensils has become outmoded because the margin of safety with steam under pressure is greater, the time required is less, and the instruments are maintained in better condition.

BOILING OF UTENSILS

The procedure given above for the disinfection of instruments by boiling also applies to utensils. It is a hazardous practice to attempt disinfection if parts of the utensils extend above the surface of the water. If the utensils are nested with parts exposed above the water it will be difficult for steam to contact all surfaces. Even when the utensils are turned bottom side up, air will be pocketed in them, thereby preventing steam contact to all surfaces. The requirement should be strictly enforced that all utensils be completely submerged during the boiling process. The exposure period should be 30 minutes from the time boiling temperature has been reached. As with instruments, dependable technique demands that the utensils undergoing disinfection be thoroughly cleaned beforehand. Do not permit the utensils to remain in the boiler for any considerable period of time after boiling. As the steam condenses and the water cools upon standing, air containing dust particles will be drawn into the chamber with the possibility of the utensils becoming contaminated.

TERMINAL DISINFECTION OF INSTRUMENTS BY BOILING

The immediate care of instruments and utensils used on septic cases is of serious concern, especially where facilities are not available for use with steam under pressure, such as the pressure instrument washer-sterilizer. At best, boiling water is a poor substitute for steam under pressure, but when an emergency occurs and the only equipment available is an instrument boiler, the most practicable procedure yielding reasonable precautionary measures must be followed. This means that some method must be used whereby the bactericidal efficiency of boiling water can be depended upon to decontaminate the instruments and to protect the nurse against the infectious hazard in later cleaning of the instruments. Immediately following the septic operation, the instruments (unlocked and open) should be transferred to the boiler and sufficient trisodium phosphate added to the water so as to make a 2 per cent solution. With the instruments completely submerged, the water should then be brought to a brisk boil and the boiling continued for not less than 15 minutes. The instruments may then be cleaned in the usual manner. The alkalinity due to the trisodium phosphate will assist in solubilizing the organic matter on the instruments and it will also enhance the bactericidal efficiency of the boiling water.

CLEANING AND SANITIZING AGENTS

Water is the universal cleaning and sanitizing agent and an adequate supply of hot water is the strongest weapon against dirt. Although water alone possesses some detergent value, it is largely ineffective for the removal of proteinaceous soil, oil and grease from the surfaces of instruments and utensils. The addition of a suitable detergent to water is, therefore, of the greatest importance for effective cleaning. The purpose of the detergent is to facilitate the exchange of a soiled surface condition for a clean surface plus a soiled detergent. This exchange process which, in effect, constitutes the cleaning operation, is dependent upon the kind of surface being cleaned, the nature and amount of soil, the composition and concentration of the detergent, time of exposure to the cleaning agent, hardness of the water, pH of the cleaning solution, and the mechanical factor of agitation or scrubbing.

Most detergents may be classified as either highly alkaline, moderately alkaline, "neutral," and acid cleaners. The highly alkaline detergents usually contain sodium hydroxide or caustic soda as the primary active ingredient, to which is added sodium metasilicate as a corrosion inhibitor. Usually trisodium phosphate or a pyrophosphate is added to the formulation to prevent calcium and magnesium salts from precipitating out when the detergent is used in hard water. One or more wetting (surface-active) agents is also added to increase the wetting, penetrating, spreading and rinsing properties of the formulation. As a rule, the highly alkaline detergents possess rapid dissolving power for dried blood or protein and for emulsifying fats and oils. They are corrosive to aluminum and will readily attack ground glass surfaces, such as syringes. They are not harmful to rubber.

The moderately alkaline cleaners, of which there are many commercially available, are of variable composition. They usually contain sodium carbonate or soda ash, sodium metasilicate and one or more phosphate compounds as the basic ingredients. A surface-active or wetting agent is also added to enhance the detergent properties. The moderately alkaline detergents are the most satisfactory for general purpose use. They are less corrosive than the highly alkaline cleaners, but they may attack aluminum and ground glass surfaces, including syringes. Representative of this class are products such as "Pyrem," "Surg-i-clean," "Calgonite," "Haemosol," "Alconox," etc.

The "neutral" cleaners are those products which in use solution develop a pH close to neutrality. They are mixtures of strong wetting agents to which are added neutral phosphate compounds or other fairly neutral builders to give the solution detergent properties in addition to the surface-active effects of the wetting agents. The synthetic (household) detergents offer many examples in this classification. Acid detergents operate in the pH range substantially below 7.0. The acid properties are usually obtained through the incorporation of a mild organic acid or phosphoric acid in the formulation to which is added an effective wetting agent. The acid detergents exhibit low-sudsing properties. They are useful for the removal of certain types of soil, such as "milkstone" from dairy equipment.

SANITIZATION OF DISHES

Wherever possible, equipment designed specifically for the washing of dishes should be used. When an efficient detergent is employed in an approved type dishwashing machine, followed by a hot water rinse, the dishes are rendered clean and the bacterial count is reduced to a safe level. The detergent solution in the washer should be in the range of pH 10-11 and at a temperature of 140°-145° F. (60°-63° C.). For rinsing, the water should

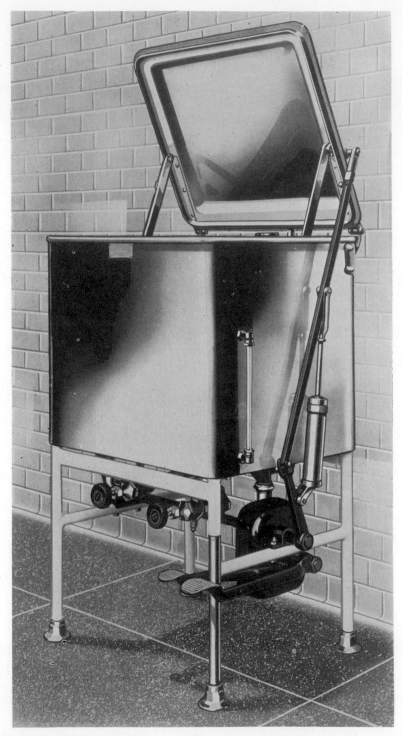

Fig. 116. Typical steam heated utensil boiler, with cover raised. Similar units heated by electricity or gas are in common use.

be maintained at a minimum temperature of 170° F. (77° C.) for 2 minutes or 212° F. (100° C.) for 30 seconds.

In the event that proper equipment is not available, the utensil boiler shown in Figure 116 may be used for sanitization or terminal disinfection of dishes. Residual particles of food must be removed from the dishes before placing them in the boiler. Plates and saucers should be stacked on edge in the tray or basket, and cups or other deep dishes should rest on their sides so that water will drain from them. All articles must be submerged in the water. A sufficient amount of low-foaming detergent is then added and the dishes are boiled for 15 minutes.

THE INDIVIDUAL PATIENT'S UTENSILS

There are various procedures in use today for the handling of the individual patient's utensils consisting of wash basin, emesis basin, mouth cup, etc. In a few hospitals these supplies are delivered to the central service department for washing, wrapping and sterilization by steam under pressure. This procedure has been criticized on the grounds that supplies of this type used by the general hospital patient do not require sterilization for safety. Also, it is difficult to maintain control over the procedure because of failures on the part of floor personnel to arrange for delivery of the utensils to central service. In other institutions adequate facilities are available for steam sterilization of the utensils in utility rooms. In many institutions it is common practice that the individual patient's utensils are not subjected to any form of sterilization following the routine washing process.

It must be acknowledged that each new patient admitted to the hospital is entitled to a freshly sanitized kit of utensils. This does not necessarily mean that the articles be subjected to a surgical sterilization process, although in certain instances autoclaving may prove to be the most convenient method. If the utensils have been thoroughly cleaned with hot water and detergent and then subjected to boiling or steaming, there is every reason to believe that the degree of sanitization is at least the equivalent of the dishes and eating utensils furnished on the food tray. Unfortunately there are few, if any, utility rooms equipped with a utensil washer-sanitizer suited for this application. The ordinary utensil boiler (Fig. 116) is largely unsatisfactory for the operation because of hard water conditions in many hospitals and the lack of a convenient hot water rinse following the boiling process. Until such time as more appropriate equipment becomes available, the recommended procedure for handling the individual patient's utensils is as follows:

When the patient leaves the hospital room, the various utensils are collected and washed with hot water and detergent in the clean-up unit of the utility room. After drying and inspection the utensils are wrapped in a double thickness muslin cover. The packaged kit is then sterilized in the autoclave at 250° F. for 15 minutes, followed by 15 minutes drying. The kit is then removed from the sterilizer, placed in clean storage in the utility room or transferred to the bedside table in the patient's room. If a pressure utility sterilizer is not available on the floor, then the utensil boiler will have to be used, but the utensils must not be wrapped. Following sanitization by boiling for 15 minutes, the utensils should be dried, wrapped in cloth or paper and then placed in storage.

DISINFECTION OF BEDPANS AND URINALS

The objective in the handling of bedpans and urinals is to dispose of the excreta under the most sanitary and least offensive conditions, and at the same time to disinfect the utensils insofar as the communicable disease organisms are concerned. Hospital personnel are well acquainted with apparatus known to the trade as "Bedpan Washers and Sterilizers." To designate such equipment as a "sterilizer" is incorrect because in normal usage no attempt is made to sterilize the utensil nor is the process capable of sterilization in the strict sense of the word. Unfortunately the term has been firmly established in the minds of hospital people as well as the manufacturers of the equipment and that name will undoubtedly continue to be used.

Modern apparatus for washing and disinfecting bedpans has been vastly improved in recent years to facilitate the completion of this most offensive duty the nurse must perform. With the automatic unit shown in Figures 117 and 118, the nurse brings the soiled pan or urinal to the fixture, presses the foot pedal to open the cover, inserts the utensil within the flexible arms and removes her foot from the pedal. The cover closes automatically and at the same time the utensil is emptied. She then touches the push-button with her forearm and this starts an uninterrupted cycle of washing and steaming. The first action is that of a cold water wash with inside and outside flushing of the utensil as well as complete flushing of the chamber. The scrubbing action of the jet stream of water is enhanced through air entrainment. After washing with cold water for ½ minute, the unit automatically shuts off the water supply and instantly admits live steam to the chamber for 1 minute. A bleeder trap is connected to the steam supply line which constantly bleeds condensate from the line, thereby assuring exposure to live steam throughout the disinfection period. The pilot light remains on during the entire cycle, warning a second operator that the fixture is in use and the door should not be opened until the cycle is completed. In a fixture of this type, steam is liberated direct from the supply line at close range against the surfaces of the utensils. The utensil heats rapidly because of its fixed proximity to the source of steam. Under these conditions a short exposure period of 1 minute is permissible for disinfection as evidenced by the following tests:

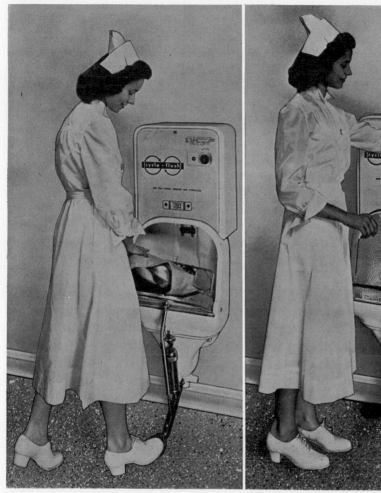
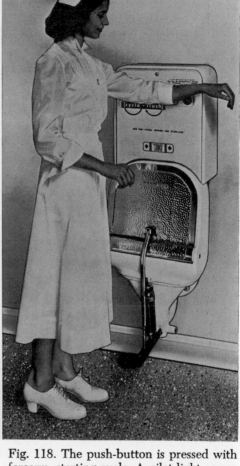

Fig. 117. Automatic bedpan washer-disinfector. The depressed foot pedal opens door and spreads locking clamps to receive bedpan or urinal.

Fig. 118. The push-button is pressed with forearm, starting cycle. A pilot light comes on and the attendant is then free to leave the unit if she so desires, returning later to remove the cleaned and disinfected bedpan or urinal.

Organisms: Micrococcus aureus and *Escherichia coli.*

Pans Inoculated: Ordinary white enamel bedpans were selected from the stock in routine use at a local hospital.

Site of Inoculation: Points of inoculation were selected that were underneath the lip of the pan in concealed locations, and in three of the tests roughened areas where the enamel was chipped off were used as inoculation sites.

Media Employed for Subculture: Plain bouillon and blood agar plates.

Exposure Time: Thirty, sixty and ninety seconds.

Tests Were Conducted as Follows: The bedpans were first sterilized by steam under pressure to free them of any spore-bearing bacteria. Different areas on the surfaces of the pans were then inoculated from fresh cultures of *Micrococcus aureus* and *Escherichia coli.* The pans were then placed in the Aeroflush fixture and flowing steam admitted for the required period. (The cold water wash was eliminated in the test series.) At the end of the steaming period the door was opened, the pans removed, and subcultures were made from the inoculated areas into the plain bouillon and on blood agar plates and these cultures were incubated for 24 hours at 37° C.

Results:

Exposure Time	Micrococcus aureus	Escherichia coli
30 seconds	Sterile	Sterile
60 seconds	Sterile	Sterile
90 seconds	Sterile	Sterile

The above tests were repeated on six different occasions, and in each case the subcultures were found sterile.

BEDPANS CONTAINING OIL

Pans containing stools from oil enema patients cannot be properly cleansed by this or any other similar washing and steaming process. The excreta will be flushed out but residual oil globules will remain in the pan. Placing paper in the bottom of the pan before use will reduce the difficulty of cleaning, but nurses are prone to forget this detail. Oily pans can only be rendered clean by use of a toilet brush and detergent. In some hospitals the brush is suspended close to the bedpan cleaning fixture and the detergent is kept on a shelf nearby. The nurse can hold the cover open with the foot pedal in position to cleanse the pan and so apply the brush and detergent. But this is an awkward procedure and proper cleaning occurs only now and then with unusually painstaking personnel. It is considered better practice to provide a clinical sink close to the bedpan washer that is used largely for this one purpose, as in Figure 119. Then when an oily pan is encountered it is taken immediately from the bedpan washer to the sink, scoured with brush and detergent, and returned to the fixture for a second cycle which renders it clean and disinfected.

ALTERNATE METHODS OF HANDLING BEDPANS AND URINALS

The procedure described above is the one most practical for any institution where steam is available for heating. Modern planning does not make provision for the installation of bedpan washing and disinfecting equipment within the utility room, unless the room is divided into soiled and clean work areas. The ideal arrangement makes provision for a sub-utility room or bedpan closet to serve each nursing unit of approximately 25 patient beds, distributed as ⅓ private room beds with toilet facilities, ⅓ semi-private room beds, and ⅓ ward beds. A typical layout for a sub-utility room is shown in Figure 120. Experience dictates that one bedpan washer-

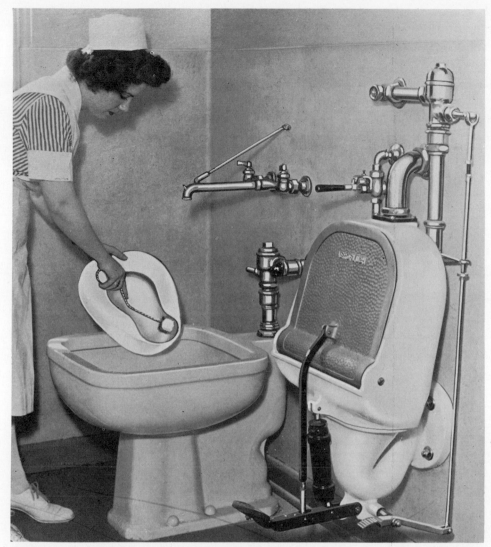

Fig. 119. The installation of a clinical sink adjacent to the bedpan washer-disinfector will be found useful, especially for the manual cleaning of bedpans with brush and detergent.

disinfector will serve about 15 patients adequately and this figure is used as a guide in the arrangement of utility rooms in new construction. In private or semi-private rooms where toilet facilities are available, the toilet should be equipped with a modern bedpan flushing attachment, as in Figure 121. The bedpan is cleaned here and retained until the patient leaves. Then it is taken to the washer-disinfector located in the sub-utility room on the floor and disinfected prior to use by the next patient. This method saves time and undesirable traffic through the corridors.

For the smaller hospitals where steam is not available for flushing of bedpans, an alternate method must be used. This requires a combination apparatus consisting of a bedpan washer, without the steaming attachment, and an electrically heated utensil boiler or steamer mounted close by, as in Figure 122. The utensil steamer contains a removable rack which holds five bedpans and a wall support is usually provided near by to accom-

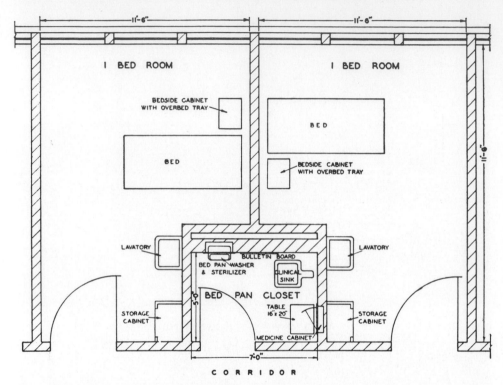

Fig. 120. Typical layout for a sub-utility room or bedpan closet to serve each nursing unit of approximately 25 patient beds.

modate two of these racks, one above the other. This is the way such apparatus is intended to be used:

The nurse disposes of the excreta in the bedpan washer and flushes the pan with cold water. If the pan is soiled with oil she scrubs it out as explained above and flushes it again in the fixture. Then she transfers the pan to the utensil steamer for disinfection. (It is assumed that the nurse who puts the fifth pan in the steamer will turn on the heat, electricity or gas, and stay with the apparatus until the pans are disinfected.) Then she removes the carrier of five pans to the wall support and returns an empty carrier from the wall support to the boiler or steamer, ready for the reception of the next pans to arrive. Maintaining this necessary technique becomes something of a problem in floor control. Nurses often forget to carry

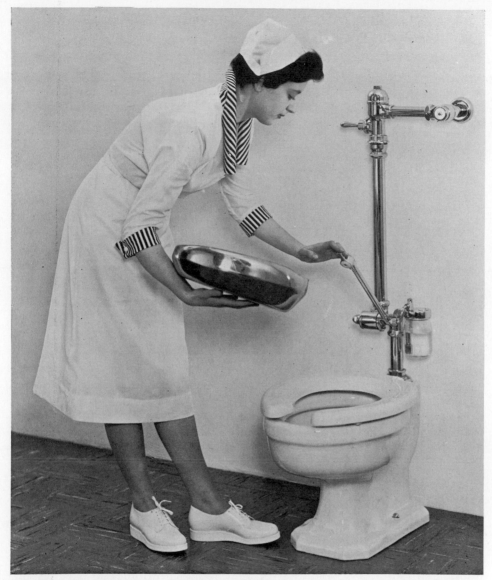

Fig. 121. The installation of a Diverter Valve with movable spray arm above the toilet, as shown, provides a convenient and effective method for flushing and rinsing bedpans.

through the disinfecting process when the carrier has been filled. Then the next nurse who arrives with a pan finds herself in an embarrassing position. She has no place to put the washed pan, must place it on something while she disinfects the loaded carrier to make room for her own pan. That sort of thing can be controlled only by rigid supervision, but it should be controlled so that the entire cycle of handling pans becomes strict routine.

ROUTINE CARE OF BEDPAN WASHER

The type of bedpan washer-disinfector shown in Figures 117 and 119 incorporates certain features of design which have done much to eliminate the serious objections inherent in earlier designs. One highly important feature is the loose fitting cover which serves a two-fold purpose. The cover

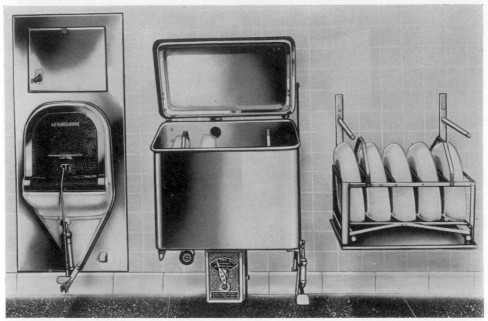

Fig. 122. A combination of bedpan washer, electrically heated utensil steamer, and a typical wall support for two five-pan racks. This kind of assembly is suitable for smaller hospitals where direct steam is not available.

is baffled on the inside so that in normal usage there is no leakage of water. The loose fitting design of cover also serves as an overflow so that pollution can rise in the chamber, under adverse conditions, not appreciably higher than the bottom of the cover. Similarly the loose fitting cover serves to admit room air to the chamber for continuous aeration. The effect is that of a chimney on any fuel consuming stove or furnace. Room air enters, entrains with odors or vapor and passes up the vent stack. Lacking the loose fitting cover or its equivalent opening for air intake, odors are trapped in the chamber offensively.

The bedpan washer-disinfector needs occasional cleaning with a toilet brush just as ordinary toilet bowls are cleaned. The white porcelain enamel finish of the hopper serves a useful purpose in making immediately apparent any soiled surfaces. Obviously the soiled surfaces can only be seen when the cover is opened, but it is a matter of good housekeeping as well

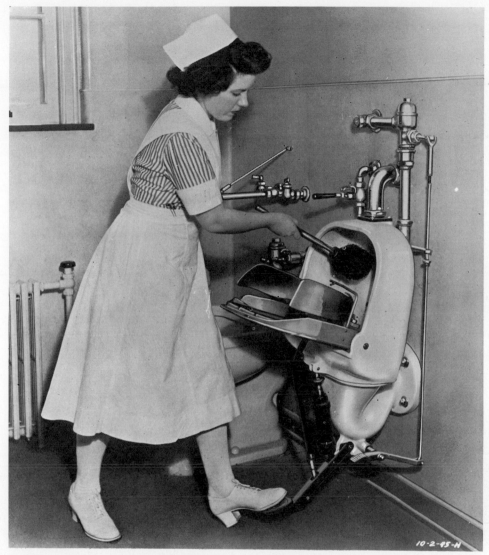

Fig. 123. The interior of any bedpan washer-disinfector becomes soiled, just as any toilet bowl does at times, and it requires the same kind of cleaning.

as sanitation, to frequently scrub the interior of the washer (Fig. 123). It is no mark of commendation, for the otherwise well managed hospital, to find bedpan washers that have never been cleaned out since installation. Strict floor supervision can surely govern the cleaning of this equipment as frequently and as thoroughly as toilets are cleaned.

In former years attempts were made to build apparatus in which the contents of bedpans and urinals could be disinfected before releasing into the sewage system. Needless to say, the equipment never proved satisfactory and sanitary protective features were largely ignored. Today the need for such equipment has been largely done away with as the result of the modern city sewage disposal plant. When it is necessary to actually disinfect feces or urine, a dependable method is to mix 1 part of compound cresol solution with each 10 parts of fecal material and allow to stand for 30 minutes.

REFERENCES

1. *The Control of Communicable Diseases in Man.* American Public Health Association. 7th Ed., 1950, p. 11.
2. Editorial: *M. Times,* New York, 79:443, July, 1951.
3. Lenard, A.: Poliomyelitis—The Possibility of Syringe Transmission. *M. Times,* New York, 79:395-399, July, 1951.
4. Mundel, O.: *Zeitschrift Hyg. u. Infektionskr., 120:*267, 1937. From *Principles of Bacteriology and Immunity,* 3rd ed., Vol. 1, by Topley and Wilson, Baltimore, Williams & Wilkins, 1946, p. 114.
5. Ecker, E. E., and Smith, R.: Sterilizing Surgical Instruments and Utensils. *Mod. Hosp., 48:*92, March, 1937.

CHAPTER XIII

Chemical Disinfection

THE NEED FOR safe and effective chemical disinfectants is of great practical importance to the hospital. They are required for the destruction of organisms present on delicate instruments and supplies which cannot be rendered sterile by other means due to their heat-sensitive characteristics. Efficient surgical antiseptics are also required to assist in the degermation of the hands and arms of the surgeon as well as the skin of the patient at the operative site. General utility disinfectants are likewise essential for institutional use in order to minimize the infection hazards from enteric, respiratory and other pathogens present on floors, walls and furniture.

DEFINITIONS

Disinfection: By definition this is any process, chemical or physical, by means of which pathogenic agents or disease-producing microbes are destroyed. It is essentially a process which will destroy the infectious agents, usually the communicable disease organisms, but not necessarily exacting to kill resistant bacterial spores. The more common disinfecting agents are chemicals, boiling water, flowing steam and ultraviolet radiation. As ordinarily employed, the disinfection process may or may not be adequate for the destruction of tubercle bacilli and for the inactivation of viruses. Disinfectants should be used on inanimate objects only. They should not be confused with the use of antiseptics as applied to the body.[1]

Sterilization: Sterilization may be defined as any process by means of which all forms of microbial life (bacteria, spores, fungi and viruses), contained in liquids, on instruments and utensils or within various substances, are completely destroyed. The word "sterile" denotes the complete freedom from or absence of all living microbes and other forms of life. In the strict sense of definition, "sterile" is an absolute term, but the word is subject to common misusage and misinterpretation by both laymen and professional people. The Council on Pharmacy and Chemistry of the American Medical Association[2] has reported on this subject as follows:

> "The Council on Pharmacy and Chemistry has formally gone on record as disapproving of the use of the terms 'sterile,' 'sterilize' and 'sterilization' in a bacteriologic sense other than in their correct scientific significance; i.e., meaning the absence or destruction of all microorganisms. These terms are not relative and to permit their use in a relative sense not only is incorrect but opens the way to abuse and misunderstanding."

Germicide: A germicide is anything that will destroy germs or microbes. Common usage involves the application of chemical agents to kill disease-producing germs, but not necessarily resistant bacterial spores. Germicides are usually employed in solution form for application to living tissue as well as inanimate objects. Other commonly used terms with similar definitions are bactericide, fungicide, virucide and sporicide.

Antiseptic: Antiseptics are substances which, when applied to microorganisms, will render them innocuous either by killing them or preventing their growth, according to the character of the preparation or the method of application.[3] They are preparations made especially for application to living tissue. If the substance is of such a nature or is used in such a way as to only prevent the growth of bacteria it may be classed as a bacteriostatic agent.

CAUSE OF DISINFECTION

The destructive processes which lead to the death of bacterial cells when in contact with a chemical disinfectant have not been satisfactorily explained. Depending upon the type of disinfectant used, certain reactions occur such as oxidation when chlorine and related compounds are used; hydrolysis in the case of acids, alkalies and hot water, and coagulation of proteins in the cell probably occurs when all potent disinfectants are employed. The relationship of chemical constitution or structure to disinfecting action is likewise imperfectly understood at the present time. It is known, however, that chemical composition does not solely account for germicidal activity. Other properties associated with the disinfectant, such as solubility, ionization and surface tension, have a marked effect upon the germicidal power. Perhaps it will suffice to say that in the disinfection process the bacterial cell is poisoned by the chemical agent. To bring this about, it is necessary to assure intimate contact of the disinfectant with the bacterial cell so that the chemical agent can be absorbed and thereby permitted to act upon the vital constituents of the cell.

FACTORS WHICH INFLUENCE DISINFECTANT ACTION

There are several factors which influence the action of a disinfectant and ultimately determine its efficiency to destroy microorganisms under practical conditions. Those of primary importance are:

1) *Cleanliness of the Surface:* Inadequate cleaning of the surface to be disinfected prevents intimate contact of the disinfectant with the bacterial cell. The presence of blood, pus, oil or grease interferes with the action of all germicides. The first requirement is absolute cleanliness of the surface.

2) *Concentration:* A weak solution is usually not as effective as a strong solution of the same disinfectant. One exception is ethyl alcohol, where 70-80% aqueous solutions are more germicidal than absolute alcohol. Where tissue irritation is not involved strong solutions can be used. The phenol coefficient should be not less than five, and the use-dilution for general

disinfecting purposes must be germicidal under the conditions of the "A.O.A.C. Use-Dilution Confirmation Test."[4]

3) *Time:* When bacteria are exposed to a disinfectant they are not destroyed instantly. Death follows an orderly process in which time and concentration are interdependent. The time required for disinfection may vary from seconds to hours.

4) *Temperature:* The rate of disinfection is accelerated with an increase in temperature. Since most disinfectants are applied at room temperature or body temperature this is relatively unimportant, except when a chemical agent is added to hot or boiling water to increase the germicidal efficiency.

5) *Type of Organism:* Some organisms are more readily killed than others. The *Pseudomonas* group are particularly resistant to the action of disinfectants, also the tubercle bacillus. Bacterial spores and certain viruses show maximum resistance to chemical agents. It is doubtful if any disinfectant suitable for routine use can be depended upon to destroy the virus of serum hepatitis. A good general disinfectant should be capable of destroying the following microorganisms in 10 minutes at room temperature:[5]

Mycobacterium tuberculosis	*Streptococcus pyogenes* var. *hemolyticus*
Shigella paradysenteriae	*Diplococcus pneumoniae*
Escherichia coli	*Corynebacterium diphtheriae*
Pseudomonas aeruginosa	*Candida albicans*

6) *Presence of Organic Matter:* The action of most disinfectants is markedly decreased and often nullified in the presence of organic wastes. Blood, pus, feces, wound debris, mucus and other heavy secretions are the common offenders. The disinfectant should retain at least 50% of its germicidal power in the presence of standard organic matter (10% horse serum) when tested by the official phenol coefficient method.

PROPERTIES OF DISINFECTANTS

Alcohols: Ethyl alcohol is widely used as a skin antiseptic. It possesses valuable wetting properties and is a fairly good fat solvent. The optimal germicidal concentration is usually given as 70 per cent by weight (81 per cent by volume), although Morton's[6] findings indicate that it has a high degree of germicidal activity in the range of 50 to 95 per cent. When properly used it will destroy vegetative organisms but is ineffective against spores. Because of its protein-coagulating action instruments must be thoroughly cleansed before contact. Its usefulness as a disinfectant for articles contaminated with acid-fast organisms—tubercle bacilli has not been well defined. Isopropyl alcohol is rapidly displacing ethyl alcohol for many uses. It exhibits slightly greater germicidal action, is a better fat solvent and has a lower surface tension. In a 50 per cent solution it is an effective germicide against non-sporulating bacteria. The degerming action is optimal when solutions of 70 per cent (by weight) and stronger are used. Price[7] has stated that "isopropyl alcohol might well be substituted for ethyl alcohol to prepare the skin of the field of operation, but it is not recommended for repeated washing of operator's hands."

Phenols and Cresols: Phenol is an extremely toxic compound and highly destructive to tissues. In germicidal concentrations it is irritant and produces local anesthesia when applied to a skin surface. When added to soap or soap solutions it has little germicidal action. It is not effective against spores. As a practical disinfectant, its use is limited. It has a high temperature coefficient, i.e., hot solutions are more effective disinfectants than cold solutions. For this reason, phenol is occasionally added to boiling water in a 2% concentration for the disinfection of contaminated instruments following a septic case. Other disinfectants, such as "Amphyl" or "O-syl" are better suited to this application. "Lysol" also is a caustic substance and not safe for application to the skin. It is widely used as a general utility disinfectant for floors and walls, although the odor is objectionable to many people.

Cresols are more valuable than phenols as practical disinfectants. The compound cresol preparations, such as Liquor Cresolis Saponatus, retain their germicidal powers in the presence of organic matter, including sputum and feces. The cresols will destroy vegetative organisms in dilutions of 1:100 to 1:300, but they are not effective against spores. They are probably the disinfectants of choice against acid-fast bacteria—*M. tuberculosis.* The virucidal powers of the cresols have not been well established. The newer synthetic phenolic disinfectants known as "O-syl" and "Amphyl" apparently display a residual antibacterial effect on disinfected surfaces[8] which should enhance their value as general utility disinfectants.

Hexachlorophene (G-11) is a phenolic derivative, currently popular as a surgical scrub. It is virtually insoluble in water, but soluble in alcohol, acetone and dilute alkali. It retains its antibacterial potency in the presence of soap. Gump[9] has stated that G-11 is a safe and harmless chemical. It is claimed that the synthetic detergent vehicle "pHisoderm" fortified with G-11 is more effective than any detergent commonly employed for the preoperative preparation of the skin.

Chlorine Compounds: The hypochlorites (sodium and calcium) are the most useful of chlorine containing compounds for practical disinfection in the hospital. Their germicidal power is dependent upon the release of free hypochlorous acid. Dakin's solution contains 0.45 to 0.50% sodium hypochlorite. Chlorinated lime contains 30 to 35% calcium hypochlorite. Commercial laundry bleaches, such as "Clorox," are solutions of sodium hypochlorite. The equivalent U.S.P. solution contains about 5% sodium hypochlorite. When diluted 1:1000 these solutions are useful for disinfection of bedpans, urinals, toilets and floors. They should not be used for disinfection of metal instruments or articles made of rubber. All hypochlorites deteriorate upon aging, either in solution or powder form. Their germicidal efficiency is reduced in the presence of organic matter.

Iodine: Iodine in tincture form is the traditional agent for preoperative skin disinfection. One or two per cent iodine dissolved in 70% alcohol is an excellent skin antiseptic. In the usual concentrations iodine displays high bactericidal efficiency and low tissue toxicity. It may be irritating to tissues and it stains badly. Two per cent aqueous iodine has been reported to be sporicidal.[10] It has been recommended as an "emergency sterilizing agent"[11] for surgical instruments, including knife blades, plastics and rubber goods. An iodine solution of 0.5 to 1 per cent in 70% alcohol is the agent of choice for disinfection of clinical thermometers. A new iodophor disinfectant ("Wescodyne") has been reported[12] to be a general purpose disinfectant, effective against viruses, fungi and bacteria, including *M. tuberculosis*.

Formaldehyde: Formaldehyde is a gas, highly soluble in water. The U.S.P. solution (Liquor Formaldehydi) contains 37% (by weight) of the gas in water. A 5 per cent solution is actively germicidal and sporicidal in the presence of moderate amounts of organic matter.[13] Formaldehyde also possesses a powerful deodorant action. It is irritating to tissues and any instrument disinfected with it must be thoroughly rinsed in sterile water before use. Because of its sporicidal activity it is probably the most reliable chemical agent for instrument disinfection. Low temperatures reduce its germicidal power. It should be used at room temperature or above.

Quaternary Ammonium Compounds: Typical of this class of germicides are "Zephiran," "Phemerol" and "Ceepryn." They are surface-active compounds and possess the useful property of lowering the surface tension of solutions. They are highly stable and non-irritating when used in recommended concentrations. They are incompatible with soap, but retain their activity reasonably well in the presence of protein. Their value as tuberculocides and virucides has not been clearly established. They cannot be depended upon to destroy spores. For instrument disinfection, the usual concentration is 1:1000 aqueous solution to which 0.5 per cent sodium nitrite is added to minimize corrosion.

CHEMICAL DISINFECTION OF INSTRUMENTS

The process of chemical disinfection of instruments is often referred to as "cold sterilization." This is confusing terminology because many of the chemical agents employed are not capable of destroying all forms of microbial life. Indeed the great majority of instrument germicides cannot be depended upon to kill the tubercle bacillus. Yet according to the strict definition of disinfection the process must destroy pathogenic or disease-producing organisms. The ideal chemical disinfectant would rapidly kill any organisms (spores, tubercle bacilli and viruses) remaining on an instrument after cleaning. It would retain a high percentage of its activity in the presence of organic matter; leave no toxic or irritating residue on the instrument; be non-corrosive and of low cost.[13] Obviously such a disinfectant has never been found. The use of chemical disinfectants should be limited to those instruments which cannot be sterilized by heat.

Cutting Edge Instruments: When facilities are not available for dry heat sterilization of delicate, sharp instruments, they may be disinfected by complete immersion for 18 hours in one of the following solutions:

> The instruments must be thoroughly cleaned beforehand to remove all blood, pus, oil and grease.
>
> I. BORAX-FORMALDEHYDE SOLUTION—
>
> Sodium tetraborate .... 50.0 gm.
> Formaldehyde solution, U.S.P. .... 100.0 ml.
> Distilled water, to ....1000.0 ml.
>
> II. BENZALKONIUM-FORMALDEHYDE SOLUTION—[14]
>
> Isopropanol, 99% .... 900.0 ml.
> Methanol (technical) .... 72.0 ml.
> Formaldehyde, 37% .... 144.0 ml.
> Zephiran concentrate, 12.8% .... 14.4 ml.
> Sodium nitrite .... 18.0 gm.
> Distilled water, to make ....1800.0 ml.

Following disinfection the instruments must be thoroughly rinsed with sterile water before use. The commercially available product known as "Bard-Parker Germicide" may be substituted for either of the above solutions. It is claimed that this product will destroy spores in 3 hours exposure, resulting in a much shorter disinfecting time.

Telescopic Instruments (Cystoscopes, Thorascopes): With the exception of the Kirwin Cystoscope, these instruments cannot be sterilized by heat. Alkaline germicides will attack the surface of the lenses and the solvent action of others may loosen the cement in which the lenses are set. Disinfection can best be accomplished by soaking in "Urolicide" solution for 30 minutes.

For the terminal disinfection of bronchoscopes and laryngoscopes it is recommended that they be soaked in 1:1000 solution of calcium hypochlorite (chlorinated lime) for 30 minutes. Following disinfection they should be rinsed in tap water and dried.

Clinical Thermometers: The method selected for the disinfection of thermometers should be effective against *M. tuberculosis.* According to Frobisher and Sommermeyer,[15] effective disinfection may be accomplished by wiping the thermometers thoroughly with cotton wet with a solution of equal parts of 95% ethyl alcohol and tincture of green soap; then immerse them for 10 minutes in a 1.0% solution of iodine in 70% (by volume) isopropyl alcohol.

Rubber and Plastic Goods: The many different synthetic materials entering into the manufacture of rubber and plastic items make it difficult to select an all-purpose agent for disinfection. In certain cases, such as for rubber sheeting, soaking in alkaline formaldehyde solution is considered satisfactory. The use of iodine solutions in strengths of 0.5 to 2 per cent may be useful. For clean plastic tubing, where spores are not a problem, soaking in 70 per cent ethyl alcohol may also be efficacious. Gum elastic catheters are best disinfected in an aqueous formaldehyde solution, after which they should be thoroughly rinsed with sterile water.

REFERENCES

1. REDDISH, G. F.: *Antiseptics, Disinfectants, Fungicides and Sterilization.* Philadelphia, Lea & Febiger, 1954, p. 25.
2. American Medical Association: Report of the Council on Pharmacy and Chemistry. Use of the Terms "Sterile," "Sterilize," and "Sterilization." *J.A.M.A., 107:*38, 1936.
3. REDDISH, G. F.: Antiseptic. *J. Am. Pharm. A., 16:*501-502, 1927.
4. Association of Official Agricultural Chemists: *Official Methods of Analysis,* 7th Ed., Wash., D.C., 1950, pp. 88-92.
5. KLARMANN, E. G.: Modern Disinfectants. *Modern Sanitation, 6:*15, Dec., 1954.
6. MORTON, H. E.: Relationship of Concentration and Germicidal Efficiency of Ethyl Alcohol. *Ann. New York Acad. Sc., 53:*191-196, 1950.
7. PRICE, P. B.: Surgical Antiseptics. From REDDISH, G. F.: *Antiseptics, Disinfectants, Fungicides and Sterilization.* Philadelphia, Lea & Febiger, 1954, p. 329.
8. KLARMANN, E. G., WRIGHT, E. S., AND SHTERNOV, V. A.: Prolongation of the Antibacterial Potential of Disinfected Surfaces. *Applied Microbiol., 1:*19-23, 1953.
9. GUMP, W.: *The Development of a Germicidal Soap.* Givaudan-Delawanna, Inc. 1945.
10. GERSHENFELD, L., AND WITLIN, B.: Iodine Solution as a Sporicidal Agent. *J. Am. Pharm. A., XLI:*451-452, 1952.
11. GERSHENFELD, L.: Iodine. From REDDISH, G. F.: *Antiseptics, Disinfectants, Fungicides and Sterilization.* Philadelphia, Lea & Febiger, 1954, p. 187.
12. BOGASH, R. C.: A New Iodophor Disinfectant. *Bull. Am. Soc. Hosp. Pharm., 12:*135-136, 1955.
13. SPAULDING, E. H.: Chemical Disinfection of Surgical Instruments. From REDDISH, G. F.: *Antiseptics, Disinfectants, Fungicides and Sterilization.* Philadelphia, Lea & Febiger, 1954, p. 525-547.
14. LAWRENCE, C. A.: A Survey and Evaluation of Germicides. *Bull. Am. Soc. Hosp. Pharm., 7:*308-313, 1950.
15. FROBISHER, M., JR., SOMMERMEYER, L., AND BLACKWELL, M. J.: Studies on Disinfection of Clinical Thermometers. *Applied Microbiol., 1:*187-194, 1953.

CHAPTER XIV

Terminal Sterilization of Instruments and Supplies Following Septic Cases

T HE NEED FOR a reliable, rapid and simple procedure for cleaning up after a septic case is apparent to all operating room personnel. In those hospitals where adequate sterilizing facilities exist in the sub-sterilizing rooms the procedure can be relatively simple, but for the institutions with one autoclave only in the operating suite, or for those equipped with non-pressure (boiling type) instrument sterilizers, the procedure becomes more difficult and proportionately less efficient. It is believed that the following technic can be adapted to the needs of most hospitals, with alternates provided to accommodate the use of sub-standard sterilizing facilities wherever they may exist:

PROCEDURE—"A"

Adapted to hospitals with adequate sterilizing facilities serving each pair of operating rooms. The equipment to consist of—

Pressure Instrument Washer-Sterilizer, with trays.

High Speed Pressure Instrument Sterilizer, 16″ x 24″, or 12″ x 16″ x 24″, with trays.

Supplies Required

Laundry bags, mesh type

Laundry bags, canvas—outer protectors

Cleaning cloths (washed gauze)

Waterproof paper bags

Waterproof paper

Needle box, perforated

Instrument tray, with cover

Instrument trays, for use in instrument washer

Suture jar, with germicide

Container for germicide

Trisodium phosphate

Germicides Required

1) For disinfection of non-expendable items such as catheters, bougies, etc.—

"Zephiran" or "Urolicide," 1:1000 aqueous solution. Exposure period: minimum of 30 minutes.

2) For disinfection of furniture—

220

"Roccal," 1:2500 aqueous solution, to which should be added 0.5% sodium nitrite as an anti-corrosive agent. Apply by scrubbing and allow to dry on surfaces.

3) If the contaminated case involves *Mycobacterium tuberculosis*, then it is recommended that "Amphyl" or "O-syl," 2% aqueous solution, be substituted for the above germicides.

4) For disinfection of unused suture tubes, ampoules, etc. Immerse in the following solution with exposure period of 18 hours:

Isopropyl alcohol, 99%	700 ml.
Formaldehyde, USP, 37%	25 ml.
Sodium bicarbonate	1.0 gm.
Sodium nitrite	1.0 gm.
Distilled water, to	1000 ml.

TECHNIC

Gloves: At the end of the operation, each member of the surgical team rinses off outside of gloves in splash basin. With the exception of the scrubbed nurse or scrubbed assistant, all gloves are removed and placed in the basin. (The feasibility of attempting to salvage contaminated gloves is a moot question. Some hospitals prefer to destroy them.)

Gowns: With the help of the circulating nurse or assistant gowns are removed from all members of the team except the scrubbed nurse or scrubbed assistant and transferred to the laundry bag, designated later as "contaminated."

Drapes and Towels: All contaminated linen from the operating field and table is collected by the scrubbed nurse and transferred to the laundry bag containing the gowns. The wet portions of linen should be rolled inwardly with the dry areas on the outside—forming a protective cover.

Instruments: The surgical instruments are collected, opened and placed in the instrument-washer tray located on the instrument table. The needles are placed in separate needle box which, in turn, is placed in instrument-washer tray.

Suture Tubes: The unused suture tubes and ampoules are immersed in the jar containing formaldehyde germicide.

Catheters and Tubing: These articles are placed in instrument pan containing appropriate germicide, making sure that all surfaces are submerged and that the solution is in contact with the lumen of the tubing.

Disposable Items: Soiled sponges, broken suture tubes, cut sutures, torn gloves, knife blades and other disposable items are collected and placed in waterproof bag. This bag is later delivered to the incinerator for burning.

Suction Bottle: The rubber tubing and stopper are removed from the suction bottle and placed on top of the instruments in the instrument-washer tray. The contents of the bottle are emptied into the hopper located in the sub-sterilizing room. The bottle is then washed with trisodium phosphate solution. (If the instrument washer-sterilizer will accommodate the suction bottle, it may be placed directly on top of the instruments in the tray, with no washing beforehand.)

Utensils: The gloves are removed from the splash basin, drained briefly, and placed in a second tray furnished with the instrument washer-sterilizer. The contents of the glove basin and other utensils are emptied into the kick bucket. The kick bucket is then emptied into the hopper, followed by washing with germicide. (If the pressure instrument sterilizer will accommodate the kick bucket, it may also be sterilized directly by pressure steam.)

Sterilization: The basins and utensils, including the suction bottle, are transferred by the scrubbed assistant to the pressure instrument sterilizer for sterilization by the circulating nurse at 270° F. (132° C.) for 3 minutes. Care should be used to place the basins on edge in the chamber and the bottle in a horizontal position so as to avoid trapping air. The trays of instruments and gloves are then transferred to the instrument washer by the scrubbed assistant.

Furniture: The nurse's instrument table is the last to be stripped. Drapes are removed and placed in the laundry bag. Germicide is applied to all contaminated surfaces of furniture, including the operating table, nurse's table, basin stands, Mayo stand, sponge rack, etc. It is best applied by saturating an absorbent cloth or gauze and then scrubbing the contaminated area. The germicide should be permitted to dry on the surface. Spots of blood or pus on the floor should be removed promptly and in the same manner before drying takes place. It is not considered necessary to wash down the walls of the operating room unless those surfaces are known to be contaminated. The floor should be mopped after each operation with an effective detergent-disinfectant.

Contaminated Linen: At the close of the clean-up the nurse's gown is removed and placed in the laundry bag containing other contaminated linens. The bag is tightly closed and transferred to a second bag made of canvas, as an outer protector. The outer bag should be plainly marked "contaminated" and then sent to the laundry. The nurse or assistant finally removes her gloves and places them in the tray of the instrument washer. Detergent is then added and the load processed according to the operating instructions.

It is no longer considered necessary to quarantine the operating room for 24 or 48 hours after a septic case. This will contribute little, if anything, to the efficiency of the decontamination process.

PROCEDURE—"B"

Adapted to hospitals with limited sterilizing facilities serving each pair of operating rooms or the entire surgical suite. The equipment to consist of—

A Dressing Sterilizer, 16″ x 24″ or 20″ x 36″ and/or

A Pressure Instrument Sterilizer, 16″ x 24″, equipped with a deep, watertight tray.

Supplies Required: In addition to the supplies listed under "Procedure A," a deep container is required, similar to an arm soak basin, unless a pressure sterilizer is available and equipped with a deep, watertight tray for holding instruments. A supply of trisodium phosphate is also needed.

Germicides Required: Same as for "Procedure A."

Technic: All steps in the handling of materials and supplies are the same as for "Procedure A," except that the instruments, gloves and tubing must be collected in the deep watertight tray, covered with water containing two tablespoonfuls of trisodium phosphate per gallon, and autoclaved for 45 minutes at 250° F. (121° C.). Caution must be exercised in removing this tray from the sterilizer to avoid scalding. The basins and suction bottle should be carefully washed with trisodium phosphate solution, placed in the autoclave and sterilized at 250° F. for 15 minutes.

PROCEDURE—"C"

Adapted to hospitals with sub-standard sterilizing facilities. The equipment to consist of—

One or more instrument boilers

One or more utensil boilers

Supplies Required: Same as for "Procedure A."

Germicides Required: Same as for "Procedure A."

Technic: All steps in the handling of materials and supplies are the same as for "Procedure A," except that the gloves and tubing should be placed in the waterproof bag and disposed of by burning. No attempt should be made to sterilize these items by boiling. The instruments should be disinfected by boiling for 30 minutes in a 2% solution of trisodium phosphate. The utensils should be treated in the same manner, making sure that all parts are completely covered with water during the boiling process. Because boiling water is not a reliable sterilizing agent, this procedure cannot be recommended except where facilities for steam under pressure are unavailable.

Handling of Contaminated Linen: The handling of contaminated linen calls for a procedure whereby no one need touch the linen after it has left the source of contamination or the isolation area. This means that at the close of the clean-up work following a septic case the laundry bags must be securely closed. If mesh bags are used they should be placed in outer bags made of canvas for proper protection. The outer bags should be plainly marked, "contaminated." They may then be transported to the laundry without concern or fear on the part of personnel. At the laundry the specially marked bags should be segregated and handled in one operation as follows:

- Open the canvas cover on the bag, and with a pair of tongs, pick up each mesh bag and deposit it in the washer.
- When the washer is loaded, treat its contents as any other load of washing.
- Deposit the empty canvas bags in a washer designed for colored garments and treat as any other similar load.
- Sterilize the tongs for future use.

For more detailed information on the handling of contaminated linen, including the public health aspects, the reader is referred to the American Hospital Association publication entitled *Hospital Laundry—Manual of Operation.*

CHAPTER XV

Sterilizer Controls, Sterilization Indicators and Culture Tests

S TERILIZATION FAILURES occur in hospitals even though personnel charged with this responsibility have instructions to correctly prepare and expose the surgical supplies to saturated steam under pressure at 250° F. for 30 minutes. As a rule, surgeons recognize that all instruments and supplies used in the performance of an operation constitute a potentially major source of contamination for operative wounds. Dandy,[1] for example, has attributed the majority of postoperative infections to inadequate sterilization of the towels, gowns, gauze and other supplies that pass through the sterilizers. The availability of the most modern sterilizing equipment as well as published methods for safe sterilization of supplies still does not entirely prevent the occurrence of fatal postoperative infections resulting from inadequate sterilization.[2] Far too few workers recognize that the organisms carried into a wound by the hands and instruments of a surgeon are apt to be more harmful and virulent than those occurring there by accident.

For the most part, sterilization failures are the result of a series of factors, either singly or combined, which make up the human equation in sterilizer operation. Those of primary importance are:

a) Failure to observe and understand the regulation of the sterilizer so as to maintain a saturated steam temperature of 250°-254° F., equivalent to 15-17 pounds pressure.

b) Incorrect methods of packaging and wrapping of supplies with little or no regard for the size and density of the individual packs.

c) Carelessness in loading the sterilizer, with disregard for the necessity of providing for complete air removal and for free circulation of steam throughout the load.

d) Failure to time correctly the proper period of exposure—usually due to ignorance or negligence on the part of the operator.

e) Failure to carry out the correct sequence of operations in the sterilizing cycle, as the result of carelessness, fatigue or distraction.

f) Attempts to sterilize materials which are impervious to steam, such as talcum powder and petrolatum.

g) Attempts to short-cut established methods of sterilization on the basis of limited bacteriological tests with organisms of unknown heat resistance.

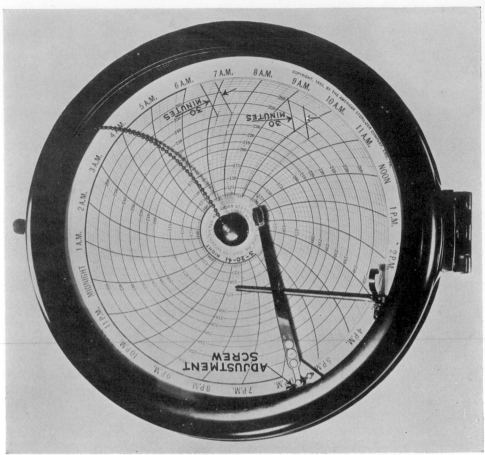

Fig. 124. Recording thermometers furnish reliable records of what transpires in the sterilizer during the day. They are invaluable in the maintenance of standards.

h) Faulty equipment resulting from lack of maintenance and lack of basic knowledge concerning the principles of operation and care of sterilizers.

RECORDING THERMOMETERS

When properly installed and used, the recording thermometer is a practical detector of faulty sterilization. This instrument (Fig. 124) contains a standard clock mechanism, electrically operated or mechanically wound, which revolves an 8-inch diameter chart once in 24 hours. It indicates and records the same temperature as that shown by the indicating thermometer located in the discharge system of the sterilizer chamber. It also records the duration of each exposure. Lacking the recorder, the operator can, and frequently does, forget to time the exposure when the temperature has advanced to 250° F. as prescribed. Without the recorder, it is difficult to maintain the required uniformity where several individuals have access to the sterilizers or to prove what has or has not been done in routine practice. If the exposure periods are greater or less than prescribed, or if the temperature has not been maintained within the proper limitations, there is a positive record of the errors, thus providing evidence needed upon which to act in correcting discrepancies.

Recording thermometers are subject to some distortion of the highly flexible pen arms but means for easy readjustment are provided on the instrument. Accuracy of the recorder should be checked at weekly intervals or oftener as follows: Operate the sterilizer in the routine manner until the temperature becomes stable at the maximum range which should not be less than 250° F., nor more than 254° F., as shown by the indicating thermometer on the sterilizer. If there is any deviation, adjust the screw on the pen arm until the temperature of the recorder is the same as that shown by the indicating thermometer.

In the author's opinion, the recording thermometer should be considered a necessary part of every surgical supply sterilizer, because its proper use most certainly promotes safer performance. It should be regarded as standard equipment, not a luxury. The ability to prove with daily chart records that definite standards of time and temperature are being maintained should appeal to those who must shoulder the responsibility for sterilization. Without the recorder, the supervisor is helpless in detecting discrepancies.

INDICATING POTENTIOMETERS

The most dependable physical method for testing the functional efficiency of sterilizers, the penetration of steam through a porous load or the rate of heat transfer through solution containers involves use of a potentiometer, an instrument for measuring temperature in the most inaccessible portion of the load during sterilization. When using this instrument, access to the load is gained through a thermocouple, two small wires of dissimilar metals (usually copper-constantan) soldered together at the ends and inserted in the load. The terminal ends of the thermocouple are brought out under the door of the sterilizer, impinging against the door gasket, and connected to the potentiometer, as in Figure 125. Any change in temperature at the joined ends of the couple develops a thermoelectric current which is immediately indicated on the dial of the instrument. A reliable potentiometer normally has an accuracy of adjustment of the order of $\pm 0.5°$ F. In this manner, the penetration of steam through a load can be followed, readings being taken at frequent intervals and the results then plotted on graph paper. With such data one can easily determine if a given sterilizing cycle provides a reasonable factor of safety.

When using the potentiometer, the chamber of the sterilizer should be filled to the maximum contemplated for routine loading. The test pack

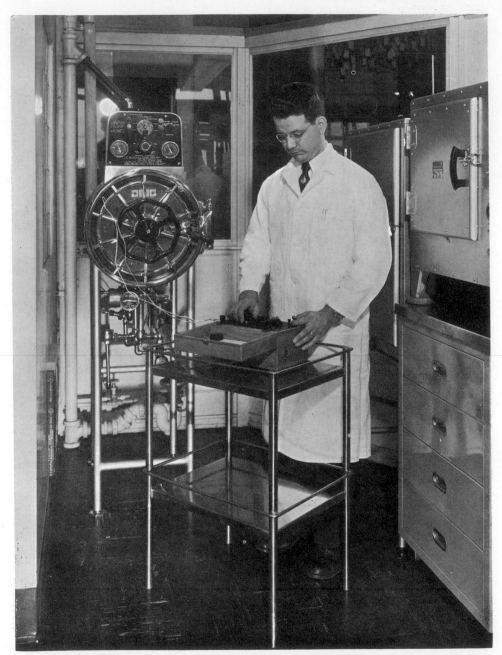

Fig. 125. The potentiometer is a useful instrument for testing the efficiency of sterilizers or in determining the rate of heating of a given load. The thermocouple leads are inserted under the edge of the door and the point is located in the center of the test pack.

selected for observation should be the largest and most densely arranged one and it should be located near the front bottom of the chamber to which point the steam will travel with the greatest lag. The thermocouple should be buried in the most compact part of the pack, usually in the center, to which steam will gain access most slowly. If the method of preparing the packs follows the standardized procedure and if the loading of the packs in the chamber is typical of routine practice, such tests are highly significant. Care should be used, however, to guard against superheating by using only freshly laundered fabrics for the test pack.

For bulk loads of surgical packs, both large and small, 30 minutes' exposure at 250° to 254° F. should show a reasonable margin of safety in time beyond that required to meet the minimum standard. For example, if the test pack with thermocouple showed that 12 minutes were required to reach 250° F., measured from the time the discharge line thermometer on the sterilizer reached this temperature, it would require an exposure of 24 minutes to meet the minimum standard. To this should then be added an additional 6 minutes for a fair margin of safety, making a total of 30 minutes exposure. If the test data shows that the pack is so dense that the minimum standard of 12 minutes at 250° F. cannot be maintained in 30 minutes' exposure, the correct procedure would be to revamp the package, perhaps remove some of the more compact articles and wrap those separately. Sterilization should not continue for much longer than 30 minutes, because added exposure becomes increasingly harmful, especially to the outer layers of fabrics.

AUTOMATIC TIME-TEMPERATURE CONTROLS

The human element must be reckoned with in order to safeguard the hospital against failures in sterilization of supplies. During the past few years sterilizer manufacturers have recognized this problem and accepted the responsibility of doing their part in bringing about better control and more effective methods for sterilization in hospitals. The development of automatic control mechanisms designed to minimize the human element in sterilizer operation is a good example of industry's attack on the problem. Typical of the class of automatic time-temperature controls is the instrument shown in Figure 41, page 86. The function of any such control should not be limited to automatic timing of the selected exposure period, but rather it should extend to all phases of the sterilizing process, to the end that all steps in the cycle normally carried out manually by the operator are conducted automatically according to a predetermined pattern established by the supervisor. This means that when the control is set for operation, it will automatically time the established exposure period at the correct temperature, exhaust the steam from the chamber, govern the process of drying, and, finally, sound an alarm announcing completion of the cycle. Since all exposure periods are based upon maintenance of a minimum standard temperature, the control should be of the type that will insure automatic re-cycling in the event that the temperature in the sterilizer falls below the standard at any time during the exposure period.

In discussing the functional efficiency of automatic controls in pressure steam sterilization, it should be understood that any such control instrument must, of necessity, have certain limitations because it cannot indicate or compensate for faulty methods used in the preparation, packaging and loading of supplies in the sterilizer. Regardless of the degree of mechanical perfection exhibited by the sterilizer and the controls which guarantee unvarying uniformity of operation, sterilization of the load is still dependent upon correct methods of packaging and strict adherence to established rules for loading the sterilizer.

The prime purpose of any automatic control is to guard against the inaccuracies of human behavior in sterilizer operation. To this end, it is essential that the instrument eliminate the mental burden of remembering the time at which the exposure period began and when it should end. Likewise, it should eliminate errors in the reading of the thermometer, insure the proper sequence of each step in the sterilizing cycle, and protect the load against under-exposure or over-exposure. The reliability of the control should merit complete confidence on the part of the operator to the extent that once it is set in operation, the exact period of continuous exposure at the correct temperature, as well as the entire cycle of performance, will be carried out with accuracy and precision not obtainable through manual operation. The use of automatic controls on sterilizers naturally presupposes the need for periodic inspection and servicing to insure peak efficiency of operation. A properly trained mechanic or serviceman familiar with the equipment should always be engaged for this work. If these requirements are met, sterilizers equipped with automatic controls can be depended upon to afford a greater factor of safety in routine sterilization with a substantial savings in personnel time, materials and supplies.

STERILIZATION INDICATORS

Authoritative opinion is seemingly divided on the actual worth of all sterilization indicators or controls of the "tell-tale" type. For long this subject has been a controversial one, and not infrequently the utilitarian value of such indicators is questioned. Ecker,[3] for example, in evaluating the efficiency of these devices found that their turning points, based on melting of the indicator substance or on color changes, had not been standardized and they varied in the time-temperature ratios required for complete change. In contrast to these findings, Hoyt[4] reported that one type of indicator, when properly used and interpreted, was found to be an adequate check on the efficacy of sterilization of rubber gloves. On the basis of hundreds of tests under widely varying conditions of application in hospitals, Underwood[5] reported that the hermetically sealed glass tube control reacted (melted) uniformly when subjected to temperatures of 248° to 252° F. for 5 to 8 minutes. At slightly lower temperature (245° F.) the time required to fuse the control ranged from 20 to 30 minutes. These results encouraged Underwood to make the recommendation that approved sterilization indicators can be used to advantage as an occasional check against faulty packaging, loading and performance of sterilizers. An evaluation of a group of tell-tale indicators by Walter[6] revealed marked discrepancies in individual controls with a sufficient number showing delayed changes in end points so as to confuse operators and to cause unnecessary resterilization of supplies.

It is the author's belief, based upon observations over a period of ten years, that all sterilization indicators possess the same general disadvantage, to a greater or lesser degree, in that a percentage will be found to react to a time-temperature ratio inadequate for sterilization or that the end points are not sufficiently clear so as to permit accurate interpretation of the results. These controls do not indicate the actual build-up of temperature in the test pack nor do they indicate how much over-exposure may have been applied. It is unfortunate for the user that the manufacturers of such controls have not attempted to bring about uniformity or standardization of end points to conform to a safe time-temperature relationship required for sterilization of supplies. Consequently, one type of indicator used in one hospital may react to a different time-temperature relationship than another type employed in another hospital.

The majority of glass tube indicators contain essentially the same material, namely, a pellet of sulfur which in the pure state has a melting point of about 248° F. (120° C.). In the process of manufacture certain changes may be introduced in the material which alter the melting point. Also, variations in the thickness or composition of the hermetically sealed glass tube affect the rate of heat transfer and the time-temperature conditions to which the control will react. It is doubtful if there is any control commercially available that can be depended upon to react exactly the same every time without failure. Studies have shown that rarely will any of the glass tube indicators melt at a temperature as low as 240° F. (116° C.) for 30 minutes. A fair percentage will, however, undergo partial or complete melting at 245° F. (118° C.) for 10 minutes. Certain of the paper indicators which undergo color change when exposed to moist heat at 250° F. for 5, 12½ and 20 minutes are fairly reliable. However, they occasionally pose a problem for the untrained operator because the color change or end point is not sharp and correct interpretation is difficult.

If sterilization indicators are to be used, the indicator of whatever form it may be should be placed in the center of the largest and most densely wrapped package in the load. This package should then be placed on the perforated tray or shelf in the front bottom of the sterilizer chamber. The correct method for placing indicators in packs is shown in Figure 126.

When indicators are used for setting up standards for sterilizing systematically prepared loads, a heavy load of supplies as large and dense as any that will be encountered in routine practice should be assembled. Then select six of the heaviest and most densely wrapped packages. Place one indicator or control in the center of each of these packs, then place the packs on edge in the bottom of the sterilizer. Add the remainder of the

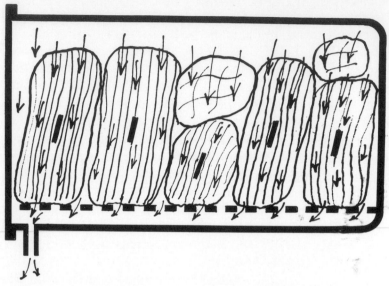

Fig. 126. The correct method for using sterilization indicators or culture tests. The controls should be located in the center of the largest packs—near the bottom and in the coolest area of the chamber. The coolest portion of the chamber is at the front bottom, near the outlet to the discharge line.

load as it will normally be placed. Sterilize for 30 minutes, timing the exposure when the thermometer shows 250° F., with the sterilizer regulated to produce a maximum of 250°-254° F. Upon completion of the cycle, remove the load and examine the controls.

Sterilization indicators, culture tests and other detectors are often placed at the extreme top of the chamber, tied to the end frames of loading cars, or located just under the covers of packages. Tests made under such careless conditions mean nothing, and may develop a false sense of security in a highly inefficient sterilizer.

CULTURE TESTS FOR DETERMINING EFFICIENCY OF STERILIZATION

The best means at our disposal to confirm the sterility of an article or to determine the efficiency of a sterilizing process are strictly of a biological nature. Bacteriological culture tests designed to confirm the presence or absence of living microorganisms constitute the most commonly employed methods. Mechanical controls or sterilization indicators of the "tell-tale" type which supposedly react to minimum standards of time and temperature do not constitute a direct approach to the lethality of the sterilizing process. Culture tests are more reassuring to bacteriologists and surgeons in general. Unfortunately, the delay entailed in determining the results of culture tests makes them somewhat impractical except for the periodic check on the maintenance of minimum standards. If they are not properly planned they may be distinctly misleading. The usual culture test is meaningless unless dry spores of established heat resistance in known populations are used.

The use of culture tests for periodically determining the efficiency of sterilizing processes in hospitals should be established as a standard procedure. If the hospital has a properly equipped laboratory and a qualified bacteriologist or trained technician to do this work, then the culture test becomes a reliable means for the periodic testing of sterility of supplies. The bacterial spore strip technic described below is a safe and practical procedure. It can be used as an effective method of control in both large and small hospitals.

SPORE-BEARING ORGANISMS

1) *Bacillus subtilis* var. *globigii*,
   U.S.D.A. Strain 1221a,
   A.T.C.C. No. 9372.
2) *Bacillus stearothermophilus*,
   N.C.A. Strain 1518,
   A.T.C.C. No. 7953.

PREPARATION OF SPORE STRIPS*

Inoculate a Kolle flask, containing nutrient agar, with a suspension of cells from a 24-hour nutrient agar slant culture of desired organism. Incubate the flask at 32° C. for *B. subtilis* or 55° C. for *B. stearothermophilus*. After 5 to 7 days incubation, prepare a smear of the growth and stain with Malachite Green spore stain. If microscopic examination shows heavy spore production, the growth is washed from the agar with a small quantity of sterile water and aseptically filtered through several layers of gauze. The suspension is then ready for standardization.

Prepare a 1:100 dilution of the suspension in sterile water, heat in boiling water for 5 minutes, and cool immediately. This will destroy the vegetative cells and the less resistant spores. From the boiled suspension prepare serial dilutions, plate on nutrient agar, incubate for 48 hours, and then make spore counts. Standardize suspension.

Small strips of filter paper, 2″ x ½″, are then inoculated with a measured

---

* A product of American Sterilizer Co., Erie, Pa.

amount of the suspension so as to give a spore count of 100,000 or more per strip. The strips are dried at room temperature for several hours, inserted in small sterilizable Glassine paper envelopes, sealed, and placed in clean storage.

HEAT RESISTANCE OF SPORE STRIPS

Contrary to popular belief, the spores of *B. subtilis* are not highly resistant to moist heat. Spores from most strains of this organism will show a

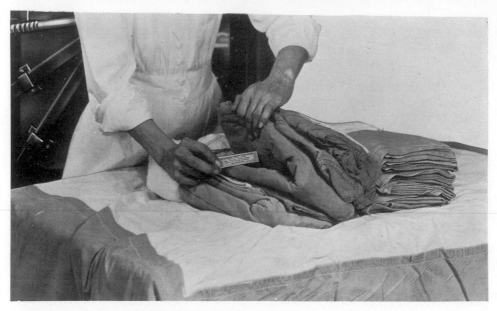

Fig. 127. Bacterial spore strips or other culture tests should be placed in the most dense portion of the test pack.

uniform resistance to moist heat equal to or greater than the pathogenic organisms, including dry spores of *Cl. tetani* and *Cl. welchii*. Strips with populations of 100,000 to 200,000 spores each will usually survive exposure to saturated steam at 215° F. (102° C.) for 5 minutes, but will be killed in 15 minutes at 220° F. (104° C.).

B. stearothermophilus is one of the most resistant organisms known. Spore strips with populations of about 100,000 will usually survive exposure to saturated steam at 250° F. (121° C.) for 5 minutes, but will be killed in 12 minutes.

USE OF SPORE STRIPS

When using bacterial spore strips for determining the efficiency of sterilizing processes, care must be taken to insure proper placement of each strip in the most inaccessible to steam portion of the test package. The correct procedure is to select two or more of the largest and most dense packs which comprise a part of the routine load of bulk supplies. Open the packs and insert two envelopes containing the bacterial spore strips in the center of each pack, as shown in Figure 127. Rewrap the packs and identify by marking with a "Venus" 6B pencil. Place the packs on edge on the bottom shelf of the sterilizer chamber, near the front, as in Figure 128. Add the remainder of the load in the usual manner and operate the sterilizer according to standard procedure. Upon completion of the sterilizing cycle, including the drying period, remove the envelopes containing the spore strips from the test packs and deliver them to the laboratory for sterility testing.

Spore strips may also be used for determining the efficiency of steriliza-

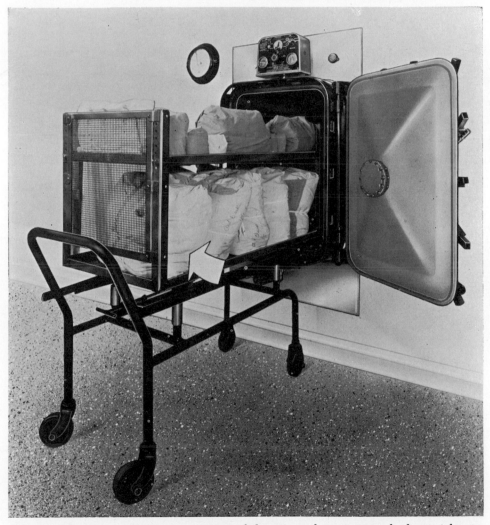

Fig. 128. This shows the correct position of the test pack containing the bacterial spore strips. It should rest on edge on the bottom shelf of the sterilizer chamber—near the front.

tion of rubber gloves. In this application it is necessary to insert the envelope containing the strip in one of the glove fingers, and then wrap in the usual manner. Do not attempt to sterilize gloves for less than 15 minutes at 250° F. The supervisor should record and file the following sterilization test data each time spore strips or other culture tests are made:

Date of test ....
Sterilizer ....
Type of load ....
Number test strips used ....
Location of test strips in load ....
Sterilizing conditions:
    Temperature (Dial thermometer) ....° F.
    Temperature (Recording thermometer) ....° F.
    Exposure period ....minutes
Test conducted by ....
Department ....

STERILITY TEST PROCEDURE

All tests for sterility should be conducted in a clean and dust-free area of the laboratory, with as nearly static air circulation as is possible. Do not work in front of open windows or in drafty areas. The bacteriologist or technician should observe rigid bacteriologic technic throughout the procedure.

1) Cut open one end of the spore strip envelope with sterile scissors, as in Figure 129. Carefully withdraw the spore strip with sterile forceps (Figure 130), and immerse it in the culture tube (25 x 200 mm.) containing 25 ml. of sterile Fluid Thioglycollate Medium, as in Figure 131.

2) Incubate the tubes for 7 days at 32° C. for *B. subtilis* strips and 55° C. for *B. stearothermophilus* strips. Observe the tubes daily during the incubation period. If turbidity develops in the medium at any time during incubation it is indicative of bacterial growth—presumably due to spores which have survived the sterilizing process.

3) Controls: One or more *positive* controls should be included in each test series, performed on a monthly or semi-monthly basis. This requires the transfer of an unexposed spore strip from the envelope to the tube of freshly prepared Fluid Thioglycollate Medium, followed by incubation at the correct temperature. A positive result indicates that the medium possesses suitable growth-promoting properties and that the spore strips contained viable spores prior to the sterilizing process. A *negative* control should also be included in each test series consisting of one or two tubes of the Fluid Thioglycollate Medium only. The absence of growth, following incubation, shows that the medium was effectively sterilized before use in the sterility test procedure.

Upon completion of the sterility test, the bacteriology laboratory should send a report to the supervisor giving the following information:

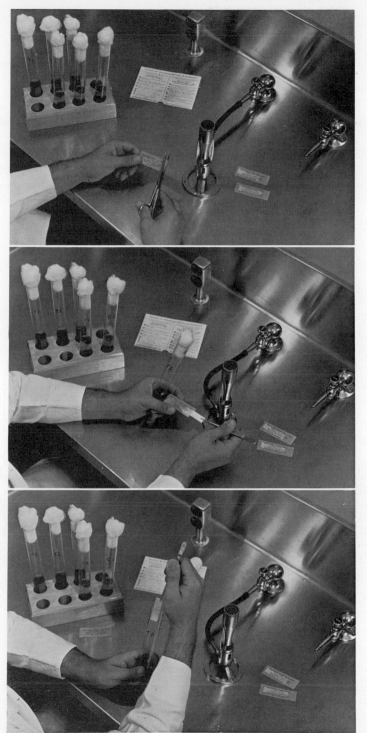

Fig. 129. The first step in culturing the bacterial spore strip is to cut open one end of the envelope with sterile scissors.

Fig. 130. Carefully withdraw the spore strip from the envelope with sterile forceps.

Fig. 131. Immerse the spore strip in the tube of sterile Fluid Thioglycollate Medium and place in incubator.

To .... (Supervisor)

Dept. ....

Date Test Strips were Cultured ....

Results of Culture Tests (Check One):

    One Strip Negative; Other Positive ☐

    Both Strips Positive ☐

    Should test be repeated? Yes ☐ No ☐

    Was Control Strip Cultured? Yes ☐ No ☐

    Control Strip Test Result:

                Positive ☐   Negative ☐

Signature ....

Date ....

FREQUENCY OF CULTURE TESTS

A standard procedure should be set up for the routine evaluation of each pressure steam sterilizer in the hospital on a monthly or semi-monthly basis by means of culture tests. If practical the procedure should also include dry heat or hot air sterilizers. Wherever possible, all bulk supplies should be sterilized with saturated steam at 250° F. for 30 minutes. The operating room supervisor and the central service supervisor should put forth every possible effort toward the standardization of sterilizing technics. Frequent checking of the sterilizing process by means of culture tests, the maintenance of exact standards for the preparation, packaging and loading of supplies in the sterilizer, plus intelligent and painstaking supervision are factors recognized as essential to the effective sterilization of surgical supplies.

REFERENCES

1. DANDY, W. E.: Importance of More Adequate Sterilization Processes in Hospitals. *Bull. Am. Coll. Surgeons,* 16:11-12, 1932.

2. SEVITT, S.: Source of Two Hospital-Infected Cases of Tetanus. *Lancet,* 2:1075, Dec. 10, 1949.

3. ECKER, E. E.: Sterilization Based on Temperature Attained and Time Ratio. *Mod. Hosp.* 48:86-90, 1937.

4. HOYT, A.: Rubber Glove Sterilization and Use of Sterility Indicators. *J. Lab. & Clin. Med.,* 19:382-390, 1934.

5. UNDERWOOD, W. B.: *Textbook of Sterilization.* Chicago, Lakeside, Donnelley, 1941, p. 100.

6. WALTER, C. W.: Evaluation of Sterility Indicators. *Surgery,* 2:585-589, 1937.—*Aseptic Treatment of Wounds,* New York, Macmillan, 1948, p. 93.

Chapter XVI

The Central (Supply) Service Department

THE CENTRAL SERVICE Department of the modern hospital, more commonly known as "central supply," is the natural outgrowth of a movement or system instituted some years ago by the American College of Surgeons,[1] for the standardization of surgical dressings and for the centralization of all surgical supplies into one unit. By definition, the central supply department comprises that service within a hospital which processes, issues and controls professional supplies and equipment, both sterile and unsterile, to all departments and floors of the hospital for the care and safety of the patients, both medical and surgical. The modern concept of sterile supply centralization has been developed by many workers, some associated directly with hospitals, others connected with government agencies and also industry. The early contributions of the late W. B. Underwood[2, 3] are particularly noteworthy. His extensive studies relating to the planning and organization of work in the central supply service department, from both the administrative and technical viewpoints, led to a number of significant and important findings. In brief, his pioneering efforts did much to establish the basic philosophy of centralization, which when put into practice later by many hospitals was proved invaluable.

In the earlier days, all sterilization for the entire hospital was centralized in the surgery, and with fewer operations to prepare for, the surgical nursing staff was able to meet the sterilizing requirements with some degree of satisfaction. Later on, as surgeries became busier, it was quite popular to relocate the sterilizers into the surgery work room, still under the supervision of the operating room supervisor. In this room, the usual surgical dressings were prepared, sterilized, and then distributed to the various wards, units or departments of the hospital. Even today, in many hospitals this still is the plan and the source of all sterile supplies for the operating rooms and the floors. Inappropriately, this work room is often referred to as "central supply." That is by no means what is implied by the modern term "central supply service" as here used.

The purpose of a central supply service is often misconstrued. In this department it is practical to prepare, sterilize and issue all professional supplies for the hospital, except instruments used in the operating and delivery rooms, supplies for the infant formula room and the laboratory. In some hospitals with facilities for steam sterilization in the operating rooms, and water, instrument and utensil sterilization on the floors, it is assumed that a perfectly satisfactory system has been achieved. With this arrangement it cannot be denied that all the necessary sterilization facilities have been provided, but who is to operate these numerous sterilizers? Under such conditions it is difficult to establish and maintain anything approaching standardization of sterilizing technics throughout the institution. In the operating room, service to the surgeon takes precedence over operation of the sterilizers. On the floors, bedside nursing care is of prime importance and operation of the sterilizers is more or less everybody's business and no one person's individual responsibility. The net result is deserving of serious consideration and it constitutes one of the valid reasons for the establishment of a comprehensive central supply service.

ADVANTAGES OF CENTRAL SUPPLY SERVICE

The recognized advantages of centralization are efficiency, economy and safety. When properly organized the system promotes efficiency through good supervision of cleaning, maintenance and sterilization of materials. The problems of standardization, uniformity, and coordination of materials and procedures are more easily controlled because the work is under constant supervision by an individual who devotes her entire time to this activity. A central supply service is also economical because it avoids duplication of equipment infrequently used. The life of materials is prolonged through more efficient handling and better methods of preparation and sterilization. Procedures do not vary from day to day with changing personnel. The use of non-professional personnel, working under competent supervision, with assembly-line methods and mechanical equipment results in marked savings for the hospital. One group of non-professional workers whose primary function is the preparation of supplies can be trained to perform exacting technics when the system is highly standardized and adequately supervised. This relieves professional personnel for other duties, not the least of which are patient care activities.

A summary of the advantages of centralization of sterile supplies would be incomplete without recognition of the element of safety. The old decentralized system of sterilization on several floors and in several departments by many people has undoubtedly been responsible for a major percentage of failures in sterilization. Many cases have been recorded where loads of supplies were inadequately sterilized, some where steam was never admitted to the chamber of the sterilizer, and in more than a few instances, the entire process of sterilization has been omitted. The evidence against over-sterilization of supplies is equally as bad, if not worse. Here no hazard is involved insofar as unsterile supplies are concerned but the destruction of materials has incurred unnecessary costs for the hospitals. These unsatisfactory practices do not always occur through the fault of the individual but rather because of interference with other, and perhaps, imperative duties. Centralization has taken the operation of sterilizers out of the class of "everybody's business and no one person's individual responsibility," and placed it in a highly specialized class with both supervision and responsibility centered on the shoulders of one responsible person, the central supply service supervisor.

PLANNING THE DEPARTMENT

In planning any department within a hospital, the functions of that department must be clearly defined; consequently, the functions of a central supply service should be carefully studied as the initial step in planning. This can best be done through the organization of a planning committee consisting of the hospital administrator, the architect, technical consultant, director of nurses, the person who will be responsible for the administration of the department and also representative members from the areas throughout the hospital which will be using the services of the central supply. Only in this way is it possible to assure inclusion of the many factors which must be considered. Schafer[4] has recently published a detailed outline of the objectives of the department which is deserving of serious study in the initial planning stage. It is reproduced here in part by permission of the publisher as follows:

1) What department will be responsible for the Central Supply Service? Very early in the planning stage it is advisable to determine where within the hospital organizational pattern the Central Supply Unit will fit. Because most of the materials supplied by the unit are used by or through the nursing department, that group usually is called upon to operate the unit. However, in some instances the pharmacist is given the responsibility for this unit.

2) What services are to be provided?

a) Sterile supplies and equipment
Hospitals vary, but most Central Supply Services include sterile supplies and equipment for treatments, surgical operations and deliveries. Routine patient care equipment is usually decentralized, but could be centralized effectively, especially in a small hospital. It is usually considered safer to decentralize the sterilization and disinfecting equipment and materials from septic or infectious patients. A system of centralization is possible, but it has not been used sufficiently to recommend it at this time.

b) Unsterile supplies and equipment, including individual items and assembled sets, can be effectively included in the Central Supply Service.

c) Apparatus
The maintenance and storage of apparatus such as oxygen tents and inhalators in the Central Supply, especially in small hospitals, is recommended. Larger hospitals may find it more practical to have apparatus storage under other departments such as anesthesia, or maintenance.

3) What departments are to be served and extent of service to each?

a) Linen

Although many hospitals have not included the preparation of linen packs for the operating room and delivery suites under Central Supply, it is now considered advisable to do so. Some sterile linen is also required for the in-patient and out-patient units. Linen inspection and folding is space and time consuming and influences area, equipment and personnel requirements.

b) Dressings

Surgical dressings, gauze and cotton supplies for all departments of the hospital can best be handled through Central Supply.

c) Gloves

It is advisable to centralize all rubber glove processing and sterilizing. The laundry may wash and dry the gloves.

d) Instruments

It is not considered advisable to include operating room and delivery room instruments in the Central Supply because of numbers required, control, and the necessity for emergency sterilization. Instruments for treatment sets on patient units can be effectively centralized.

e) Syringes and needles for all units can best be handled through a centralized system. Recent studies on the causes of infectious hepatitis have emphasized the importance of efficient sterilization of syringes and needles.

f) Centralizing the processing of treatment trays and sets for all in-patient and out-patient units provides improved service.

g) Unsterile supplies and equipment for the in-patient and out-patient units include such items as non-sterile treatment trays, bandages, pads, hot water bottles, ice bags, heating pads, communion sets, and morgue sets.

h) Operating Room and Delivery Room Suite apparatus are usually not kept in a Central Supply Unit. The apparatus normally stored in Central Supply includes such items as inhalators, suction machines, oxygen tents, and drainage equipment.

i) Other services could include certain drugs or solutions, but it is generally accepted that these should be included under the pharmacy.

4) What items will be purchased ready made?

a) It is usually considered more economical for hospitals to purchase surgical dressings ready made.

b) Parenteral solutions

Manufacturing parenteral solutions in a hospital reflects a substantial monetary saving but for safety reasons should only be done under the supervision of a qualified pharmacist.

c) Sterile disposable parenteral administration sets are now used by many hospitals. They assure safety and savings in personnel time.

5) What preparation will materials receive in other departments?

a) Some hospital laundries prepare linen packs for surgery and obstetrics and send them to Central Supply ready for sterilization.

b) Some hospital laundries efficiently wash and dry rubber gloves, but doing them in the Central Supply Unit eliminates the necessity of transporting the gloves from one department to another and centralizes the entire procedure in one area.

6) How frequently raw supplies are received from central stores will determine the storage space required. Usually materials are issued to Central Supply about once a week in quantities required for the week or in carton lots as supplied by the manufacturer. The Central Supply Unit should not be used for a Central Store Room.

7) What method of distribution will be used, i.e., dumb waiter, truck or messenger? Since any centralized service is only as effective as its distribution system, careful study and attention should be given to this aspect of operation. To provide good patient care, supplies and equipment must be available whenever and wherever needed with a minimum of delay. When a minimum stock of frequently used items are delivered to the various hospital units where they are used, the inefficient and costly practice of unit personnel making frequent trips to Central Supply and the numerous interruptions for the Central Supply workers to issue materials is eliminated or at least minimized. A dumbwaiter, properly located, is also helpful.

8) Where will supplies and equipment prepared in Central Supply be stored? Except in a small hospital where the distance to Central Supply is minimal, it is usually better to stock a minimum quantity of items routinely used on the particular units and keep only a reserve of these items (usually 24 hour stock), and materials infrequently used in Central Supply storage.

9) What sterilizing equipment is available in other areas of the hospital? The number, kind and location of sterilizers throughout the hospital may influence the Central Supply Unit functions.

10) Where will the Central Supply Service be located?
In an existing hospital available space usually dictates the location. In a new hospital ease of distribution to various hospital units is a very important factor. In a small hospital an area adjoining the operating room suite is often selected.

11) The size of staff required to operate the department will be determined by the services included, organization and training of personnel, and the utilization of mechanical equipment. It has been estimated that a 100-bed hospital, furnishing sterile material for treatments, surgical operations and deliveries, and some unsterile supplies, equipment, and apparatus will require approximately four workers provided mechanical equipment is used and work simplification practiced.

12) Are personnel facilities such as lockers and toilets nearby? Since all workers should change to clean uniforms to work in Central Supply, locker facilities should be available.

13) Are housekeeping facilities such as a janitor's closet nearby? Housekeeping facilities may be included outside the Central Supply Unit, but provision for a mop and some cleaning supplies within the unit is desirable.

14) What type of record system is planned? Some hospitals make a direct charge to patients for equipment obtained from Central Supply, others prepare charges from the patient's record on the basis of services given or have

inclusive rates for care. Many hospitals have printed or mimeographed requisition forms which promote uniformity and simplify "paper work." An exchange system is also sometimes used. A procedure book and card file or Kardex for various procedures is also helpful. Requisitions may be received by messenger or by a pneumatic tube system.

15) Teaching programs should make provision for adequate instruction and training of staff.

16) What work stations should be planned?

The work stations should provide a continuous work flow of all materials and equipment through the Central Supply Unit from dirty to clean to sterile, without back tracking for maximum efficiency and to avoid contaminating sterile supplies which could be disastrous.

FLOW OF WORK

Materials are received into the Central Supply Unit by dumbwaiter, truck or messenger from

Central Stores
Hospital Units and
Laundry

Materials from Central Stores are put in Bulk Storage area and removed as required. Used materials go to disassembly where they are taken apart and sorted for cleaning.

The first step in processing all used materials and some new materials brought into the unit is a thorough cleaning.

Clean materials, including linen from the laundry, go to the processing and assembly area where they are inspected, put in proper condition, assembled, and packaged for sterilization or stored clean ready for use. Sterilized goods are either distributed directly to the departments where they are used or stored in the storage area in Central Supply. Four storage areas are required, sterile, unsterile, apparatus and bulk (raw storage). Bulk or unsterile storage can be safely included in the processing area but it is advisable to provide a separate sterile storage area.

Materials are distributed by dumbwaiters, carts, trucks, or messenger to hospital units.

In order to operate the department, office space, employee and housekeeping facilities must also be provided.

SPACE ASSIGNMENT FOR DEPARTMENT

The total area allotment in square feet per hospital bed (including bassinets) will vary with the size and type of hospital. Experience has shown that the following areas can be relied upon to provide adequate space in most instances:

```
 75- 99 Beds ........................... 7  Square feet per bed
100-149 Beds ........................... 6  Square feet per bed
150-199 Beds ........................... 5½ Square feet per bed
```

200-249 Beds .... 5 Square feet per bed
250-300 Beds .... 4½ Square feet per bed
300 Beds and up .... 4 Square feet per bed

Proper distribution of the appropriate area for a basic department is normally accomplished in this manner:

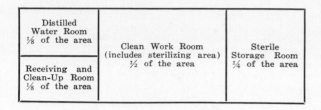

RECTANGULAR PLAN

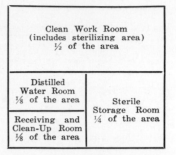

SQUARE PLAN

The above conditions fulfill the requirements of a basic department only. Additional space must be provided for a more comprehensive service when:

1) All surgical packs, dressings and utensils are to be prepared in this

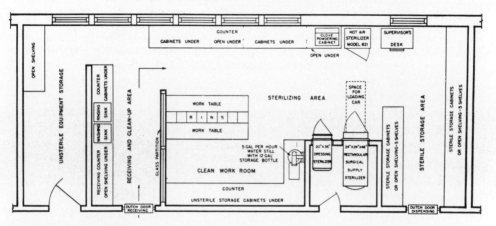

Fig. 132. Typical layout of a central supply room for a 100-bed hospital. The dimensions of the space allotted are 42 feet long by 16 feet wide. This provides an area of about 6 square feet per bed, including space for unsterile equipment storage.

department. Add ½ square foot per bed to the "clean work room" area for this additional service.

2) All delivery room packs, dressings and utensils are to be prepared in this department. Add ½ square foot per bed to the "clean work room" area for this additional service.

3) The department is required to prepare parenteral solutions for the

hospital. Add ¼ square foot per bed to the "distilled water room" for this service.

4) An unsterile equipment room is required for the storage of apparatus, such as oxygen tents, gas evacuators, heating cradles, etc. Add 1 square foot per bed in the form of an additional room for this service.

5) A separate area for the processing of gloves is required. It should be

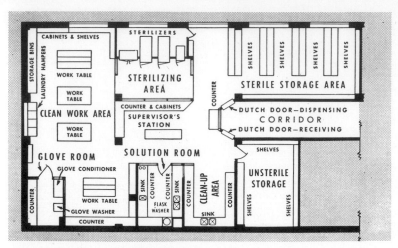

Fig. 133. This central supply department layout is representative of modern planning for a hospital of 400 beds. The entire department comprises an area of 2600 square feet, equivalent to 6½ square feet per bed. Note how planning permits a continuous work flow from receiving to dispensing sections, without back-tracking. Figures 134 to 139 illustrate individual sections of this department.

located within the "clean work room," completely enclosed with a glass partition. The glove room should be equipped with washer, dryer and powdering apparatus. A work counter for glove repairing and wrapping is also essential (see Fig. 63, p. 118). An area of approximately 100 square feet will usually suffice for this service.

A typical layout of a central supply room for a 100-bed hospital is shown in Figure 132. The space allotted is 42½ feet long by 16½ feet wide, including space for unsterile equipment storage. The layout shown in Figure 133 is for a hospital of 400 beds. It represents an area of 2600 square feet, with all facilities for a comprehensive department included. Figures 134 to 139 inclusive also apply to this plan.

LOCATION OF DEPARTMENT

Since the goal of central supply service is perfection of sterilization techniques and economy in centralized control of professional equipment, actual location in relation to distance from departments is of secondary importance. Whether in new construction or in existing buildings, the place most isolated from other functions of the hospital will usually bring the

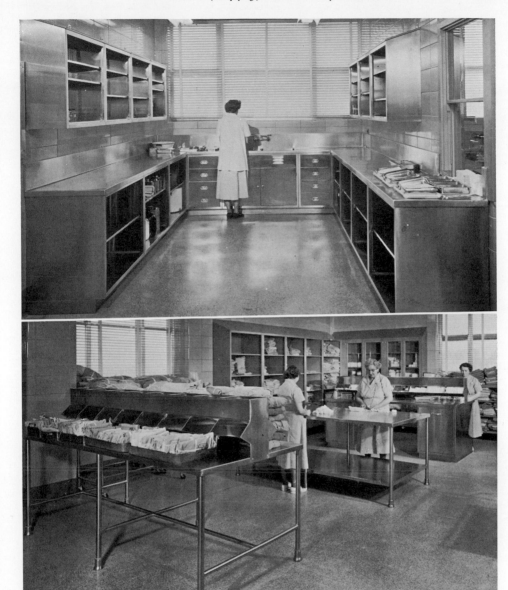

Courtesy Georgia Baptist Hospital, Atlanta, Ga.

Fig. 134. General clean-up area where soiled supplies are received, disassembled, cleaned, then sent to the clean work area.

Fi₋. 135. Clean work area. Table in left foreground is used for making up various trays. The other tables are used for preparing surgical and obstetrical packs.

best results. Any floor or even the basement where the traffic to and from the department will not seriously interfere with general hospital operation is considered an acceptable location. It should not be located in the surgery corridor or in the delivery room suite. However, in certain cases it may be

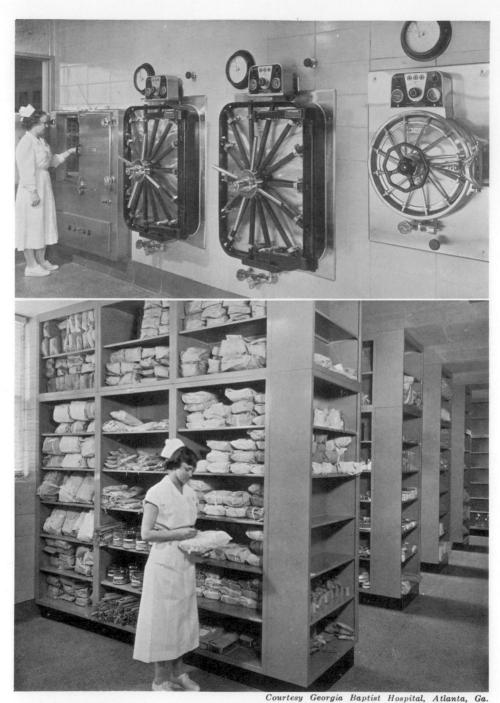

Courtesy Georgia Baptist Hospital, Atlanta, Ga.

Fig. 136. Sterilizing area. The large rectangular sterilizers, equipped with automatic controls and recording thermometers, are used for bulk loads. The cylindrical sterilizer at right is for emergency and small loads. Hot air sterilizer at left is for needles, syringes, oils, etc.

Fig. 137. Sterile storage area. Sterile supplies are kept here for distribution upon requisition. This section is conveniently located adjacent to the dispensing door.

on the same floor with these departments. In the basement there is least traffic, patient and otherwise, and least confliction with and interference from other departments. As a rule, space does not come at as high a premium in the basement as it does on other floor levels. The location selected should be a sanitary and reasonably dust-free area with good lighting, ventilation, access to vertical transportation and possibilities for expansion, if required.

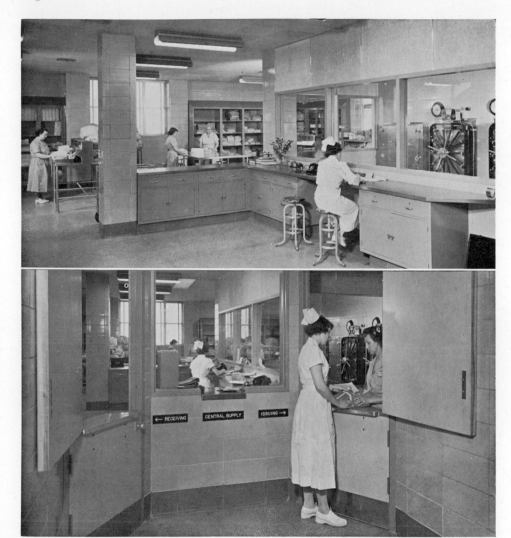

Courtesy Georgia Baptist Hospital, Atlanta, Ga.

Fig. 138. Supervisor's station. Here all clerical work is performed in connection with control and operation of central supply.

Fig. 139. Receiving and dispensing stations. Returned materials are received through Dutch door at left. Entire door opens to admit linen carts from laundry. Supplies are issued through dispensing door at right upon presentation of a charge slip.

ESSENTIAL EQUIPMENT FOR DEPARTMENT

Receiving and Clean-up Room: The stationary equipment in this area should consist of a receiving counter with three open shelves under, two sinks, one for washing and the other for rinsing, with storage cabinets under; also a clean equipment counter with storage cabinets under. Stainless steel is the metal of choice for fabrication of the equipment (see Fig. 134).

Distilled Water or Solution Room: The units in this room should also be fabricated of stainless steel, all-welded, seamless construction. The clean-up unit should consist of an unclean equipment counter with three open shelves under, two sinks, one for washing and one for rinsing, with storage cabinets under; also a clean equipment counter with storage cabinets under. A water still and distilled water storage bottle should be mounted integrally above this unit.

The preparation unit should have at least one small sink with removable grille and storage cabinets under. A water still and distilled water storage bottle should be mounted integrally above this unit. Complete facilities for the cleaning and preparation of needles, tubing and syringes should also be provided. If parenteral solutions are to be prepared here, the following additional equipment is required:

Flask washer	Flask drainage carriage
Hot plate (two burners)	Solution-making equipment and glassware

The Solution Room should be a strictly sanitary area, enclosed with a glass partition to keep out dust and lint which may arise from the handling of dry goods and fabrics in other areas of the department (see Figs. 147 and 148, p. 263).

Clean Work Room: The equipment in this area may be of enameled steel construction with all work surfaces made of stainless steel. Depending upon the size of the room, the essential items are as follows:

Unsterile storage cabinets with glass doors (six feet high) or open shelving.	Work table with bins across top and tilting bins on sides.
Work counters, with cabinets, drawers and knee space under.	Portable carriages (double deck).
Work table with flat top.	Supervisor's desk.

The sterilizing area which comprises a part of this room should have sterilizers of the appropriate types and sizes to meet the peak requirements of the department (see Fig. 136).

Sterile Supply Storage Room: Here again the various cabinets may be of enameled steel. The normal requirements include storage cabinets with glass doors (six feet high), some cabinets with open shelving, others with doors above and drawers below. A record counter with drawers under is also an essential item.

Unsterile Equipment Storage Room: The only equipment required for this room is an adequate number of open shelving racks (six feet high) of enameled steel construction. The room should be located adjacent to the receiving and clean-up area, if possible, at least on the unsterile end of the department.

STAFFING THE DEPARTMENT

The problem of selecting personnel for operation of the central supply service begins with the supervisor. In a few cases supervision of this department has been placed under the direction of the hospital pharmacist. However, most hospital administrators[5] agree that it should be under the direction of a registered nurse who would act as supervisor. The selection of this nurse with responsibility as supervisor is a highly important factor in determining the ultimate success of the department. In addition to being a topflight nurse with thorough experience in her profession, she should possess more than average executive ability, be capable of supervising the activities of others, and at the same time have the faculty of grasping problems quickly and to see that the duties of the department are carried out in the most efficient manner. Granted that a nurse with this degree of executive ability may not be readily found in some hospitals, but usually one can be selected, who, after being sent to other hospitals to familiarize herself with organization and operation of the department, will become a successful supervisor. The supervisor should also have a well grounded sense of economy and a firm but personable disposition. Technically she should have a thorough knowledge of hospital requirements covering the diagnostic and therapeutic armamentarium, and an ever present sense of responsibility toward safe and efficient patient care. The supervisor needs an assistant, preferably a registered nurse, to relieve her and act as supervisor during vacation periods and in emergencies.

Beyond these two key persons, the personnel of central supply service may differ with each hospital. However, nursing students and lay personnel are commonly employed in the department. Male and female attendants can be used. A female attendant is usually found more efficient for the daytime periods when the bulk of meticulous work is to be done. In the average general hospital of between 100 and 250 beds the staff of this department will consist of five to seven persons. The supervisor, her assistant and one or two attendants will be on duty during the hours from 7 A.M. to 3 P.M. One or two attendants will work from 3 P.M. to 11 P.M. If a nurse or other qualified and responsible person is available for night duty, it may be advantageous to keep the department open from 11 P.M. to 7 A.M. In addition to these employees there is needed one clerk who can work part time on the clerical duties and the remainder as a general attendant.

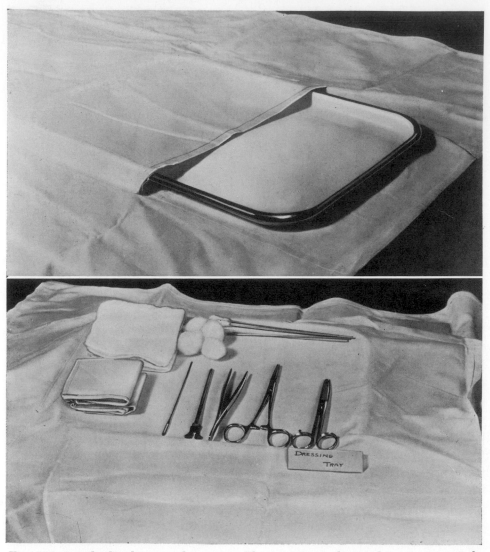

Fig. 140. Standardized tray and wrapper. The wrapper is designed in size to suit the tray and includes a pocket into which the tray slips freely as shown. This provides the liner for the tray and is convenient to use.

Fig. 141. Typical dressing tray. Instruments are not harmed when handled in this manner, but for effective sterilization the jointed instruments must not be locked.

PREPARATION AND STERILIZATION OF TREATMENT TRAYS

The preparation and sterilization of treatment trays is normally a function of central supply service. In certain hospitals it is not unusual to find a total of 40 to 50 different trays carried in stock in varying quantities. Other hospitals, where the requirements have been carefully studied with the aim of eliminating unnecessary work without the sacrifice of any important article, require only about half that number of trays. The suggestion is

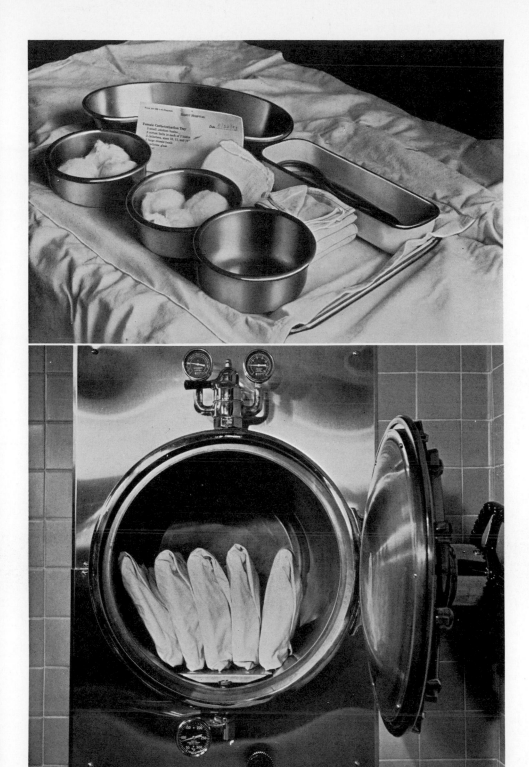

Fig. 142. Female catheterization tray. The catheters should be flushed with distilled water just before wrapping. The tray should be placed on edge in the sterilizer, never right side up, since in that position air would be trapped in the basins.

Fig. 143. Correct method of loading trays in the sterilizer. All are resting on edge, with no interference from other packs or supplies.

made, therefore, that the actual requirements be studied on the basis of elimination of those trays in which the contents are so similar to others that possibly certain ones can be combined and still serve the needs adequately.

Wherever possible, shallow trays similar to the one shown in Figures 140 and 141 should be used. The purpose of the shallow tray is to minimize the hazard in sterilization in the event that it is carelessly loaded in the sterilizer. If a deep tray is placed in the sterilizer right side up, air will be trapped in it and the sterilizing process will be ineffective. A shallow tray largely eliminates this hazard, merely because it is shallow and can trap very little air. Similarly, if the tray includes any vessel such as a medicine glass or Kelly flask, as shown in Figure 69, the arrangement should be such that when the tray is placed in the sterilizer, any water that might be contained in the vessel would all drain out. If this is done the air in the vessel will gravitate from it and steam will promptly take its place. Otherwise, as with the deep tray resting right side up in the sterilizer, the air will be trapped within and sterilization will be ineffective. The assembling of trays is greatly facilitated by keeping on file a photograph of each type of tray, plus a list of items on the tray. The 6 x 8 inch cards may be used for listing the items and also for giving specific instructions for processing each item.

When rubber tubing is included in the tray contents, care must be used to avoid contact with other materials, such as glassware and instruments. During the process of sterilization used tubing will frequently stick to these surfaces. Just before wrapping, the tubing and its attachments must be flushed with freshly distilled water and the interior surfaces left moist. This also applies to catheters (Figure 142). Avoid kinks in the tubing because they are harmful to rubber and make sterilization difficult. Wrapping of the trays can be greatly simplified by preparing covers of suitable size, as shown in Figure 140. The tray slides into the pocket provided and eliminates the need for any other liner over the tray. The correct method of loading trays in the sterilizer is shown in Figure 143. All are resting on edge, with no interference from any surrounding packs or supplies. Effective sterilization calls for 30 minutes exposure to saturated steam at 250° F., followed by 15 minutes drying.

LENGTH OF TIME SUPPLIES MAY BE CONSIDERED TO REMAIN STERILE

The data reported in the literature on this subject is indeed scanty. It is known that protection against contamination of sterile wrapped supplies is largely dependent upon the porosity of the wrapper and the method of wrapping. The most serious aspect of contamination is that due to insects and vermin (ants, roaches and silverfish), which may gain access to the interior of a package through the folds of the wrapper. In general, the storage areas for sterile supplies in hospitals can be depended upon to be free of insects and vermin. In the tropics the problem of insect control may be more difficult, and occasionally it has been found necessary to institute rather elaborate methods, such as specially designed containers, to protect the supplies against insect contamination.

Aside from the problem of insect contamination, there is a possibility, however remote it may seem, of bacteria eventually penetrating the muslin or paper barrier. Just when this will occur or under what conditions is difficult to determine in hospital practice. Changes in atmospheric conditions surrounding the packages, handling the packages so as to force air in and out, are contributing factors to possible contamination. In the author's laboratory studies have been made to determine how long syringes and needles will remain sterile when wrapped in muslin as compared to packaging in paper bags and then held in clean storage. The results indicated that bacterial contamination does not gain access to syringes or needles packaged in either muslin or paper bags for at least four weeks. Certainly under normal conditions of clean storage supplies properly wrapped in double thickness muslin, comprising four layers, can be depended upon to remain sterile for at least four weeks. There is no need to resterilize supplies at the end of one week or even two weeks' storage. Beyond this period most articles will have been issued for use.

REFERENCES

1. "Preliminary Report of a Survey and Study of Surgical Dressings and Materials," Research and Information Dept. *Am. Coll. Surgeons,* Oct., 1928.
2. UNDERWOOD, W. B.: Notes on the Planning and Organization of the Central Sterile Supply, *The Surgical Supervisor,* Vol. 4, Sept., 1944.
3. UNDERWOOD, W. B.: More About That Central Sterile Supply, *The Surgical Supervisor,* Vol. 5, Nov., 1945.
4. SCHAFER, M. K.: Central Supply—Economy and Efficiency. *Hospital Topics, 30:27-30,* April, 1952.
5. ROSENBERGER, D. M.: Administrative and Communication Factors of Central Sterile Supply, Paper delivered before Institute on Development of Hospital Plans. *Am. Hosp. A.,* New York City, Feb. 13, 1952.

CHAPTER XVII

The Rectangular (Bulk Supply) Sterilizer

THE RECTANGULAR bulk supply sterilizers are used extensively in hospitals for sterilization of heavy loads of supplies, in laboratories for sterilization of apparatus, including animal cages, and in industry for sterilization of surgical dressings and various proprietary products. For many years bulk sterilizers were piped to carry the full steam supply line pressure in the jackets, pressure ranging from 40 to 60 pounds or higher. With this method of piping, a reducing valve was supplied, by means of which the high jacket pressure could be reduced automatically to the common sterilizing range of 15 to 20 pounds for the chamber. It was formerly thought that the high jacket pressure was of special value in the drying of materials. Later it was found that the increased pressure serves no useful purpose. In fact, it is definitely harmful, because it develops a high degree of superheat in the chamber which is injurious to fabrics and other materials. The superheating of steam detracts from its microbicidal properties because it dries out the steam—reduces its moisture content. Internal temperatures in such sterilizers may range as high as 280° to 300° F., while the chamber pressure is only 15 to 20 pounds, which should develop a temperature no greater than 250°-259° F. For this reason, bulk type sterilizers have occasionally been criticized because of the destructive effect on fabrics, mattresses, etc.

The modern rectangular surgical supply and bulk type sterilizers have controlled jacket pressure of 15-17 pounds, which develops adequate sterilizing temperature of 250°-254° F., and no superheat is produced by the jacket. The details of construction, piping and valving for a typical bulk sterilizer are shown in Figure 144. All pressure sterilizers should be designed, constructed and stamped to meet the requirements of the "Unfired Pressure Vessel Code" of the American Society of Mechanical Engineers. This assures the purchaser that the equipment meets acceptable standards of safety.

One of the most uneconomical practices the hospital can indulge in is the selection of sterilizers of small capacity, or perhaps several units of small size rather than one or two large sterilizers. This handicaps the central supply department especially, because with limited capacity the personnel may be unable to conscientiously sterilize the full quota of supplies within the working hours. Every hospital should have one or two large sterilizers with sufficient capacity so that 75% of the bulk supplies required daily can be sterilized in three or four loads. There is also a limit in size and capacity of sterilizers for hospital use. The very large chambers with dimensions of 36 x 42 x 84 inches (75 cubic feet) and greater are cumbersome from the standpoint of loading and unloading. Nurses also experience difficulty in the opening and closing of the large doors. The most desirable sizes of sterilizers for routine hospital use, particularly in central supply, are those with dimensions of 24 x 36 x 48 inches (24 cubic feet) and 24 x 36 x 60 inches (30 cubic feet). Adequate capacity, ease of loading, economy of operation and reduction of labor are the essential factors in determining sterilizer sizes.

DISINFECTION OF MATTRESSES, BEDDING AND CLOTHING

There is a need for disinfection of mattresses, bedding and clothing in communicable disease units, psychiatric hospitals and penal institutions. As a rule, the organisms responsible for communicable diseases are rather easily destroyed. The usual sanitization processes of boiling and laundering appear to be adequate for terminal disinfection of blankets and linens. However, these methods are not considered practical for the treatment of mattresses and pillows. Also, when these materials become infested with parasites associated with pediculosis or scabies effective methods of control must be enforced. Steam under pressure has been widely used for the disinfection and sterilization of mattresses for many years, but not without difficulty. Oversterilization and extreme carelessness in handling have been responsible for the ruination of many mattresses in institutions. If the disinfection process is to be successful and the materials preserved, then an efficient method of handling must be devised, the operator must be properly trained and someone in authority should supervise the work. Only under these conditions can reasonably satisfactory results be obtained.

The mattress disinfector should be of the correct size for efficient loading. Chambers with dimensions of 42 x 48 x 84 inches and 48 x 54 x 84 inches are suitable for the reception of the commonly used mattresses when resting on horizontal shelves, as in Figure 145. Do not place more than one mattress on each shelf because stacking of mattresses together will seriously interfere with steam penetration and drying. Bedding should be rolled in loose bundles, the materials from one bed only in each bundle. These can be wrapped in one of the sheets from the bed. Clothing should be placed loosely in fish-netting bags. When loaded in the sterilizer, the bundles must be restricted to no more than one layer deep. Using the shelf-type carriage, alternate shelves can be removed to give sufficient space.

Lower temperatures are utilized for disinfection than are required for sterilization. The regulator valve controlling steam to the sterilizer should be adjusted to provide pressure at 4 to 6 pounds, no higher. This should produce a maximum temperature in the chamber of 220° to 230° F. (104°-110° C.). An exposure period of 30 minutes is required at this temperature. At the end of the exposure period, the steam is exhausted from the chamber and a partial vacuum created in the chamber either by means of a steam

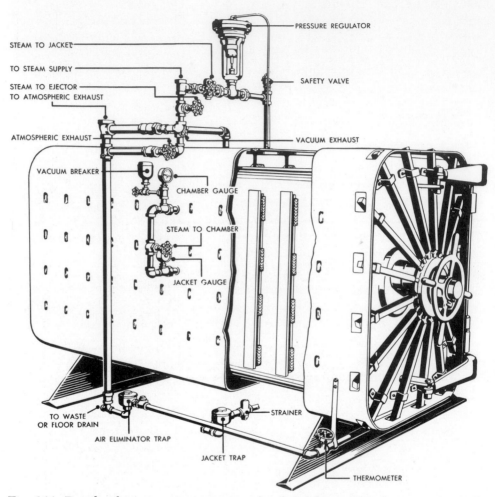

Fig. 144. Details of construction, piping and valving for a typical rectangular bulk sterilizer.

ejector or a vacuum pump. When the chamber gauge shows about 20 inches of vacuum, the vacuum breaker valve should be opened, leaving the ejector and chamber exhaust valves open also. This will admit room air into the chamber for entrainment with the remaining vapor and odors, which will then be exhausted to the atmosphere. This aerating and drying process should be continued for at least 15 minutes, after which the load may be removed from the chamber. If a large amount of vapor or odor escapes into the room when the door is opened, that will indicate that the drying process

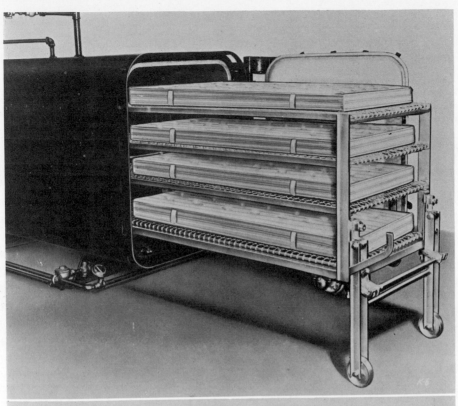

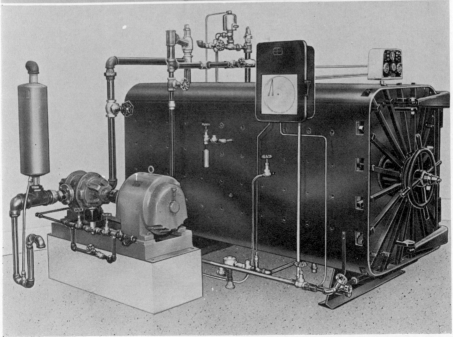

Fig. 145. Mattress disinfector with drop wheel loading car.

Fig. 146. Rectangular bulk sterilizer and vacuum pump for commercial sterilization of packaged dressings, cotton, etc.

should have been continued for a longer period. Do not permit mattresses, bedding or clothing to remain in the chamber following the disinfection process, unless the door is wide open. Otherwise, wet materials may be expected. Preferably remove the load to ventilated shelving to avoid sweating.

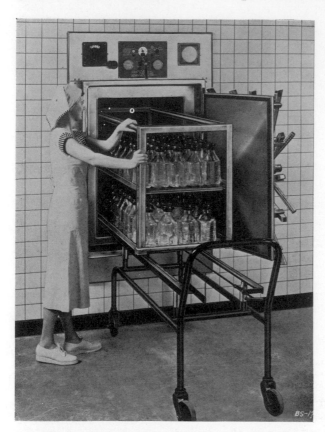

Fig. 146A. One of the latest developments in rectangular sterilizer design. The corrosion resistant nickel clad steel of the chamber interior is welded to the solid Monel metal end ring. The instruments and controls are flush mounted in the finishing panel. This type of sterilizer for recessed installation functions ideally in the sterilization of bulk loads of fabrics or solutions.

Under the most efficient method of operation, the disinfection of mattresses by steam leaves much to be desired. The process is not satisfactory for the treatment of innerspring mattresses because of the problem of corrosion. It also has an adverse effect upon foam rubber mattresses or materials. Repeated disinfection will result in discoloration, hardening, loss of elasticity and tensile strength. Hair and feathers commonly used in mattresses and pillows are subject to hydrolytic decomposition by steam which releases active sulfur-containing substances. These substances have a particular affinity for the metallic surfaces of the chamber and the loading carriage, resulting in the accumulation of a dark, greasy deposit. A newer process for "cold" disinfection of mattresses, bedding and clothing utilizing ethylene oxide gas in the form of "Carboxide" shows promise of being a superior method.

COMMERCIAL STERILIZATION

The problem in commercial sterilization of packaged dressings, cotton, etc. is to permeate bulk loads of material with moist steam, carefully avoiding too much moisture, and to accomplish sterilization in an economical period of exposure. The process invariably requires an efficient vacuum pump, one capable of producing not less than 26-28 inches (mercury) vacuum in the sterilizer in a brief period (Fig. 146). This method of air discharge from the sterilizer is used in preference to the gravity process because of its speed and efficiency. The larger bulk sterilizers usually have two drain outlets from the bottom of the chamber, each individually fitted with a thermostatic trap to facilitate rapid drainage. Provision is also made for a by-pass around the pressure control valve to the jacket by means of which the delivery of steam to the chamber can be considerably expedited. The method of operation is as follows:

First the steam is admitted to the jacket until the pressure becomes stable at 15-17 pounds. Then the vacuum pump is turned on to create an initial vacuum of 26-28 inches in the chamber. Steam is then admitted to the chamber for a brief period of what is termed "preheating." This continues for about 15 minutes during which the load is heated to about 212° F. The vacuum pump is turned on again to discharge the initial (preheating) steam and to draw out the excess moisture deposited on the goods, but leaving them hot. The actual sterilizing steam is then admitted to the chamber, and since the materials are essentially dry and hot, very little additional moisture is deposited. Exposure for 30 minutes to a temperature of 250° F. then follows, after which a final vacuum is drawn to dry the load. Aeration of the chamber is accomplished by opening a vacuum breaker valve containing an air filter and the load is then removed from the chamber sufficiently dry for immediate storage. The refinements of the system usually cause very little distortion of cartons or discoloration of labels.

Apparently some commercial processes for sterilization of packaged market cotton are not always as effective as they should be. Silliker and Hess[1] found 14 samples of market cotton, labeled "contents sterile until package is opened," out of 415 samples taken to contain viable organisms. This represents a rather small percentage of contamination which could have escaped standard control measures. However, the conclusion was drawn that the cotton itself was the source of the bacteria.

REFERENCE

1. SILLIKER, J. H. AND HESS, E. P.: Sterility of Market Cotton. *J.A.M.A.*, *149*:1374-1376, 1952.

Chapter XVIII

Preparation of Parenteral Solutions

THE SUBJECT of parenteral therapy is of the utmost importance to clinicians and hospitals. The word "parenteral" is derived from the Greek, meaning "other than the intestinal tract."[1] In normal usage the term parenteral therapy is applied to the method of administering fluids through veins. The purposes of parenteral therapy are to maintain or replace body stores of water, electrolytes, calories, vitamins, and protein; to restore acid-base balance; and to restore blood volume. Safe intravenous solutions are, therefore, required to achieve these purposes and to meet the individual needs of each patient.

There are two courses available to hospitals to meet the widespread demand for safe parenteral solutions. The institution may purchase the commercially prepared products or it may manufacture its own solutions. The latter method is particularly attractive because the economics of hospital manufacture results in a marked savings for the institution. Many hospitals currently prepare their own solutions and there is a steadily increasing body of evidence to show that these solutions are safe, economical and practical.[2, 3, 4, 5] Other hospitals are also desirous of reducing costs of solutions used in parenteral therapy, but they are reluctant to undertake the manufacturing program because of fear of untoward allergic or febrile reactions. This fear complex is founded largely upon unsatisfactory past experiences in certain hospitals where the solutions were prepared under conditions believed to be safe and practical at the time. It is now known that these past failures to produce satisfactory solutions were almost invariably due to inadequate cleaning facilities, lack of control on quality of distilled water, improvised equipment, and lack of skilled supervision.

The preparation of chemically pure, sterile, and pyrogen-free solutions is not a difficult matter, providing the materials used in manufacturing are of high purity, and if the personnel responsible for cleaning of the apparatus are thoroughly reliable. A dependable system for hospital-made solutions comprises the following major elements:

1) *Proper Planning of the Solution Room:* Adequate space should be provided in a room designed specifically for this purpose. It may be located as a part of or adjacent to the Pharmacy or in the Central Service Department. (See Figs. 147 and 148.)

2) *Adequate Cleaning Facilities:* Efficient methods must be used for the cleaning of all apparatus, bottles and closures entering into the manufacture of solutions.

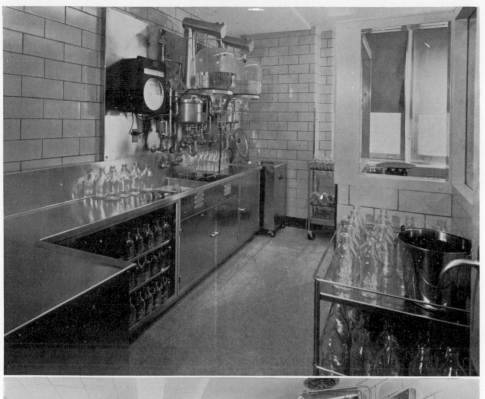

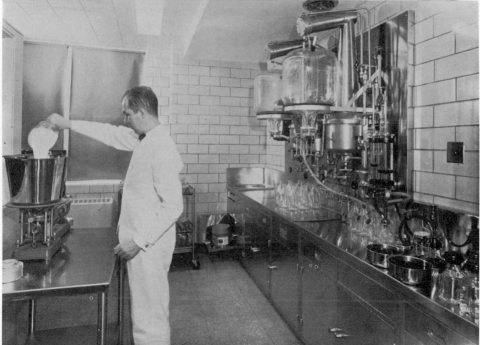

Courtesy The Reading Hospital, Reading, Pa.

Fig. 147. Intravenous and external solution equipment clean-up room.

Fig. 148. Intravenous and external solution preparation room.

3) *Purity of Distilled Water:* A source of high purity, pyrogen-free distillate is essential. Water stills should be equipped with conductivity recorders for a continuous check on the purity of the distillate.

4) *Purity of Chemicals:* All chemicals used in making the solutions must be of high purity and free from pyrogenic substances.

5) *Disposable Intravenous Administration Sets:* It is no longer considered safe or practical for the hospital to employ reusable intravenous sets. The availability of disposable commercial sets which are sterile, non-toxic and pyrogen-free is an added incentive to the hospital-made solution program.

6) *Needle Cleaning Facilities:* Chemical cleanliness of needles is essential for safe, reactionless infusions.

7) *Skilled Supervision:* Centralized responsibility for the preparation of solutions should be delegated to the hospital pharmacist or the pathologist.

PYROGENS

Familiarity with the basic facts concerning pyrogens is essential to the successful preparation and handling of parenteral solutions. The term "pyrogen" means "fever-producing." Although the chemical composition of pyrogens has not been definitely established, the latest evidence suggests that they are complex polysaccharides apparently attached to another radical containing nitrogen and phosphorus.[6, 7] It is generally accepted that pyrogens are by-products of bacterial growth or metabolism. They may be closely related chemically to bacterial antigens.[8] It is known that pyrogens occur only in media which have been contaminated with bacteria. Many species of bacteria, including air-borne contaminants, yeasts and molds, produce pyrogens.[9] They have been shown to be of a particulate nature, larger than 50 millimicrons, but smaller than 1 micron.[10]

The concept of a pyrogenic substance produced by bacteria was established by Seibert,[11] who showed that the substances designated "pyrogens" were products of bacilli usually found in river water. Rademaker[12] also found them in varying numbers in tap water in numerous cities, their number varying with the seasons. Pyrogens are extremely soluble in water and they cannot be removed by passage through a Berkefeld filter. They may, however, be removed by adsorption on an activated asbestos filter or on activated charcoal.[13, 14, 10, 15] Pyrogens cannot be destroyed by autoclaving except at very high temperatures for a prolonged period of time. Banks,[16] for example, found that pyrogenic water was rendered innocuous by heating to a temperature of 284° F. (140° C.) for 30 minutes. Sterilization is of no practical value in removing pyrogen from solutions intended for parenteral administration. According to Wylie and Todd,[17] the ordinary process of sterilization by autoclaving at 240° F. (116° C.) for 30 minutes will destroy about 25 per cent of the pyrogenic activity of a concentrated solution, yet this process will have little effect on a dilute solution such as might arise from accidental contamination of water.

One major source of pyrogens is distilled water which has become contaminated with air-borne pyrogenic bacteria. A poorly designed water still or one that is operated incorrectly may also produce distillate containing pyrogenic substances. Although pyrogens are non-volatile, they are still capable of passing through the ordinary distillation process by means of entrainment or carry-over with mineral impurities to the distillate. Tap water is the usual source of contamination, and any glassware or tubing rinsed or washed in tap water will produce pyrogen unless sterilized within an hour. Rademaker[18] found that pyrogen can be developed within two hours at room temperature in the drying films of moisture remaining in such tubing and equipment. Similarly, a sufficient amount of pyrogen can be formed within an intravenous needle rinsed in tap water to produce a reaction.

A pyrogenic or febrile reaction may occur any time from 15 minutes to 8 hours following the injection of a solution containing pyrogenic substances. Such reactions from intravenous solutions occur in hospitals even though the means to eliminate them entirely are well known. In the opinion of certain authorities,[19, 4] these reactions are inexcusable in the light of present day knowledge. The precautions necessary for the prevention of reactions in routine parenteral therapy are:

1) Use only freshly distilled water from an efficient still in the preparation of solutions and for the rinsing of all apparatus.

2) Provide for intelligent and reliable operation of the water still. Discard the first fraction of distillate at the beginning of each day's operation. Frequent cleaning of the water still at regular intervals is necessary.

3) Prepare solutions and sterilize the final products within a few hours after the water has been distilled.

4) Immediately sterilize all tubing, needles and glassware after rinsing with distilled water to prevent production of pyrogens in residual moisture films.

5) If nondisposable intravenous sets are used, permit 50 to 100 ml. of pyrogen-free solution to be run through the set and wasted, before inserting the needle into the vein.

WATER STILLS

Modern usage of the term "distilled water" signifies a process involving evaporation of raw water by boiling, followed by immediate condensation of the liberated steam or water vapor. The quality or purity of the condensate produced by this process can vary greatly and still conform to the basic characteristics of distilled water. If the distilled water is to be used in critical applications demanding unusual quality, such as for the preparation of injectables or intravenous infusions, it must be substantially free from impurities of a mineral, metallic or organic nature and, above all, free from pyrogenic substances. Of the methods currently available for the preparation of low residue water, that of distillation when carried out in a properly designed and correctly operated still stands unequalled as the best method for producing pyrogen-free water of the highest purity. Evidence confirming the superiority of the distillation process is not always easily

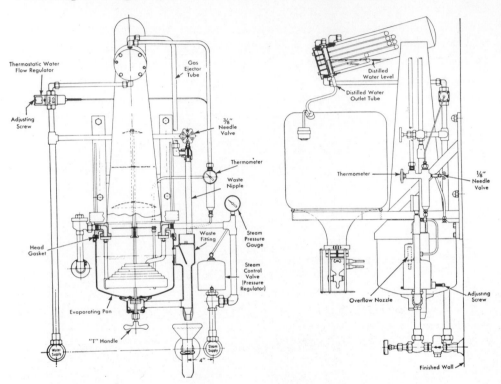

Fig. 149. Sectional view of water still designed for the production of pyrogen-free distillate, 10 gallons per hour capacity.

Fig. 150. Side view of still with storage carboy mounted directly in front.

obtainable because of the mediocre performance of the average water still.

The principle upon which all water stills operate is essentially the same. The source of heat may be either steam, electricity or gas, depending upon the type of still. The larger capacity stills ranging from 5 to 50 gallons per hour output are usually heated by steam, while those of small capacity from 1 to 5 gallons per hour are usually heated by electricity. The basic parts of the still consist of an evaporator pan or boiler, a medium of heating, a vapor tower, and a condenser. In operation, the raw water is fed into the evaporating pan where it is heated and converted into steam (see Figs. 149 and 150). The steam rises in the vapor tower where it contacts a series of baffle plates, the purpose of which is to eliminate entrainment of droplets of spray or foam from the rising steam. After passing the baffle plates, the dry steam continues upward to the condenser where it contacts a cooling coil, is condensed into water, and finally flows by gravity to the collecting vessel or storage bottle.

The mechanical design features of any still will largely determine its efficiency in producing distillate of high purity. The cross-sectional area or diameter of the evaporating pan is an important factor. The larger the

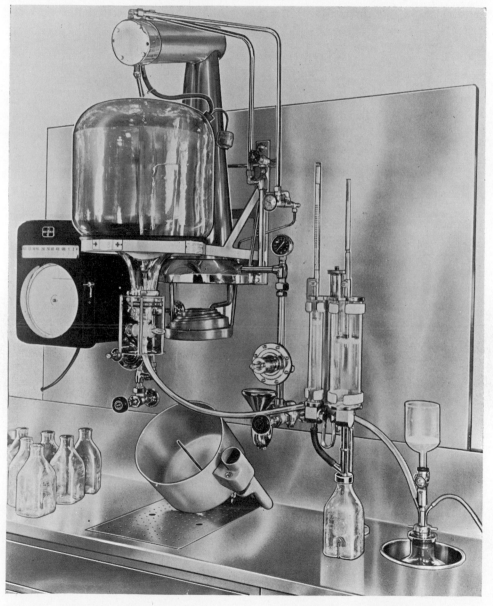

Fig. 151. Still with evaporator pan removed and steam coil exposed for daily cleaning.

water area in the evaporator pan with generous allowance for steam space above the water surface, the less opportunity there is for violent boiling. When the water boils violently there is proportionately more carry-over of non-volatile substances than when the water is subjected to moderate controlled boiling. In addition, the evaporator pan should be easily removable without the use of tools, within convenient reach of the operator, to facilitate daily cleaning of the pan and heating coil, as in Figure 151.

The height of the vapor tower is another important factor in the design of the still. This determines the disengaging distance between the water level in the evaporating pan and the condenser. It has a direct bearing on the amount of entrainment or possible carry-over of droplets of raw water into the condenser. The vapor tower should also be of wide cross-section so that the velocity of the steam can be maintained at a low level, thereby discouraging entrainment. The 30-inch rise of the vapor tower on the 10 gallons per hour still shown in Figure 149, including the proper placement of baffles, insures optimum conditions for the prevention or removal of entrained spray or foam from the steam.

One of the most difficult problems to cope with in any water still is the removal of released gases from the condenser. Unless some positive and efficient means is incorporated on the still to promptly remove liberated gases ascending from the evaporator, such as carbon dioxide, chlorine, ammonia, etc., it is difficult to prevent their reabsorption into the distillate. When this occurs in the average still the purity of the distilled water is markedly lowered as can be demonstrated by means of the conductivity meter. If these foreign gases are forcefully and continuously ejected from the condenser a water of higher purity is obtained. Most water stills depend on a slight emission of steam vapor from the condenser to force ejection of the foreign gases and to visibly indicate that the gases are not stratified in the condenser. A more efficient method is the installation of a controlled jet evacuator, which introduces a slight negative pressure on the condenser, thereby assuring automatic removal of the gases as rapidly as they collect in the condenser.

All water stills should be equipped with a deconcentrator or bleeder device on the evaporating pan to permit continuous formation of steam from a flowing stream of water. This prevents concentration of impurities, which in the case of hard water, may produce excessive foaming with resulting entrainment of droplets to the distillate. Stills should also be provided with automatic regulating valves on both water and steam lines to prevent priming or surges in boiling, and to maintain the correct balance between water supply to evaporator and the rate of heating.

The metals used in the construction of a still also influence the quality of distillate. Monel, nickel, aluminum, copper and brass are the commonly used metals. Copper and brass should be plated with pure block tin if it is anticipated that these metals will come in contact with the distillate. A still fabricated of corrosion-resistant monel metal with nickel condensing coil probably represents the most satisfactory combination. Aluminum is not a suitable material for fabrication of the evaporating pan because of its susceptibility to attack by alkaline water.

The selection of suitable tubing for the transmission of distilled water from the source to various locations frequently poses a problem. Block tin tubing has long been recognized as a satisfactory material for this purpose because of its low solubility characteristics. Stainless steel (316) tubing may also be used with a fair degree of certainty that the distilled water will not become seriously contaminated with metallic substances. Aluminum pipe or tubing has likewise been used successfully for the transmission of distilled water. However, small amounts of aluminum will be dissolved in the water until a substantial aluminum oxide coating has formed on the interior of the tubing and fittings. The product known as "Uscolite," a rigid plastic pipe, is probably as safe as any available material for the transmission of distilled water. It is insoluble in water and can be threaded to accommodate fittings in much the same manner as ordinary pipe.

OPERATION AND MAINTENANCE OF WATER STILLS

The water still must be kept clean. This point has been recognized by authorities for years, but too frequently stills are put into service and operated for long periods of time with no cleaning of the interior parts until something goes drastically wrong. Practice has clearly demonstrated that the distillate from a single effect still of good design is entirely suitable for parenteral solutions when, but only when, the still is clean. Frequent cleaning is a fundamental requirement in the operation of any still. The frequency of cleaning will depend upon the quality of the raw water supply.

When parenteral solutions first came into extensive use, serious difficulties were experienced with distillate collected from inefficient or foul stills. In an effort to solve the problem, double or triple stills were widely advocated, users forgetting that while double or triple distillation might postpone the day, that ultimately these stills would also become foul and their product unfit for use. Cleaning double or triple stills involves twice or three times the labor, expense and delay needed for cleaning a single effect still. Any still in continuous service will become increasingly foul until, regardless of all the protective baffles and intricate passageways with mysterious names, the product becomes unfit for use. Ultra refinements in the performance of a clean still are not significant. The intent should be to provide an apparatus instead which will produce initially water of satisfactory purity, with the all-important provision of means for maintaining that quality by easy daily cleaning.

The still shown in Figure 149 has been designed specifically for production of distillate for parenteral fluids. Repeated tests in various laboratories have shown the distillate to be pyrogen-free, with the average purity ranging from 400,000 to 800,000 specific ohms resistance. Interior parts of the still are easily accessible for inspection and cleaning, without the use of tools. The evaporating pan is attached to the body of the still, or detached, by loosening the tee handle and then applying a twisting motion which actuates a bayonet joint. This pan should be removed daily for thorough rinsing, to remove sludge and scale. Hard scale adhering to the steam coil will slow down the performance and cause the still to produce less than its rated capacity. When the coil becomes badly coated, it should be disconnected and a clean (spare) coil put in its place. The coated coil can then be treated with a dilute (5%) hydrochloric acid solution to remove the scale, after which it is retained as a spare. When handled in this manner no great delay occurs as the result of the cleaning process.

PURITY OF DISTILLED WATER

All distilled water entering into the production of parenteral or intravenous solutions must be pyrogen-free and meet the requirements of the Pyrogen Test, as outlined in the Pharmacopoeia of the United States. The water must also contain no more than 10 parts of total dissolved solids per million parts of water. To meet these requirements a continuous and accurate check on the purity of the distillate is required. The simplest over-all check on the quality of distilled water is the measurement of specific conductance. Electrolytic or solution conductivity is a measure of the ability of a solution to carry an electric current. Specific conductance is defined as the reciprocal of the resistance in ohms of a 1-cm. cube of the liquid at a specified temperature. The unit of specific conductance is the reciprocal ohm or mho. Since this is a very large value of electrolytic conductivity, the practical unit commonly employed is 1 millionth of a mho or 1 micromho. In practice, conductance measurements are usually made in terms of resistance since resistance is the reciprocal of conductance. Resistance is measured in ohms, and the term "specific resistance" is, therefore, ohms per centimeter cube.

Aqueous solutions of acids, alkalies and salts have high conductivity because these chemicals, when dissolved in water, dissociate into positively and negatively charged ions which carry electrical current as they migrate through the solvent. In the process of distillation or deionization, there is a reduction in the number of ions both positive and negative in the water resulting in poorer conductivity or, the reverse, higher resistance. The relationship of parts per million of sodium chloride in solution to specific resistance and specific conductance is as follows:

P.P.M. Sodium Chloride	Specific Resistance in Ohms (18° C.)	Specific Conductance in Micromhos (18° C.)
0.1	1,010,000	0.99
0.5	578,000	1.73
1.0	377,400	2.65
2.0	222,200	4.50
3.0	157,500	6.35
4.0	122,000	8.20
5.0	99,500	10.05
6.0	84,000	11.90
7.0	72,700	13.75
8.0	64,100	15.60
9.0	57,300	17.45
10.0	51,800	19.30

Absolutely pure water would have a conductance of about 0.05 micromhos or 20,000,000 specific ohms resistance at 25° C. Water of this purity cannot be produced by the distillation process but it has been obtained by the deionization process. Actually, the production of 20, 10 or even 5 million ohms water is chiefly of academic interest, since water exceeding 1 million ohms is of adequate purity for almost every application. It is obviously not difficult to meet the requirements of the Pharmacopoeia for distilled water with total dissolved solids of less than 10 parts per million. In terms of ionizable solids this would mean a distillate of approximately 50,000 ohms resistance. Almost any still, even one that is carelessly operated, will produce distillate of this purity. The problem is to provide assurance that the water shall be pyrogen-free. To measure conductance or resistance in terms of specific ohms is a direct function of the quantity of electrolytes or ionizable impurities present in the water. Admittedly this does not constitute a direct measurement of pyrogenic content, but it should be understood that pyrogens are nonvolatile and their presence in freshly distilled water is proportional to the amount of entrainment or carry-over of droplets of raw water from the evaporating pan of the still. Therefore, measurement of the ionizable (mineral) impurities by means of the conductivity meter affords a continuous check on the performance of the still and also a reliable indication of the possibility of pyrogen contamination.

A convenient and accurate method for determining the purity of distilled water is shown in Figure 152. The recording conductivity meter is attached to the wall, adjacent to the still. The conductivity cell with self-contained thermistor (automatic temperature compensator) is sealed into the draw-off cock of the Pyrex glass storage bottle. This feature assures the operator of known purity of the distillate at the point of use. When water is drawn from the bottle, it passes through the conductivity cell, and the specific resistance is indicated on a 10-inch horizontal scale located at the top of the conductivity meter. The resistance is also recorded on the 12-inch circular chart which rotates once each 24 hours.

Distilled water acceptable for use in preparation of parenteral solutions should have a purity equal to or better than the following characteristics:

Resistance (specific ohms) 500,000
Specific conductance (micromhos) 2.0
pH 5.7-6.0
Residue after evaporation (1 hr. @ 105° C.) .... 1.0 p.p.m.
Chloride (Cl) .... 0.1 p.p.m.
Ammonia (NH₃) .... 0.1 p.p.m.
Heavy metals (as Pb) .... 0.01 p.p.m.

As a general rule, it is advisable to reject all distilled water which gives a reading of 250,000 specific ohms or less on the conductivity instrument. This is equivalent to about 2 parts per million of electrolytes.

The reaction of ordinary distilled water is always acid, because of the absorption of carbon dioxide. Water which has taken up carbon dioxide from the air until equilibrium has been established, will contain about 0.03 per cent of carbon dioxide by volume, and the calculated pH should be 5.7. In fact, this is the value usually found in distilled water which has been freely exposed to the air. Water from an efficient still, collected and stored in closed, nonsoluble glass containers, will usually have a pH of 6.0 to 6.4.

CHEMICALS

All chemicals used in the preparation of parenteral solutions must be of a high degree of chemical purity and free from pyrogenic substances. The standard of purity of each chemical should conform to the requirements of the U.S. Pharmacopoeia, or preferably the American Chemical Society Specifications for Reagent Chemicals. Wherever possible, the chemicals should be purchased on a tested, pyrogen-free and known chemical assay basis in pre-weighed quantities, protected against contamination in well closed containers. The acceptance of any particular lot of chemical also depends upon the quantity of foreign matter present. Excessive dust or dirt is evidence of careless handling prior to packaging and sufficient cause for rejection. The presence of foreign particles such as parts of insects indicates serious contamination.

Only the highest purity dextrose should be used for the preparation of solutions. Certain lots of dextrose may contain acid dehydration products or protein split products formed by side reactions during the course of manufacture. These impurities may give rise to a yellow color, often mistaken for caramelization, upon sterilization of the dextrose solutions. They may also lead to the formation of white, flocculent precipitates in the final solutions.[4]

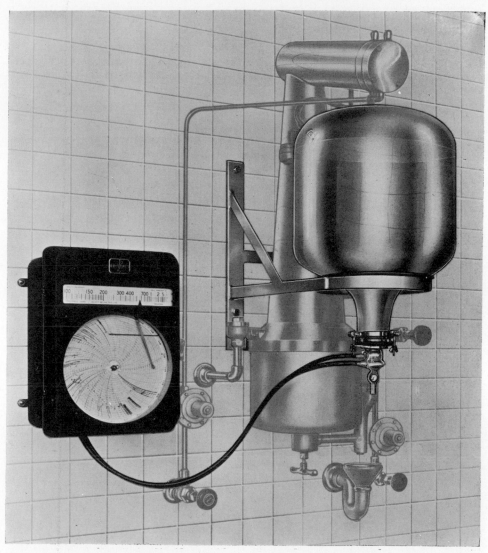

Fig. 152. Recording conductivity meter and storage carboy. The conductivity cell is sealed into the draw-off cock of the glass storage carboy.

GLASS CONTAINERS

The solution containers should be made of non-soluble, borosilicate, heat-resistant glass. Pyrex (Corning) glass has been found most satisfactory for this purpose. Its low expansion coefficient minimizes breakage due to thermal shock, its physical hardness resists breakage due to careless handling, and its chemical stability resists hydrolysis by the solutions when subjected to repeated use. The containers should be designed for heavy, thick-wall fabrication so as to withstand repeated use, moderately rough

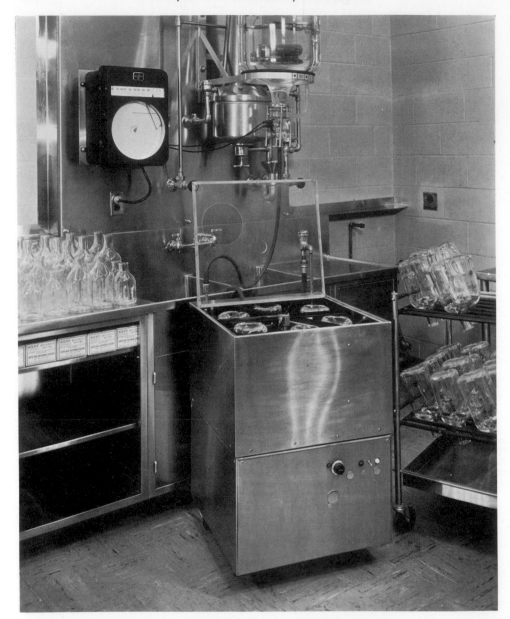

Fig. 153. Automatic flask washer and rinser. This unit has an index drive mechanism with 6 stations: loading, tap water rinse, two wash stations, tap water rinse and final distilled water rinse. Accommodates flasks from 75 ml. to 2000 ml. capacity. It will clean about 360 flasks per hour. Washing action is accomplished by forced jets, operated from a centrifugal pump. An automatic detergent dispenser is built into the chamber.

handling, and both positive and negative pressures created during the sterilization and cooling process. All surfaces must be smooth and free from depressions or crevices which would hinder thorough cleaning.

Solution flasks of square design, as shown in Figure 154, offer several advantages over the round or pear-shaped types. The square shape provides an almost flat contact surface between flasks when placed side by side, thus avoiding pressure cracks or fractures when the flasks are forcibly bumped against each other. The square shape also permits a greater number of flasks to be sterilized per load and requires less storage space in shelf area following sterilization.

The thorough cleaning of flasks and all other items of glassware is essential to the successful preparation of safe solutions. The cleaning process should be conducted as follows:

1) Rinse each flask with tap water to remove any residue of solution.

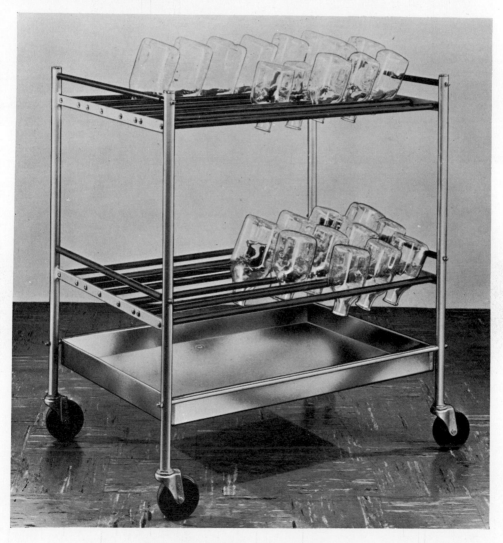

Fig. 154. Portable flask drain carriage.

2) Wash in solution of 0.5 per cent Calgonite or other equally effective detergent in distilled water. Rinse three times with freshly distilled water. (The use of an automatic flask washer and rinser as shown in Fig. 153 provides a more efficient method of cleaning.)

3) Inspect each flask for "water breaks." The interior should be crystal

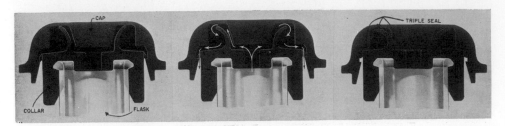

Fig. 155. Automatic sealing closure. This shows position of cap on collar before sterilization.

Fig. 156. Position of cap on collar showing pathway for escape of air from flask when 1½ pounds pressure has developed in flask during sterilization.

Fig. 157. Position of cap automatically sealed on collar by vacuum after solution has been sterilized.

clear with no spots in the film of distilled water left on the glass after the final rinsing.

4) Invert on portable flask drain cart for draining, as in Figure 154.

5) The flasks should be filled with solution as promptly as possible after washing. If they are permitted to stand for several hours before filling, the final rinsing process with freshly distilled water must be repeated.

FLASK CLOSURE

An automatic self-sealing closure should be used on all parenteral solution flasks. The combination closure consisting of collar and cap when applied to the glass container must provide safe storage of the sterilized solution under hermetically sealed conditions. The collar should be of molded, nontoxic, heat-resistant neoprene or equal which retains its resiliency after repeated sterilization. It should not become tacky nor should it stick to either the container or the cap. The cap should be fabricated from a heat-resistant plastic, such as Durez, with smooth surfaces accurately formed to fit perfectly and securely over the top and flanged edge of the companion collar. All collars and caps must be free of easily detached fragments or particles of neoprene or plastic.

A typical example of one kind of self-sealing closure is shown in Figures 155, 156 and 157. Figure 155 illustrates the collar in position on the flask with the cap engaged. The cap locks on the collar and it will not fall off when the flask is moved about. The lip of the collar is slightly compressed by the cap when in proper position, thus sealing out possible airborne contamination.

Figure 156 shows the position of the cap and collar during sterilization. Due to the rise in temperature and pressure during sterilization, the liquid and air in the flask expand and when an internal pressure of 1½ pounds is reached the seal between the lip of the collar and the top of the cap is broken, thus permitting the trapped air to escape. In this manner all excess vapor and air are evacuated from the flask during sterilization.

Figure 157 shows the collar and cap after sterilization. When the internal pressure of the flask drops below 1½ pounds, the seal between the lip of the collar and cap will again be in effect. In the process of cooling the liquid in the flask will revert to its original volume less the amount lost by vaporization. Since the primary seal between the lip of the collar and the cap will not permit entry of air, a vacuum results which draws the cap down tightly onto the collar forming a triple seal as illustrated.

All collars and caps must be thoroughly cleaned and rinsed with freshly distilled water before placing on flasks.

SOLUTION PREPARATION UNIT

In general, there are two systems available to hospitals for the preparation of parenteral solutions. The first, and most widely used system, employs the principle of initially preparing a solution concentrate which is then filtered. An appropriate aliquot of this concentrate is delivered to the final container together with the required volume of distilled water so that the final solution is of the correct concentration. This procedure is accomplished with the aid of automatic burettes or the safety filler device, as shown in Figure 158. The safety filler device uses two graduated Pyrex glass cylinders with adjustable, locking pistons which are set for a predetermined quantity of concentrate solution and distilled water. The safety filler is adjustable for any size flask by simply raising or lowering the suspension bar which is attached to the counter top. The concentrate bottle of 9 liters capacity with dispensing tube and fritted glass filter is also shown in Figure 158. The concentrate dispensing tube has openings for the attachment of a rubber tubing connection to the concentrate cylinder and also for the application of pressure or vacuum to the concentrate bottle.

The bulk system or batch method for the preparation of parenteral solutions is shown in Figure 159. This necessitates the use of a large mixing tank equipped with facilities for bulk dilution, filtration, and semi-automatic dispensing of the finished solution into flasks. The portable pre-mix tank of 200 liters capacity is fabricated of stainless steel. All parts coming in contact with the solution can be readily disassembled for cleaning and sterilization. Mixing is accomplished by means of a circulating centrifugal pump which operates from a ¼ h.p. motor attached to the exterior of the tank. The solution level in the tank is easily determined by indicator knobs permanently located on the pump support tube. This permits the convenient preparation of quantities of solution ranging from 40 to 180 liters. The bottles are filled by means of pressure from the pump which also circulates the solution through an unglazed porcelain filter. The correct volume of solution is automatically delivered to each bottle when

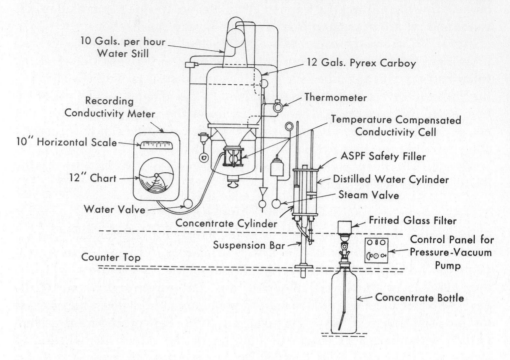

Fig. 158. Diagram of solution preparation unit, similar to the assembly shown in Figure 148.

the hand lever is depressed. When filling, the bottle is completely closed and air escapes through an automatic vent. With the pre-mix tank system, it is practical to fill about 200 bottles per hour.

PROCEDURE FOR MAKING PARENTERAL SOLUTIONS
(Safety Filler Apparatus—Fig. 158)

1) Open water supply valve on still. Then open steam supply valve. Open draw-off cock on storage bottle to permit initial distillate to drain to waste.

2) Prepare concentrate solution with freshly distilled water as per directions given in Table 11. Insert fritted glass filter into top of dispensing tube in the concentrate bottle. Attach rubber tubing to the opening in the concentrate dispensing tube and the vacuum side of the pump. Apply vacuum to bottle. Then pour concentrate into the filter.

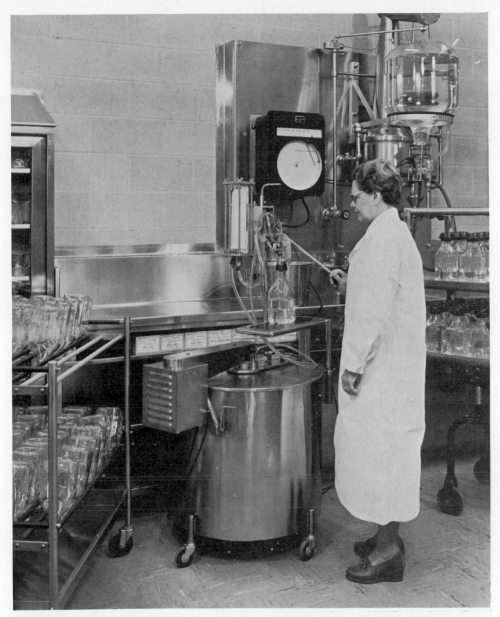

Fig. 159. Portable Pre-mix tank of 200 liters capacity. For use with bulk system or batch method for preparation of parenteral solutions.

3) Frequently check the reading on the Recording Conductivity Meter. When the pointer indicates a resistance of better than 250,000 specific ohms, close the draw-off cock and permit the distillate to accumulate in the 12-gal. storage bottle.

4) After the concentrate is filtered, change the rubber tubing connection on the vacuum side of the pump to the pressure side. Remove glass filter

and insert cap in opening. Attach rubber tubing from draw-off cock on storage bottle to large cylinder inlet on the Safety Filler. Set adjustable pistons on Safety Filler for the desired volumes.

5) With the pump applying approximately 2 pounds pressure on the concentrate bottle and the draw-off cock on the distilled water storage bottle open, raise the valve handle on the Safety Filler to the horizontal position. This will permit both cylinders to fill simultaneously, the concentrate cylinder by pressure and the distilled water cylinder by gravity.

6) Have clean supply of flasks, collars and caps prepared. Collars and caps should be placed in a shallow tray of freshly distilled water conveniently positioned near the operator. Tag or label flasks with proper identification of solution.

7) Raise hood of Safety Filler and position flask under it; then lower hood over the mouth of the flask. Lower valve handle of Safety Filler to the vertical position, causing both cylinders to empty into flask.

8) After draining of cylinders, raise valve handle on Safety Filler to the horizontal position. This will again permit both cylinders to fill. Meanwhile, operator can attach collar and cap to the filled flask and position another flask under the hood.

9) Continue until desired number of flasks are filled.

10) After the desired number of flasks are filled and closures applied, transfer to the sterilizer loading carriage. Immediately sterilize at 250° F. for 30 minutes. At the end of the exposure period, steam should be exhausted slowly from the chamber of the sterilizer to avoid violent ebullition. If sterilizer is equipped with automatic control, selector switch should be set at "slow exhaust." When chamber pressure gauge shows zero, door of sterilizer is opened and load removed.

11) After cooling, check each flask for vacuum seal. To test for proper seal, grasp the flask firmly in one hand and jar the flask by tapping the cap with the other hand. A water-hammer click gives evidence that the sterilized flask has the proper degree of vacuum and is hermetically sealed.

STERILIZATION OF HEAT-SENSITIVE SOLUTIONS

Careless operation of the sterilizer, use of too much heat or an unduly prolonged exposure period will destroy or seriously impair the quality of certain solutions. When difficulty is encountered the cause is almost invariably "over-sterilization." The exposure period selected must be adequate for each individual flask or bottle in the sterilizer. The total number of flasks placed in the sterilizer is not important. The time required for the sterilizer to reach 250° F. will vary with the size of the load but exposure at this temperature should not vary. For example, 1000 ml. flasks of dextrose solution are normally and properly sterilized in 30 minutes exposure, with the sterilizer operating at maximum controlled temperature of 250°-

TABLE 11

Directions for Making Concentrate Solutions

Desired Solution	*Weight of Chemical in Concentrate Solution	Weight of Distilled Water in Concentrate Solution	Total Weight of Concentrate	Total Volume of Concentrate	Piston Setting On Safety Filler — Concentrate Solution	Piston Setting On Safety Filler — Distilled Water	Volume of Finished Product After Sterilization
5% Dextrose in Distilled H$_2$O	900 gm. Dextrose	1414 gm.	2314 gm.	2000 ml.	50 ml. / 100 ml. / 75 ml.	475 ml. / 950 ml. / 700 ml.	500 ml. / 1000 ml. / **1500 ml.
10% Dextrose in Distilled H$_2$O	900 gm. Dextrose	1414 gm.	2314 gm.	2000 ml.	100 ml. / 200 ml. / 150 ml.	425 ml. / 850 ml. / 625 ml.	500 ml. / 1000 ml. / 1500 ml.
5% Dextrose in Isotonic Saline	900 gm. Dextrose / 180 gm. NaCl	1350 gm.	2430 gm.	2000 ml.	50 ml. / 100 ml. / 75 ml.	475 ml. / 950 ml. / 700 ml.	500 ml. / 1000 ml. / 1500 ml.
10% Dextrose in Isotonic Saline	900 gm. Dextrose / 90 gm. NaCl	1382 gm.	2372 gm.	2000 ml.	100 ml. / 200 ml. / 150 ml.	425 ml. / 850 ml. / 625 ml.	500 ml. / 1000 ml. / 1500 ml.
0.9% Isotonic Saline	90 gm. NaCl	964 gm.	1054 gm.	1000 ml.	50 ml. / 100 ml. / 75 ml.	475 ml. / 950 ml. / 700 ml.	500 ml. / 1000 ml. / 1500 ml.
Ringer's Solution	86 gm. NaCl / 3.3 gm. CaCl$_2$.2H$_2$O / 3.0 gm. KCl	963 gm.	1055 gm.	1000 ml.	50 ml. / 100 ml. / 75 ml.	475 ml. / 950 ml. / 700 ml.	500 ml. / 1000 ml. / 1500 ml.

* All chemicals should be C.P. or A.C.S. grade, and the anhydrous form of dextrose used for all concentrates.
** For dispensing 1500 ml. quantities draw concentrate solution and distilled water twice.

Procedure for preparation of concentrate.
1) Pour approximately 80 to 90% of required weight of distilled water in appropriate container and heat almost to a boil.
2) Add required weight of chemical or chemicals and stir until dissolved.
3) Add the balance of distilled water to correct total weight.
4) Filter into concentrate bottle.

254° F. The average small bottle or flask of procaine solution (one or two ounces) will receive the same sterilizing effect in 12 to 15 minutes at this temperature (see p. 319). Obviously the two containers should not be sterilized in the same load, unless the procaine solution is of the correct pH which increases heat stability.

Murphy and Stoklosa[20] have studied the effect of autoclaving on the stability of solutions of alkaloidal salts, including procaine hydrochloride. Their findings indicated that such solutions may be sterilized by autoclaving, under properly controlled conditions, without significantly affecting their potency. The optimum pH range for maximum stability of solutions of alkaloidal salts was found to be from 2.9 to 4.8, before and after sterilization. According to Bullock and Cannell,[21] procaine hydrochloride solutions are most stable at a pH of 3.0 to 3.5. In this range they may be autoclaved at 250° F. for as long as two hours with only 2.5% decomposition.

After sterilization, pressure in the sterilizer must be exhausted slowly. Otherwise, violent ebullition will take place which will result in blown stoppers and an undue loss of fluid. At best, under the most careful regulation of exhaust, there will be a loss of 3 to 5% of the fluid by vaporization. This establishes a general rule for making up solutions which should be observed. Add an extra 5% of distilled water to each flask so that the sterilized product will have the concentration intended. This factor has been included in the directions for preparing solutions given in Table 11.

The practice of permitting the entire sterilizer to cool down slowly after solution sterilization prolongs exposure to excessive heat. In the case of heat-sensitive solutions, this may be detrimental, as evidenced by discoloration. The most satisfactory method calls for some skill and care in regulation of the exhaust, as follows: At the close of the exposure period, turn off all heat to the sterilizer. Close the valve admitting steam to the chamber, and then adjust the chamber exhaust valve slightly open to a degree that will permit exhaust of pressure to zero in not less than 10 to 15 minutes. With this method, the heat of the solution will be dissipated without violent ebullition, and at about the same rate at which the pressure is reduced.

THE SIGNIFICANCE OF TESTS TO DETERMINE QUALITY OF PARENTERAL SOLUTIONS

Can hospitals make satisfactory solutions without an elaborate testing program? This question is frequently asked by administrators, medical and surgical staffs and other professional workers who concern themselves with the problems of parenteral therapy. Many of these people labor under the impression that it is essential to maintain a biologics testing laboratory, including an animal colony, in order to make pyrogen and sterility tests on each batch of solutions prepared in the hospital. Such an understanding is not entirely correct. To be sure, if pyrogen tests are to be performed routinely on solutions, it is necessary to have available a sufficient number of test animals. Sterility tests can usually be performed in the clinical laboratory of the hospital. The basic reasons for concern about the element of testing stem from unsatisfactory experiences in certain hospitals in the past when solutions were made under adverse conditions with makeshift equipment, and more recently from "scare-selling" on the part of biased individuals trying to prevent hospitals from making their own intravenous solutions.

The significance of tests to determine the quality of solutions should be thoroughly understood. Certainly it is not the author's intent to discourage the testing of solutions in any hospital providing that suitable facilities are available. Rather, it is the intent to point out that the hospital need not institute an elaborate testing program to safeguard the production of intravenous solutions. It is acknowledged, however, that in the beginning and for the first few months' operation of a new solution room, the quality of the solutions produced should be firmly established, in order to convince doubtful persons as to the safety and quality of product. This factor of safety and assurance is as much a responsibility of the manufacturer of the equipment as it is of the hospital. When a new solution room is opened, it should be the responsibility of the equipment supplier to thoroughly instruct the hospital personnel in the preparation of solutions, as well as to periodically collect samples of the solutions for pyrogen test, sterility test and chemical assay. These tests should be made by some responsible laboratory and a report issued in writing to the hospital as substantial proof of the safety of the system and to show that the quality of the solutions meets the requirements of the U. S. Pharmacopoeia in every respect.

When parenteral solutions are properly prepared from freshly distilled water and high purity chemicals, it is not necessary to routinely test each lot for pyrogenic reactions. Of the approximately 200 hospitals now making their own solutions, very few routinely perform pyrogen tests. There are a few authorities, however, who insist upon a biologic test as an additional safeguard in establishing the quality of the product or as an occasional check on a lot of material which may be under suspicion. Even then it must be admitted that the biologic test for pyrogens is not conducted routinely but rather on a periodic basis, either monthly or semi-monthly, on random samples taken from the stock of freshly prepared (sterile) solutions made on the day of the test. If an occasional pyrogen test is required it should be conducted as follows:

Use rabbits (1500 gm. or more) maintained at least one week on an unrestricted diet and which are not losing weight. Animals which have been previously used for pyrogen tests must have a rest period of at least two days. Use clinical thermometers previously tested to determine time required to record a maximum temperature. Two days before test take four temperature readings every two hours and reject animals with temperatures above 39.8° C. House test animals in individual cages and keep them at uniform environmental temperature ± 5° for at least 48 hours before the test day.

Performance of Test

1) Perform test at the same temperature as the animal quarters.

2) Use three animals for each test.

3) Withhold food one hour before test is started and for the duration of the test. Water may be allowed.

4) Take a control test 15 minutes before injection of test material. Animals may be used if the control temperature is above 38.9° C. and below 39.8° C.

5) Warm product to be tested to about 37° C. and inject through ear vein 10 ml. per kg. (Use only syringes and needles known to be pyrogen-free by heating in a muffle furnace at 250° C. for 30 minutes.)

6) Record temperature every hour for three hours.

7) A positive test for pyrogens is demonstrated if two of the three rabbits show a temperature rise of 0.6° C. or greater. If only one animal shows such a rise, or if the sum of the temperature rises of the three animals exceeds 1.4° C., the test must be repeated using five rabbits. The test shall be considered positive if two or more of the group of five rabbits show an individual rise in temperature of 0.6° C. or more above the normal established for these animals.

REFERENCES

1. DORLAND, W. A.: *The American Illustrated Medical Dictionary.* Philadelphia, Saunders, 1950, p. 1068.

2. LARSEN, F. L.: Considerations in the Preparation of Parenteral Solutions—A Case Study. *Bull. Am. Soc. Hosp. Pharm.,* 10:210-219, 1953.

3. LISWOOD, S. AND FINER, N. S.: The Best "Buy" in Parenteral Solutions? *Modern Hospital,* pp. 90-94, May, 1955.

4. WALTER, C. W.: The Relation of Proper Preparation of Solutions for Intravenous Therapy to Febrile Reactions. *Ann. Surg., 112:*603-617, 1940.

5. ZUGICH, J. J.: Parenteral Fluids in the Hospital. *Pharmacy International,* 4:9-48-54, 1950.

6. NESSET, N. M., MCLALLEN, J., ANTHONY, P. Z., AND GINGER, L. G.: Bacterial Pyrogens. I. Pyrogenic Preparation from a Pseudomonas Species. *J. Am. Pharm. A.,* 39:456-459, 1950.

7. WALKER, J.: A Method for the Isolation of Toxic and Immunizing Fractions from Bacteria of the Salmonella Group. *Biochem. J.,* 34:325, 1940.

8. MORGAN, H. R.: Preparation of Antigenic Material Inducing Leucopenia from E. Typhosa Cultured in a Synthetic Medium. *Proc. Soc. Exper. Biol. & Med.,* 43:529, 1940.

9. COTUI, F. W., AND SCHRIFT, M. H.: Production of Pyrogen by Some Bacteria. *J. Lab. & Clin. Med.,* 27:569-575, 1942.

10. LEES, J. C., AND LEVVY, G. A.: Emergency Preparation of Pyrogen-Free Water. *Brit. M.J.,* 1:430-432, 1940.

11. SEIBERT, F. B.: Fever Producing Substance Found in Some Distilled Waters. *Am. J. Physiol.,* 67:90-104, 1923.

———: The Case of Many Febrile Reactions Following Intravenous Infusions. *Am. J. Physiol.,* 71:621-651, 1924.

12. RADEMAKER, L. A.: The Cause of Elimination of Reactions After Intravenous Infusions. *Ann. Surg.,* 92:195-201, 1930.

13. CoTui, F. W., McCloskey, K. L., Schrift, M., and Yates, A. L.: New Method of Preparing Infusion Fluids Based on Removal of Pyrogens by Filtration. *J.A.M.A., 109:*250, 1937.

14. CoTui, F. W., and Wright, A. M.: The Preparation of Nonpyrogenic Infusion and Other Intravenous Fluids by Adsorptive Filtration. *Ann. Surg., 116:*412-425, 1942.

15. Brindle and Rigby: Preparation of Nonpyrogenic Water and Infusion Fluids, Using Activated Charcoal. *Quart. J. Pharm. & Pharmacol., 19:*302, 1946.

16. Banks, H. M.: Study of Hyperpyrexia Reaction Following Intravenous Therapy. *Am. J. Clin. Path., 4:*260, 1934.

17. Wylie, D. W., and Todd, J. P.: An Examination of the Sources and the Quantitative Methods of Testing Pyrogen. *Quart. J. Pharm. & Pharmacol., 21:*240-252, 1948.

18. Rademaker, L.: Intravenous Solutions: Facts and Fancies. *J. Internat. Coll. Surg., 11:*194-199, 1948.

19. Rademaker, L.: Reactions to Intravenous Administration of Solutions. *J.A.M.A., 135:*1140-1141, 1947.

20. Murphy, J. T., and Stoklosa, M. J.: Effect of Autoclaving on the Stability of Solutions of Certain Thermolabile Substances. *Bull. Am. Soc. Hosp. Pharm., 9:*94-97, 1952.

21. Bullock, K., and Cannell, J. S.: The Preparation of Solutions of Procaine and Adrenaline Hydrochlorides for Surgical Use. *Quart. J. Pharm. & Pharmacol., 14:*241-251, 1941.

Chapter XIX

The Infant Formula Room

PREPARATION AND TERMINAL HEATING OF INFANT FORMULAS

THERE IS PROBABLY no subject of greater importance to the hospital than that which deals with the immediate care of the newborn infant and its relation to neonatal mortality. Medical science supported by accurate statistical data has shown that infections constitute one of the leading preventable causes of infant deaths under one month of age. Just what percentage of this annual toll of infants' lives is due to infections acquired as the result of inadequacies within the hospital nursery, formula room and facilities for the segregated care of premature and infected infants is apparently not known. It is generally recognized, however, among the various regulatory bodies and public health authorities passing upon appointments for maternity service, that certain basic standards should be adopted to insure decontamination or sterility of all supplies, such as food, water, clothing, etc., which represent a potential means of mass spread of infection. One of the more common causes of outbreaks of diarrhea in hospital nurseries is believed to be contamination of milk preparations and equipment used in the feeding of infants.

Milk and milk mixtures are excellent culture media for bacteria and consequently they are preeminently fitted to convey the germs of infectious disease. It has long been known that the changes which take place in milk to the extent of adding or detracting from its nutritive value are due largely to bacterial growth. As the result of this relationship of milk to infectious disease, the commercial pasteurization process has been adopted by most of the dairies serving the larger cities and communities throughout the country.

Experience has proved, however, that it is not advisable for a hospital to rely entirely upon the efficiency of commercial pasteurization of milk as delivered from local dairies for the feeding of infants. In fact, it would seem logical to consider that a disease in the community may be the possible source of a nursery infection due to a contaminated milk supply. Such a condition was reported by Ensign and Hunter[1] in an epidemic of diarrhea among 24 newborn infants in which there were 9 deaths. The infants were apparently secondarily infected by mothers and nurses who drank the contaminated milk in the hospital.

DIARRHEAL DISEASES OF THE NEWBORN

It is the belief of certain public health authorities[2] that nearly every hospital, at one time or another, encounters epidemics of diarrheal disorders. When but few fatalities occur, it is highly possible that the condition may not be recognized as epidemic. It may be said, however, that in the aggregate, diarrheal diseases constitute one of the major preventable causes of infant morbidity and mortality.

The recognized pathogenic bacteria frequently associated with such disorders are for the most part located in the intestines and they are spread principally by person-to-person contact (in the case of infants a third party assists) of a sort which permits transfer of human excreta. A virus has long been suspected as the cause of many of these disorders and at least five epidemics with specific virus etiology have been proved.[3, 4, 5]

Rubinstein and Foley[6] have reviewed nineteen outbreaks of epidemic diarrhea of the newborn as reported to the Massachusetts Department of Health from 1935 to 1945. Of 768 newborn infants who were exposed during the course of these outbreaks, 258 developed symptoms and 85 died, resulting in a case fatality rate of 33 per cent. Investigation of nursing techniques and methods of formula preparation where these outbreaks occurred revealed many inadequacies. Overcrowding, insufficient personnel, general use of a common rectal thermometer and inadequate supervision of formula making were frequently encountered. Laboratory examinations of so-called sterilizing solutions, including alcohol hand solution and thermometer dips, formulas, nipples and utensils showed heavy bacterial contamination. These authors concluded that supervision of nursery room technics and of formula preparation constitutes a factor in the hospital care of newborn infants that merits serious attention from hospital administrators.

Although diarrheal diseases of the newborn are incompletely understood at the present time, it is still possible to establish basic standards designed to minimize the introduction and spread of infectious agents in nurseries. To this end it is important to note that the American Academy of Pediatrics Committee on Fetus and Newborn has published a report covering "Standards and Recommendations for Hospital Care of Newborn Infants—Fullterm and Premature."[7] Similarly, the American Hospital Association has prepared a manual embodying the physical facilities, procedures and precautions necessary to the efficient production of formulas by the terminal heating process.[8] Also, certain states[9] have established by regulation what are considered to be the minimum precautions to be observed for the control of diarrhea of the newborn. These standards and recommendations have contributed greatly to progress in a nation-wide program sponsored by hospital, medical and public health groups to better the care of newborn infants.

Important among these standards are procedures to assure decontamination or sterility of supplies such as food, water, clothing, etc., which constitute a potential means of mass spread of infection. Major attention must also be given to the space, equipment and facilities available for the preparation of infant formulas. The need for a strict formula room technic together with a reliable method for terminal heating of formulas cannot be overemphasized. The method employed must provide positive protection against contamination in later handling of the formulas up to the time of feeding. Furthermore, a scrupulous technique must be developed for the control of cross-infections within the nursery.

PLANNING THE FORMULA ROOM

The location of the formula room and supervision of the work of preparing the formulas will vary with the type of hospital, its personnel and its special administrative problems. Suggested locations are the dietary, the maternity and the pediatrics departments. The advocates of the dietary department location are usually of the opinion that preparation of formulas is primarily the dietitian's responsibility, therefore the formula room should be located near the general diet kitchen. However, if this location is selected, it is important to make sure that the formula room is completely separated from the diet kitchen and food storage room. The maternity specialists feel that, since they are most directly concerned with the welfare of newborn infants, the formula room should be under their supervision on the maternity floor. Also, when a separate pediatrics department exists, some pediatricians are of the opinion that the formula room should be under their direction. Certain hospitals have located the formula room near the central supply department and so far as can be determined this has not proved to be a disadvantageous location. The final selection of a location can, as a rule, be decided only after consultation with the hospital administrator, director of nurses, the pediatrician and the dietitian. Whatever the circumstances may be, it is essential that the formula room be located where the danger of contamination is the least and where the most adequate supervision can be rendered by a nurse or dietitian who is experienced in formula room and sterilizing procedures. It is also essential that a separate room be provided for preparation of the feedings and that this room be used for no other purpose.

Many formula rooms are too small to effectively accommodate the preparation of the normal complement of feedings each day. Operating efficiency is largely dependent upon the provision of ample space, proper arrangement of counters, cabinets and sinks so that the important details of preparation can be accomplished without confusion. Wherever possible, the formula room should be divided into two sections, a clean-up area and a preparation area, separated by means of a full-length partition wall in which there is located a visual communication window and a double door formula sterilizer extending into both sections, as in Figure 160. This arrangement provides positive segregation and permits the exclusive use of the clean-up area for receiving and washing of the bottles, nipples and

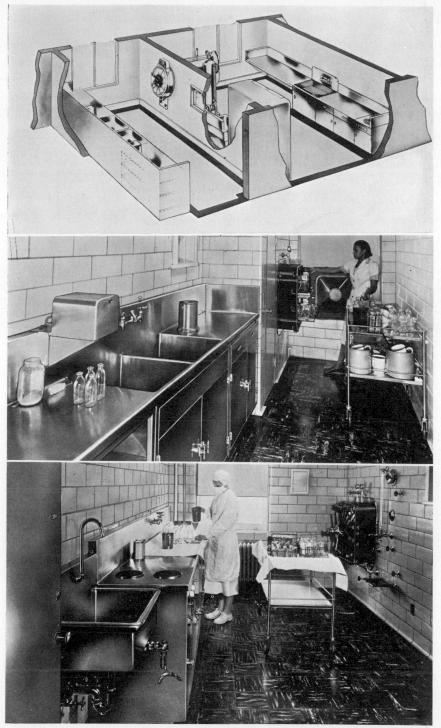

Courtesy Shadyside Hospital, Pittsburgh, Pa.

Fig. 160. A highly practical arrangement for the formula room, suited to the needs of the average hospital. The clean-up area shown at the left is segregated from the preparation area by means of a partition wall.

Fig. 160A. Receiving and clean-up area of modern formula room (approximately 7' x 17').

Fig. 160B. Formula preparation room (approximately 9' x 17').

utensils, and the other section for preparation, terminal heating and storage of the formulas. With the aid of the double door sterilizer it becomes convenient to establish an exacting technic within the preparation area which insures presterilization of the washed supplies (bottles, nipples and utensils) and thus precludes the entrance of potentially contaminated equipment into the preparation room.

Formula Room Flow Chart: The continuity of procedures or work flow of

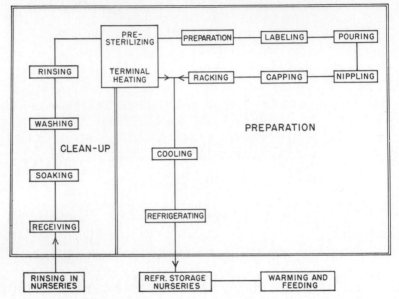

Fig. 161. Formula room flow chart.

supplies through the formula room is illustrated in Figure 161. The activity naturally begins at the receiving entrance of the clean-up room where used bottles, nipples, racks, utensils, etc., are returned for cleaning. Then follows in correct sequence the operations of soaking, washing, and rinsing of the supplies, after which they are placed on the counter or a portable carriage for subsequent movement to the sterilizer. From this point, the materials and supplies may be transferred directly to the double door sterilizer, observing the usual precautions for racking of bottles, use of containers or wrappers for supplies when required.

After sterilization, the load of empty bottles, nipples, etc., is withdrawn in the preparation room and placed upon the appropriate counter section. With clean, presterilized equipment now available, the formula ingredients are measured and mixed, bottles labeled, filled, nipples attached, protective caps applied, and the assembled bottles placed in racks. The completed formulas are then transferred to the sterilizer for the terminal heating process, after which they are permitted to cool for a short time at room temperature. Finally, they are placed in a large refrigerator located in the preparation room or preferably transferred to smaller refrigerators serving each nursery unit.

Allocation of Space: In selecting a space for the formula room consideration must be given to the maximum number of bottles of formula and water to be prepared each day, with due allowance for future expansion, if contemplated. The total area to be allocated will vary somewhat with the type of layout and the equipment selected for the service. Experience gained in formula rooms using the segregated type of plan and the double door sterilizer (Figures 160A and 160B) supports the recommendation that the area should be adequate for the installation of a sterilizer of sufficient capacity to permit processing of the total number of bottles in no more than three and preferably two cycles of operation. This statement is based upon a total processing time of approximately one hour for each load of formulas, including loading and unloading of the sterilizer, and irrespective of whether the nonpressure or pressure method is used for terminal heating. The following table gives suggested space requirements for formula rooms based upon current planning data:

Total Number of Bottles Per Day (Formula and Water)	Suggested Space for Formula Laboratory			Size of Sterilizer
	Clean-up Room	Preparation Room	Total Area Sq. Ft.	
Up to 66	8' x 12'	(one room)	100	16" x 24"
72 to 180	6' x 13'	9' x 13'	200	20" x 36"
186 to 360	6' x 15'	10' x 15'	250	24" x 24" x 36"
366 to 600	8' x 15'	12' x 15'	300	24" x 36" x 36"
606 to 900	8' x 16'	17' x 16'	400	24" x 36" x 48"

Almost without exception it can be said that the two-section segregated type of plan is the layout of choice for the infant formula room. However, it is also recognized that there are many small hospitals, with requirements approximating 6 to 12 formulas (36 to 72 bottles) daily, desirous of establishing a safe formula room technique but obviously unable to allocate space and to provide equipment to conform to the ideal and more refined features of planning because of limited facilities and economic reasons. For these hospitals it is suggested that serious consideration be given to the single room type of plan as shown in Figure 162. The over-all dimensions of this layout are 8' x 12' and a minimum of equipment is specified. A formula room so planned can function with efficiency, speed and safety under competent supervision, providing the procedures of cleaning and preparation are segregated by the proper time and space and with due regard for the necessity of terminal heating of all formulas.

In discussing the various aspects of formula room planning and technique, it is important to note that certain states[9] have established by regulation what are considered to be the minimal standards required for the control of diarrheal diseases of the newborn. Therefore, it is essential where

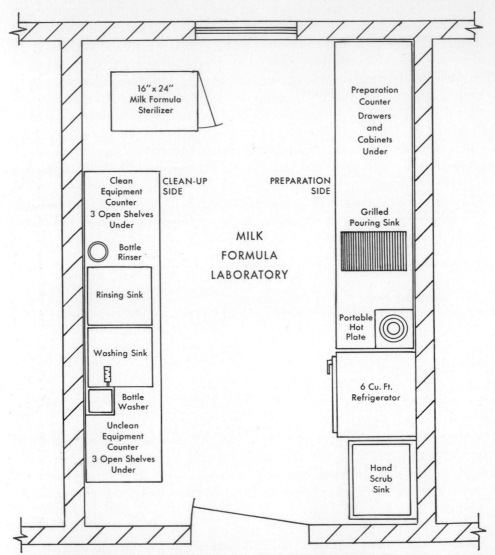

Fig. 162. Suggested formula room layout for the small hospital.

such regulations are in force that the hospital secure approval from the proper health authority (usually the State Department of Health) on all proposed construction plans and equipment to insure that they comply with the regulations or sanitary codes applicable to the hospital and formula room.

ESSENTIAL EQUIPMENT FOR THE HOSPITAL FORMULA SERVICE

In listing essential equipment for the formula service it is important to give consideration to the installation of counters, cabinets and sinks fabricated of noncorrosive metal, preferably stainless steel. The features of construction should be of high quality in order to be assured of functional efficiency and so as to permit easy cleaning of all working surfaces. Operating efficiency in any formula room is largely dependent upon the provision of adequate space, proper arrangement of work counters and appropriate equipment so that the important details of cleaning and preparation can be accomplished without confusion. The following items are usually regarded as essential equipment for the average hospital formula service:

Clean-up Room

1) A work counter of appropriate size, with open shelving under the receiving end for the temporary storage of used bottles, racks, supplies, etc. It should be equipped with two sinks, motor-driven bottle (brush) washer and bottle rinser as individual units. Such equipment should preferably be fabricated of a noncorrosive metal (18-8 stainless steel), all-welded, seamless construction, offering no possibility of drainage or seepage collecting in cracks which might serve as harbors for bacteria or vermin propagation.

2) One or more portable bottle carriages, double or triple deck, for the conveyance of bottles and utensils within the formula room.

3) Wherever space permits, a hand scrub sink or lavatory should be installed in the clean-up room. This unit should be equipped with a knee-operated water supply valve and liquid soap dispenser operated with arm control.

4) A janitor's closet or cabinet for the storage of room cleaning supplies and mops should be located in the clean-up room or adjacent to it. This feature permits the exclusive use of cleaning equipment in the formula unit.

Preparation Room

1) A formula preparation unit, consisting of a work counter of suitable size, with storage cabinets under, fabricated of stainless steel. Standard construction usually features one compartment sink with removable grilled cover and a two-burner (electric) hot-plate conveniently located along the counter section. Since this unit must be used for the preparation of bulk formulas, mixing of ingredients, filling of bottles, etc., care should be taken to insure that the counter section is of sufficient length and width to permit the various operations to be conducted efficiently.

2) Wherever space permits, consideration should be given to the placement of a central work table within the preparation room. This item is im-

portant to the busy formula room in order to maintain the proper continuity of work flow and to provide additional counter space for the filling, capping and racking of the bottles of formula. The table need not be more than 2½ or 3 feet wide and 6 feet long, fabricated preferably of a noncorrosive metal.

3) The presence of a hand scrub sink or lavatory is regarded by all authorities as an essential item for every formula preparation room. It should be equipped with a knee- or foot-operated water supply valve and located near the entrance to the preparation room. A liquid soap dispenser with arm-operated control should also be included.

4) Formula sterilizer, for recessed or open mounting, double door construction, of sufficient size and capacity to permit terminal heating of the total number of bottles in no more than three and preferably two cycles of operation. The sterilizer should be equipped with suitable controls, valving and piping for rapid and precise terminal heating of formulas by either the nonpressure (streaming steam) process at 212° F. (100° C.) or the pressure steam method at 230° F. (110° C.). In addition, the sterilizer should permit, without mechanical adjustment, the pressure steam sterilization of empty bottles, nipples, dry goods and other supplies common to the formula room.

The sterilizer shown in Figure 160 fulfills the most exacting requirements in that positive segregation of the clean-up room from the preparation room can be maintained simply by building the partition wall around the sterilizer. The double door feature with controls on the clean side permits presterilization of the washed bottles, nipples and utensils and precludes the entrance of potentially contaminated equipment into the preparation room.

5) It has long been recognized that the human element is of considerable importance in the development of a safe formula room technique. The physical and chemical changes produced in formulas in the event of overexposure or excessive heat treatment and the degree of manual control and attention required during the sterilizing cycle should definitely not be minimized. Success in obtaining uniform results, day after day, in terminal heating processes is largely dependent upon the simplicity of the process and the amount of attention required from the operator for correct operation of the sterilizer.

The human element in formula sterilizer operation can be markedly relieved by the installation of an efficient automatic time-temperature control such as illustrated in Figure 166. The functional efficiency of the automatic control in formula sterilizer operation may be summarized as follows:

a) The human error attendant with manual operation of the sterilizer is minimized.

b) The conventional method of timing the exposure period is eliminated —a safeguard against possible underexposure or overexposure of the load.

c) The manual opening and closing of valves on the sterilizer are eliminated.

d) Operating instructions are simplified.

e) Conserves power, materials and personnel time.

6) A pressure water sterilizer, single tank, is also considered an essential item for the formula preparation room. It not only assures a convenient and adequate supply of sterile water for certain types of feedings which cannot be subjected to terminal heating, but it also promotes sanitation and provides a constant and controlled quality of water for use in the preparation of routine formulas. The water sterilizer filter system removes particulate matter from raw tap water; sterilization process reduces mineral content of hard water, thereby preventing further precipitation of lime salts on inside of formula bottles. (The flask system may be substituted for the water sterilizer with equal or greater efficiency.)

7) Adequate refrigeration is a necessity for the proper cooling and storage of formulas. Extraordinary load conditions are imposed by attempting to cool rapidly the hot bottles at a temperature of approximately 200° F. (93° C.) to the holding temperature of 40°-45° F. (4°-7° C.) in a minimum of time and without excessive wear and strain on the equipment.

Care should be used in the selection of a refrigerator for this application because repeated tests have shown that the average commercial refrigerator cannot be depended upon for prompt and efficient cooling of formula bottles. The performance specifications are such as to require a specially designed refrigeration system equipped with a heavy duty compressor, equalizer tank, oversize coils and a forced air evaporator.

The size of the refrigerator and the net cubic capacity will vary with the average requirements of the nursery and whether the prepared formulas are to be stored and dispensed from one large refrigerator located in the formula room or stored in a smaller refrigerator located in each nursery work-room.

8) Portable bottle carriages, double or triple deck, stainless steel, with rails surrounding each deck to prevent bottles or racks from sliding off. These carriages are used for the conveyance of bottles and utensils within the formula room and for transporting prepared formulas to nurseries.

9) Formula bottle carriers, fabricated of corrosion-resistant metal, either 6, 8 or 12 bottles capacity.

Nursery

1) Portable bottle warmer fabricated of Monel metal, with thermostatic control and thermometer. This unit should be of sufficient capacity to accommodate the heating of 12 or 24 formula bottles of either 4-oz. or 8-oz. size from the normal refrigerator holding temperature of 45° F. (7° C.)

to the normal feeding temperature of 100° F. (38° C.) within approximately 20 minutes.

2) Scrub sink or lavatory, equipped with knee-operated water supply valve and liquid soap dispenser.

3) Refrigerator, with adequate capacity for cooling and storage of formulas. This unit is usually located in the workroom adjoining the nursery and need not be more than 10 cubic feet capacity.

FORMULA ROOM TECHNIC

Even though there may exist some diversity of opinion with respect to the various details of formula room procedure, it is generally recognized that the combined application of a strictly clean technique with an approved method of terminal heating offers the greatest promise of success in producing formulas that are uniform in quality and bacteriologically safe.

The procedure outlined below is especially recommended for the preparation and terminal heating of formulas and water for infants. It overcomes unconditionally the problems attendant with the sterilization of solutions by means of pressure steam as well as the uncertainties of the outmoded pasteurization process. It makes available a precision method that not only insures positive destruction of all communicable disease-producing organisms but, in addition, provides a maximum of protection against contamination in later handling of the formulas—up to the time of feeding.

A) Formula Preparation

Step 1. Before performing any duty in the Formula Preparation Room the nurse should employ the conventional three-minute scrub.

Step 2. All bottles, nipples and utensils are to be thoroughly washed with hot soap suds or some other effective detergent, rinsed in hot water and sterilized by pressure steam at 250°-254° F. (121°-123° C.) for a period of 15 minutes. (See "Care of Bottles and Nipples," Sections D and E.)

Step 3. Formula ingredients (milk, sugar or modifier, such as Dextri-Maltose, corn syrup, etc.) and sterile water should be placed in sterile containers, mixed and then transferred to previously washed sterile bottles. (Caution—Do not fill bottles beyond last graduated line, indicating maximum volume.)

Step 4. Sterile nipples are then attached to bottles and each nipple completely covered with a previously sterilized paper cap, extending well over the shoulder of the bottle and held firmly in place with a rubber band. Label bottles and place in appropriate racks or carriers. (If paper caps are used, the infant's name or number can be written directly on the cap.)

B) Terminal Heating of Formulas

Feedings prepared with whole milk, skim milk, evaporated milk and/or water should be subjected to this process. Lactic acid formulas prepared with Mead's Powdered Lactic Acid Milk No. 1 (with Dextri-Maltose), Lactic Acid Milk No. 2 (Plain), Powdered Protein Milk, and Mead's Powdered Lactic Acid Milk, Half Skim, may also be subjected to terminal heating.

Step 1. Following preparation, the formulas are immediately placed in sterilizer and subjected to nonpressure steam for 30 minutes at 212° F. (100° C.). The period of exposure is timed when the thermometer indicates 210° F. (99° C.) in its advance toward the maximum. Exposure continues for 30 minutes (no longer), after which the steam is turned off and the door opened immediately. Detailed instructions for operation of formula sterilizer are given on page 307.

Note: Certain public health authorities[9] and other regulatory bodies require that terminal heating shall be conducted as follows: "The entire product shall then be subjected to terminal heating by steam under pressure of not less than 15 pounds (250° F. or 121° C.) for not less than 5 minutes, or at a pressure of not less than 6 pounds (230° F. or 110° C.) for not less than 10 minutes, or by flowing steam at a temperature of not less than 212° F. (100° C.) for not less than 30 minutes. The temperature of the formula or fluid, as determined by periodic examination, shall be not less than 200° F. (93° C.) at the end of the heating process. The nipple cap shall remain on the bottle until the time of feeding. If fruit juices, or formulas containing lactic acid, meats or cereals are given to newborn infants, they may be offered without such terminal heating, but shall be prepared with and stored in presterilized equipment."

Step 2. Remove formulas from sterilizer and allow to cool at room temperature for one to two hours. Finally, transfer formulas to refrigerator maintained at a temperature of 40°-45° F. (4°-7° C.) where they remain until feeding time.

C) Feeding of the Infant (Nursery)

Step 1. At feeding time, the nurse, with scrubbed and disinfected hands, removes from the refrigerator a bottle of formula for each infant and places it in the bottle rack or carrier. The rack is then placed in the "bottle warmer" containing water at the correct level and allowed to remain there for a short period of time (15-20 minutes) until the formulas have attained a temperature of 100° F. (38° C.).

Note: The "bottle warmer" should accommodate 24 formula bottles of either 4 or 8 ounces capacity and it should automatically maintain the correct temperature of 100° F. (38° C.). Care should be taken to insure that the level of water in the bath does not come in contact with the paper cap protecting the nipple and upper portion of the bottle. It is important that the warmer be emptied, washed with soap and water, and resterilized daily. The constant warm temperature is conducive to bacterial growth. Unless it is cleaned and sterilized daily, it may harbor bacteria which could adhere to the bottles and be carried to the infant.

Step 2. The feeding nurse (masked, hands and arms scrubbed and disinfected) selects from the rack or carrier the formula labeled for the infant, checks and records the amount of milk in the bottle. Finally, the paper cap is removed from the nipple and the infant elevated for the feeding.

D) Care of Bottles

Immediately after feeding, rinse the bottles well with cold water. All bottles should then be returned to the clean-up section of the formula room and carefully washed in hot water containing some efficient detergent. (The bottles, nipples and caps from isolation and suspect nurseries should be disinfected by boiling before being returned to the formula room.) The use of a bottle brush or preferably a mechanical washing unit to remove any particles of milk protein or sediment that may adhere to the glass is recommended. Rinse bottles thoroughly in hot running water (mechanical rinser), invert in stainless steel carriers and sterilize by pressure steam at 250°-254° F. (121°-123° C.) for a period of 15 minutes. After sterilization, bottles may be placed on preparation work counter and covered with a sterile sheet.

E) Care of Nipples

Remove nipples from bottles immediately after feeding and rinse inside and out with cold running water, followed by careful washing in hot water containing some efficient detergent, upon return to the formula room. Rinse thoroughly with hot running water. Place nipples in muslin bag and sterilize by pressure steam at 250°-254° F. (121°-123° C.) for a period of 15 minutes. Longer exposure should be avoided.

F) Care of Utensils

Following completion of the formulas, the various utensils and containers used in their preparation should be delivered to the clean-up section of the room for thorough washing, rinsing and sterilization. When loading utensils, large graduates, quart milk bottles, jars and other containers in the sterilizer, care should be taken to insure that the containers are inverted or at least rest on their sides, never in the upright position, otherwise sterilization may not be accomplished.

G) Miscellaneous Supplies

The same sterilizer used for terminal heating of formulas should be so adapted that it can be also utilized for the pressure steam sterilization of gowns, table covers, face masks and other supplies common to the formula room and nursery. The recommended periods of exposure at a temperature of 250°-254° F. (121°-123° C.) for these various supplies are as follows:

Empty nursing bottles, always bottom side up .... 15 minutes
Nipples, in muslin bag .... 15 minutes
Utensils, spoons, measuring devices .... 15 minutes
Paper caps, loosely packed in tray with perforated bottom .... 15 minutes
Rubber gloves in muslin wrapper .... 15 minutes
Water in 1000 or 2000 ml. flasks .... 30 minutes
Table covers, gowns, face masks in muslin covers .... 30 minutes

H) Bacteriologic Testing of Formulas

For hospitals with adequate laboratory service and a competent bacteriologist it is considered essential that an assembled bottle of formula, taken at random, after 24 hours of refrigeration at 40° F. (4° C.) be sent daily to the laboratory for examination. Such examination should include a bacterial plate count of the formula according to "Standard Methods for Examination of Dairy Products." The nipple should also be checked for bacterial contamination. Formulas having less than 25 organisms per ml. are considered acceptable.

For hospitals without adequate laboratory service, arrangements should be made to have a sample of terminally heated formula tested at least once a week by some recognized laboratory.

NECESSITY FOR PRESTERILIZATION OF SUPPLIES

With the technic outlined above for terminal heating of formulas in bottles with nipples attached, it might be argued that presterilization of bottles, nipples and utensils is an unnecessary step and that thorough washing of the equipment should suffice as a preparatory measure. Theoretically that is true. However, the important point is, one cannot always be sure of the thoroughness of the washing process, especially if milk has been permitted to dry on the inside of bottles and nipple surfaces. Even then it is acknowledged that neither presterilization of bottles and equipment nor terminal heating of the formulas can altogether compensate for poor cleaning. It has been shown experimentally[10] that formula bottles used day after day without thorough cleaning eventually can produce contaminated formulas in spite of a terminal heat treatment of 230° F. (110° C.) for 10 minutes.

There is no substitute for good cleaning of bottles, nipples and utensils used in preparing infant formulas. The extra precaution of presterilization is, nevertheless, considered to be good practice if for no other reason than to prevent the entrance of potentially contaminated equipment into the formula preparation room. Also, when special formulas are required that cannot be subjected to terminal heating, the feature of presterilization as a part of the standard formula procedure makes it unnecessary to set up a special technique. Since authorities are in agreement that nipples especially must undergo presterilization as an extra precaution, it is only logical that the bottles and utensils should likewise be presterilized and thereby effect a standard procedure.

Preventing Nipple Clogging: When certain types of formulas prepared from whole milk, powdered milk or evaporated milk are subjected to terminal heating a scum frequently forms on the surface of the milk. Unless this scum is broken up it will almost invariably clog or plug the holes in the nipples during the course of feeding. To guard against difficult scum formation it is good practice to shake lightly each bottle of formula as soon as it is removed from the sterilizer and again during the period the formulas are permitted to cool at room temperature before transferring to the refrigerator.

A rigid rule should be established to prohibit change or removal of nipples from formula bottles for any reason during the feeding of an infant. Another bottle of formula should be substituted rather than risk contamination by changing the nipple. Since clogging of the nipple is probably the most prevalent reason for making the change, it has been recommended by the American Hospital Association[8] that nipples with crucial incisions be used rather than those with ordinary punctured holes. The crucial cut consisting of two 4 mm. incisions made in the rubber at right angles forming a cross provides a valve-like action which closes as soon as pressure of the infant's mouth is released. Peto[11] has summarized the advantages and disadvantages of the crucial cut nipple for uniform flow of formula. Nipples with this type of opening appear to function satisfactorily for about five weeks of daily use. Most of the commercial manufacturers of nipples have now added the crucial cut type to their lines.

APPROVED METHODS FOR TERMINAL HEATING

The terminal heating of formulas should be universally adopted in hospitals. Under practical conditions of operation and competent supervision, the method can assure bacteriologically safe milk mixtures for infants. The time-temperature relationship of the process must be adequate to destroy pathogens, including the inactivation of viruses. Whereas sterility of the formula is highly desirable, it is not always obtainable. The amount of heat that can be applied is limited by the fragile character of milk which, if heating is too severe, will undergo both physical and nutritional damage.

According to Light and Hodes,[12] the filtrable virus isolated from stools of infants with epidemic diarrhea is regularly inactivated by 10 minutes' boiling. Smith *et al.*[13] also showed that formulas maintained at 212° F. (100° C.) for 15 minutes were sterile and complete destruction of various pathogenic test organisms was obtained when formulas were inoculated with substantial numbers of these organisms. These workers also demonstrated that the nonpathogenic, spore-forming organism, *B. globigii*, was completely destroyed in the majority of samples tested, and in the remaining samples the counts were reduced to less than 10 organisms per ml. Similar data has been reported by Finley *et al.*[10] on formulas processed at 230° F. (110° C.) for 10 minutes.

For preservation of nutritive value of formulas, terminal heating must be controlled as regards time and temperature so as to avoid undesirable chemical changes in the milk. The nutrients which are more easily damaged by excessive heat treatment are the amino acid, lysine, and certain of the vitamins, particularly ascorbic acid and thiamine. Studies by Hodson[14] have shown that proper treatment of formulas by either of the approved methods of terminal heating does not produce deleterious changes to a significant degree.

At the present time public health authorities and other regulatory bodies recognize two methods for terminal heating of formulas—the nonpressure (flowing steam) process and the pressure steam method. Although experience has demonstrated that on the whole the nonpressure method is more dependable and less troublesome, it should be understood that both methods are regarded as satisfactory for terminal heating if conducted properly in sterilizers designed and constructed for this purpose.

The nonpressure terminal heating process, described above, was developed with full appreciation of those factors which form the basis for heat treatment of infants' formulas, namely, to render formulas bacteriologically safe; of uniform quality without producing significant chemical or physical changes; and simplicity of the process so that the technic may be entrusted to the relatively untrained personnel, with full assurance that the formulas will be subjected to the same sterilizing influence day after day. Research on the part of various investigators has shown that nonpressure terminal heating at a temperature of 212° F. (100° C.) for 15 to 30 minutes not only yielded formulas bacteriologically safe, but fewer complications were encountered than when using pressure steam at abnormally high temperatures. Space will not permit a detailed explanation of the known advantages and disadvantages of the two methods. Therefore, the characteristic data has been summarized as follows:

Pressure Method

1) Time-temperature relationship—
   a) 250°F. (121°C.) for 5 minutes.
   b) 230°-232°F. (110°-111°C.) for 10 minutes.
2) Bacteriologically safe.
3) Chemical changes produced—
   a) Partial destruction of vitamins B_1 and C.
   b) Caramelization—resulting in partial destruction of lactose (milk sugar).
   c) Coagulation of milk proteins, apparent in formulas prepared with whole milk.

Nonpressure Method

1) Time-temperature relationship—
   210°-212°F. (99°-100°C.) for 30 minutes.
2) Bacteriologically safe.
3) Chemical changes produced—minimum of untoward effects. Some destruction of heat-labile vitamins, apparent in any method of heat treatment including that of pasteurization.

4) Boiling of formulas may occur with some loss due to evaporation. Nipples may be blown off bottles, holes in nipples clogged and/or outer surfaces of nipples contaminated with dried milk.

5) Requires careful mechanical control and attention during sterilizing cycle.

6) Total processing time—30 to 40 minutes.

7) Overexposure of formulas—produces undesirable physical and chemical changes.

8) Requires slow exhaust of pressure from sterilizer—10 to 15 minutes.

9) Plugging of chamber drain line of sterilizer. This usually occurs if formulas boil over and coagulated milk gains access to the outlet valve.

4) Formulas do not boil. No engendered pressure within bottles.

5) Minimum of attention required from the mechanical or operator's standpoint.

6) Total processing time—35 to 40 minutes.

7) No undesirable changes produced in formulas as result of moderate overexposure.

8) Nonpressure steam in chamber of sterilizer. Load may be removed immediately upon completion of period of exposure.

9) Plugging of chamber drain line of sterilizer does not constitute a problem with nonpressure method.

With the above factors forming the basis for investigative work on this subject, the author has no hesitancy in recommending the nonpressure method as the superior technic for the terminal heating of formulas. The recommended period of exposure for 30 minutes after the thermometer indicates 210°-212° F. (99°-100° C.) allows an ample factor of safety that will automatically compensate for normal variations in load characteristics. Furthermore, even though the temperature of the vapor surrounding the bottles is 212° F. (100° C.) the formulas will not boil. This point has been determined by carefully conducted tests utilizing a Leeds & Northrup potentiometer with thermocouples extending into the bottles of formula during the entire period of exposure. Figure 163 shows a typical temperature chart performance curve of the nonpressure terminal heating process.

An inspection of Figure 163 will reveal that in the environment of flowing steam at a temperature of 212° F. (100° C.) the formula itself will develop a maximum temperature of 212° F. (100° C.) for not less than 20 minutes. From the time when the thermometer indicates 212° F. (100° C.), the formula requires approximately 8 minutes to reach maximum temperature. In addition, it has been determined that the nipple attached to the bottle and protected by a paper cap reaches a temperature of 212° F. (100° C.) at the same time as the thermometer located in the chamber drain line of the sterilizer.

Boiling of the fluid is definitely and intentionally avoided for more than one reason, but specifically to avoid forcing some of the formula out through the nipples, to clog the nipples, and to leave a film of dried milk on the outer surfaces which might promote later contamination. It matters not at all whether the chamber of the sterilizer is large or small or whether it is completely filled or only partly filled, the exposure period should always be the same—and the sterilizing results will be the same.

In evaluating any method for the heat treatment of formulas, whether by nonpressure or pressure steam, the path to the elimination of contamination is beset with pitfalls. If the technique set up does not eliminate the

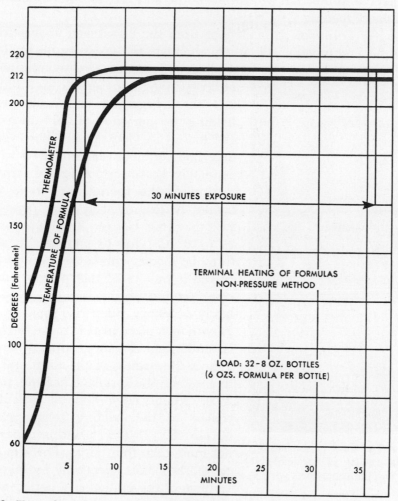

Fig. 163. Typical temperature chart performance curve of the nonpressure terminal heating process.

numerous and obvious opportunities for recontamination of formulas, exteriors of bottles and nipples, between heat treatment and feeding, all other refinements will be lost or most certainly minimized in value. For this reason, the short paper bag or cap has been proposed as a protective medium against contamination in later handling of the formulas. This feature, shown in Figure 164, represents a distinct advance, in the author's opinion, over the conventional glass or metal nipple protectors which interfere to some extent with immediate and complete contact of the steam to all surfaces of the nipple. Steam readily permeates the paper covering, thus assuring decontamination of all surfaces of the nipple. As long as the paper cap remains intact and held firmly in place by means of a rubber band, it provides effective protection against air-borne and contact contamination up to the time of feeding.

Cooling of Formulas: It is obvious from the data given above that the terminal heating process will largely eliminate the necessity for immediate cooling and permit a reasonable amount of laxity in getting the processed formulas into the refrigerator and cooled to the holding temperature of 40° to 45° F. (4° to 7° C.). Occasionally, however, one may find formulas contaminated with an extremely heat-resistant sport-bearing organism of the thermophilic type which cannot be destroyed at a temperature of 212° F. (100° C.) for 30 minutes or 230° F. (110° C.) for 10 minutes. In certain formula rooms where this condition occurred it was found that prompt and efficient cooling of the formulas was absolutely necessary, otherwise rapid bacterial growth took place so as to make the formulas undesirable for the feeding of newborn infants. Regardless of the form and effectiveness of the terminal hearing process, it is recommended that all formulas be cooled to the holding temperature of 40°-45° F. (4°-7° C.) within a period of not more than four hours. This can be accomplished most effectively by taking advantage of the preliminary period of cooling at room temperature for one hour followed by adequate refrigeration.

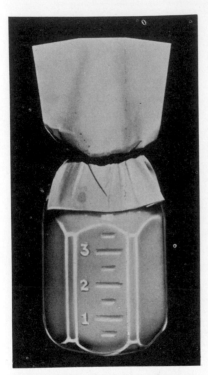

Fig. 164. The short paper bag applied as shown is an effective nipple protector.

Whereas the most rapid method for cooling formulas is by means of a circulating cold water bath, this process does not necessarily represent safe practice for milk formula rooms even though the cooling (tap) water has previously been subjected to some form of chlorination. Outbreaks of intestinal disease attributed to water supplies which have presumably conformed to the United States Public Health Service standards for water have raised the question as to whether present criteria for evaluation of potability of water might not be profitably re-examined. To be sure, the tap water used for this cooling process comes in contact only with the exteriors of the nursing bottles, but it is not difficult to visualize that the wet bottles, as removed from the bath, may in certain instances constitute a potential means of contamination carried to the refrigerator and thence to the nursery. Another reason why the cold water bath is not recommended for the

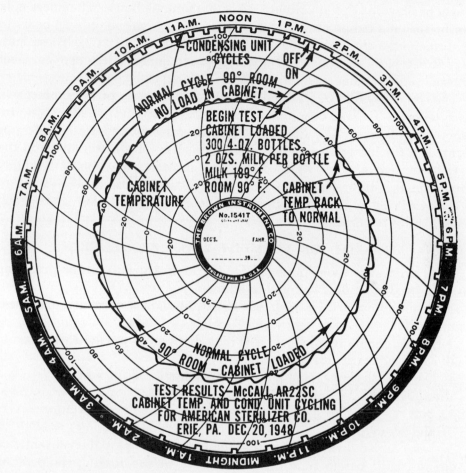

Fig. 165. Refrigerator test results in cooling load of formula bottles from 189° F. to 45° F.

cooling of formulas is the possibility of a contaminated water supply through cross-connections or defects in the hospital's plumbing system. Such defects in plumbing systems are not altogether infrequent even though present day practice requires the elimination of all submerged inlets and direct connections to drains on all plumbing fixtures.

Adequate refrigeration becomes, therefore, a necessity for the proper cooling and storage of the infants' formulas. The average commercial refrigerator cannot be depended upon for prompt and efficient cooling of formula bottles within a maximum of four hours' time. The performance specifications are such as to require a specially designed refrigeration system equipped with a forced air evaporator and an extra heavy duty compressor and condensing unit. Suitable refrigeration equipment is available for this application as shown by the test results given in Figure 165. Here it will be observed that a normal load of 300 formula bottles (2 ounces milk per bottle) at a temperature of 189° F. (87° C.) required only 2½ hours to cool the bottles to the holding temperature of 45° F. (7° C.). These findings are typical of suitable refrigeration equipment designed to meet unusual requirements encountered in the cooling of formulas.

The size of the refrigerator and the net cubic capacity of the cabinet will vary with the average requirements of the nursery and whether the prepared formulas are to be stored and dispensed from one large refrigerator located in the formula room or stored in smaller refrigerator units on the various nursery wards. Whatever the circumstances may be, it is highly important that the refrigerator be equipped with a forced air evaporator and an extra heavy duty compressor and condensing unit, designed specifically for this application.

APPRAISAL OF FORMULA ROOM PROCEDURES

1) Is a separate room provided for the exclusive purpose of preparing formulas and other fluids offered to infants?

2) Is the formula room situated where the danger of contamination is minimized?

3) Is the formula room supervised by a dietitian or nurse experienced in milk room and sterilizing procedures?

4) Does the formula room contain as minimum equipment:

Sterilizer	Refrigerator
2 Sinks	Work Table and Counters
Hand Scrub Sink	

5) Does each individual preparing the formulas employ the conventional 3-minute scrub before performing any duty in the formula preparation room?

6) Are formula ingredients placed in sterile containers, mixed, and the formula then dispensed into previously washed sterile bottles?

7) Are individual feeding bottles covered with sterile nipples and paper caps after filling?

8) Are formula bottles placed in racks or containers each providing the 24-hour supply of feeding for an individual infant and labeled with the name of the infant?

9) Are the bottles of formula then placed in a sterilizer and subjected to terminal heating at a temperature of 212° F. (100° C.) for 30 minutes or 230° F. (110° C.) for 10 minutes?

10) Are formulas allowed to cool at room temperature for about one to

two hours after terminal heat treatment—or is a safe method of water cooling utilized?

11) Are formulas then placed in a refrigerator and maintained at a temperature of 40° F. (4° C.) until feeding time?

12) Does the individual who removes the bottles of formula from the refrigerator at feeding time scrub her hands before touching the bottles?

13) Does the feeding nurse wear a mask and scrub her hands and arms?

14) Is the nurse prohibited from changing the nipple or the size of the holes in the nipple?

15) Are bottles and nipples from isolation and suspect nurseries disinfected by boiling for 15 minutes before being returned to the formula room?

16) Are bottles and nipples rinsed well with cold running water in the nursery immediately after feeding and before being returned to the formula room?

17) In the formula room are all bottles, nipples and utensils washed with an effective detergent, using a bottle brush or mechanical washing unit?

18) Are nipples inverted in the cleaning process to remove any coagulated material?

19) Are bottles and nipples rinsed in hot running water and presterilized before use?

20) Is a bottle of formula taken at random sent daily to the laboratory for bacteriologic testing?

FORMULA STERILIZER OPERATING INSTRUCTIONS

(Refer to Fig. 166)

1) *Daily Before Heating Sterilizer:* Remove plug screen from bottom of chamber and clean lint and sediment from pores of strainer.

2) *Operation of Cyclomatic Control:* Always set "Selector" and "Timer" before turning "Valve Handle" (located in center of control panel). Turn "Timer" counterclockwise only. The small white light indicates when "Timer" is operating. When "Valve Handle" is turned to "Ster." the red light will come on. At completion of timed sterilizing period, the valve automatically turns to "Exhaust." Yellow light comes on and red light goes out. When load is completely processed, green light comes on and alarm will sound until operator turns "Valve Handle" to "Off." Load now may be removed from sterilizer. To permit excess vapor to escape from sterilizer, open door slightly (about ½″) for 5 minutes. Then open door fully and remove load.

Terminal Heating of Formulas: Terminal heating may be conducted by either Nonpressure (streaming steam) Method or Pressure Method. Do not subject lactic acid formulas or protein milk formulas to terminal heating

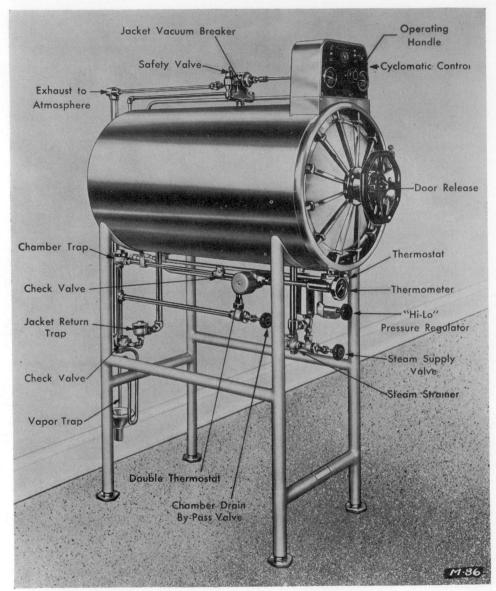

Fig. 166. Typical formula sterilizer, equipped with automatic control.

unless it is known that the preparation will withstand such heating without evidence of curdling.

3) *Recommended Method—Nonpressure (Streaming Steam) Sterilization at 212° F. (100° C.)* With "Valve Handle" at "Off," turn handle on "Pressure Regulator" to left ("Low" position) as far as it will go. Open "Steam Supply Valve." Place racks of bottles in sterilizer and lock door. Then open "By-Pass Valve." Set "Selector" at "Slow Exh." and "Timer" to 30 minutes'

exposure. When "Jacket Gauge" indicates 5-7 pounds pressure, turn "Valve Handle" to "Ster." Operator may now leave the sterilizer and return only when cycle has been completed.

The thermostat and pressure regulator are set at factory for streaming steam operation unless otherwise specified.

4) *Alternate Method—Pressure Sterilization at 230° F. (110° C.)* Set "Pressure Regulator" to obtain 5-7 pounds jacket pressure. The control thermostat also should be adjusted by mechanic for operation at 230° F. (110° C.). Turn handle on "Pressure Regulator" to left ("Low" position) as far as it will go. Open "Steam Supply Valve" and allow jacket pressure to build up to 7 pounds. Place racks of bottles in sterilizer and lock door. Set "Selector" at "Slow Exh." and "Timer" to 10 minutes' exposure. Close "By-Pass Valve" and turn "Valve Handle" to "Ster." Operator may now leave sterilizer and return only when cycle has been completed.

5) *To Sterilize Empty Bottles, Nipples, Utensils and Wrapped Supplies.* With "Valve Handle" at "Off," turn handle of "Pressure Regulator" to right ("High" position) as far as it will go. Open "Steam Supply Valve." Allow jacket pressure to build up to 15-17 pounds. Place load in sterilizer and lock door. Close "By-Pass Valve." Turn "Timer" counterclockwise to desired exposure period. Then turn "Selector" to the appropriate position of:

"Fast Exh." if drying is not required.

"Fast Exh. and Dry" for wrapped supplies.

Turn "Valve Handle" (clockwise only) to "Ster." Operator may now leave sterilizer and return only when cycle has been completed.

RECOMMENDED PERIODS OF EXPOSURE
At 250° F. (121° C.)   *Minutes*

Utensils, containers and measuring devices	15
Nursing bottles, inverted in racks	15
Nipples, in muslin bags	15
Paper caps, loosely packed in tray with perforated bottom	15
Rubber gloves, in muslin wrapper	15
Table covers, gowns, face masks, in muslin wrapper	30

6) *Manual Operation.* In the event of electrical current failure, sterilizer may be operated manually by simply turning "Selector" to "Manual," and then turning "Valve Handle" (clockwise only) to that position on the dial which corresponds to the proper sequence of operations in the sterilizing cycle.

7) *Shut Off "Steam Supply Valve."* Unless sterilizer is to be used again within a short time, close this valve and permit sterilizer to cool.

REFERENCES

1. ENSIGN, P. R. AND HUNTER, C. A.: Epidemic of Diarrhea in Newborn Nursery Caused by Milk-borne Epidemic in Community. *J. Pediat.*, 29:620-628, 1946.
2. LEMBCKE, P. A.: Prevention and Control of Epidemic Diarrhea Is the Administrator's Responsibility. *The Modern Hospital*, 60, No. 3, March, 1943.

3. Light, J. S. and Hodes, F. L.: Studies on Epidemic Diarrhea of the Newborn. *Am. J. Pub. Health, 33:*1451-1454, 1943.

4. Buddingh, G. J.: Virus Stomatitis and Virus Diarrhea of Infants and Young Children. *South. Med. J., 39:*382-388, 1946.

5. Clifford, S. H.: Diarrhea of the Newborn, Its Causes and Prevention. *New England J. Med., 237:*969-976, 1947.

6. Rubinstein, A. D. and Foley, G. E.: Epidemic Diarrhea of the Newborn in Massachusetts: Ten Year Survey. *New England J. Med., 236:*87-120, 1947.

7. *Standards and Recommendations for Hospital Care of Newborn Infants—Full-term and Premature.* American Academy of Pediatrics, 1801 Hinman, Evanston, Ill., 1948.

8. *Procedures and Layout for the Infant Formula Room,* American Hospital Assoc., 18 East Division Street, Chicago, Ill., 1949.

9. New York State Dept. of Health, Sanitary Code, Chapter II, Regulation 35: Precautions to Be Observed for the Control of Diarrhea of the Newborn, Health News Supplement, *25,* No. S-7, Feb. 16, 1948.

10. Finley, R. D., Smith, F. R. and Louder, E. A.: Terminal Heating of Infant Formula. II. Bacteriological Investigation of High-Pressure Technique. *J. Am. Dietet. A., 24:*760-763, 1948.

11. Peto, M.: Preventing Nipple Clogging. *Am. J. Nursing, 50:*487, 1950.

12. Light, J. S. and Hodes, H. L.: Studies on Epidemic Diarrhea of Newborn: Isolation of Filtrable Agent Causing Diarrhea in Calves. *Am. J. Pub. Health, 33:*1451-1454, 1943.

13. Smith, F. R., Finley, R. D., Wright, H. J. and Louder, E. A.: Terminal Heating of Infant Formula. I. Bacteriological Investigation of Low-Pressure Technique. *J. Am. Dietet. A., 24:*755-759, 1948.

14. Hodson, A. Z.: Terminal Heating of Infant Formula. III. Retention of Heat-Labile Nutrients. *J. Am. Dietet. A., 25:*119, 1949.

CHAPTER XX

The Laboratory Sterilizer (Autoclave)

I T IS NO LONGER advisable to attempt to confine the subject of bacteriological sterilization to the use of a single type of laboratory sterilizer. The development of new laboratory techniques, resulting from research in infectious diseases and allied fields, has necessitated the design of highly specialized sterilizing equipment to meet the unusual requirements of these rapidly expanding sterile techniques and processes. Many of these sterilizers are of the combination type for use with either saturated steam under pressure or "Carboxide" gas (page 329). The latter method is relatively new as a sterilizing process and it can be used to advantage as a substitute for steam in the sterilization of a variety of heat and moisture sensitive materials and apparatus. Also deserving of mention are the many double door laboratory sterilizers in routine use, which operate under automatic control, for applications where the transfer of material from an unsterile room to a sterile room without introduction of contamination is the prime requisite. Space will not permit detailed explanations of the form and functions of these different types of laboratory sterilizers employed in bacteriological research and industrial process control. Only basic principles of sterilization can be covered in this book. The more complex equipment and accompanying techniques will have to await the appearance of a more advanced work on the subject.

It is regrettable that in more than a few laboratories, otherwise equipped with highly efficient apparatus, one still finds autoclaves retained in use that are hopelessly obsolete. Some of them are 20 to 30 years old—built at a period when the fundamentals of steam sterilization as we now recognize them were not thoroughly understood, certainly not applied. With such sterilizers, dependable operation and uniformity of results cannot be expected. Reference is made specifically to those sterilizers from which air is discharged, if at all, by some type of hand regulation and in which the thermometer, if one is provided, is located at the top of the chamber. It is true that these sterilizers can be operated so that air will be satisfactorily eliminated from the chamber, but accurate, dependable performance requires expert knowledge of the control and a degree of close supervision that is commonly impractical to apply. Another common fault found in old sterilizers, especially those heated by gas or electricity, is the slow rate of heating which makes it almost impossible to sterilize heat-sensitive fluids and media in them without destructive effect. Such sterilizers have been responsible in a large measure for the erroneous assumption that lower pressures and temperatures or fractional sterilization must be resorted to for all heat-sensitive fluids.

MODERN LABORATORY STERILIZERS

The fundamental principles under which late models of sterilizers function were applied in this country about 1933, at which time rather radical changes were made by the manufacturers. For several years following these changes in design, the most commonly used laboratory sterilizer was the single jacketed pressure chamber as illustrated in Figure 167. This type of sterilizer with minor modifications is still widely used with either direct steam, gas or electric heat. It will function satisfactorily for the sterilization of bacteriological media and solutions. It is not well adapted, nor is any single-walled chamber, to the sterilization of wrapped supplies or any type of load that requires drying after sterilization. Because of the single wall construction, the chamber will contain an excessive amount of moisture following sterilization, and without the aid of radiant heat from a steam jacket, the residual moisture cannot be eliminated. Another disadvantage found in the single jacketed autoclave is that in continuous service, one load after another, it is necessary to cool down the entire autoclave each time a load is withdrawn.

Today, the more generally useful and certainly more efficient laboratory sterilizer is of the type shown in Figure 168. This is constructed with a steam jacket which surrounds the side walls of the chamber, exactly the same as provided on all surgical supply sterilizers. Pressure is first generated in the jacket prior to admission of steam to the chamber, and this pressure is maintained constant at 15-17 pounds throughout the cycle of operation or the entire day. With hot side walls no condensate forms on them, and the load will absorb only that amount of moisture from the steam that is required to heat the load. This feature permits the sterilizer to function just as efficiently for the sterilization and drying of wrapped or porous supplies as does any surgical dressing sterilizer. The drying process may be accomplished either by means of the vacuum dryer device, which operates in conjunction with the automatic control, or by the "cracked door" method (see p. 111). Since pressure is maintained in the steam jacket continuously throughout working hours, the sterilizer remains ready for immediate and more rapid use than is possible with the single wall chamber from which pressure and heat must be exhausted each time a load is withdrawn.

The discharge of air and the movement of steam through the laboratory sterilizer is the same as in any modern pressure steam sterilizer. When steam is admitted to the air-filled chamber, it immediately rises to the top, compressing the air at the bottom. As the pressure builds up in the chamber the air is gradually forced out through the screened outlet leading to the

chamber discharge line, past the thermometer bulb, through the thermostatic trap and finally to the atmospheric vent. This flow will continue until

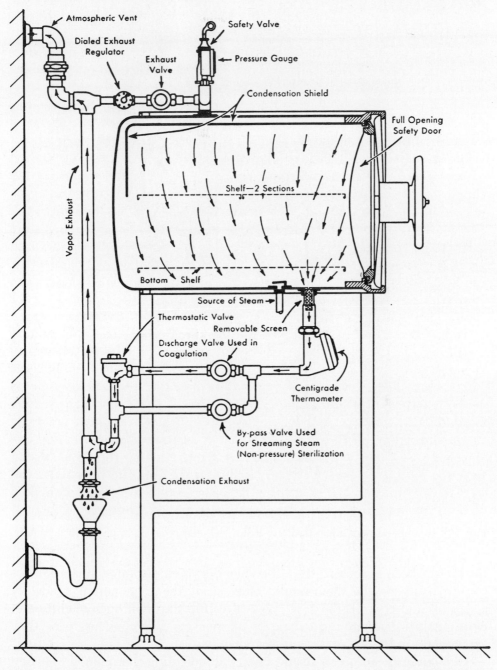

Fig. 167. Diagrammatic illustration of single wall laboratory sterilizer. The arrows
indicate movement of air and steam through the chamber. This type of sterilizer is
now almost obsolete.

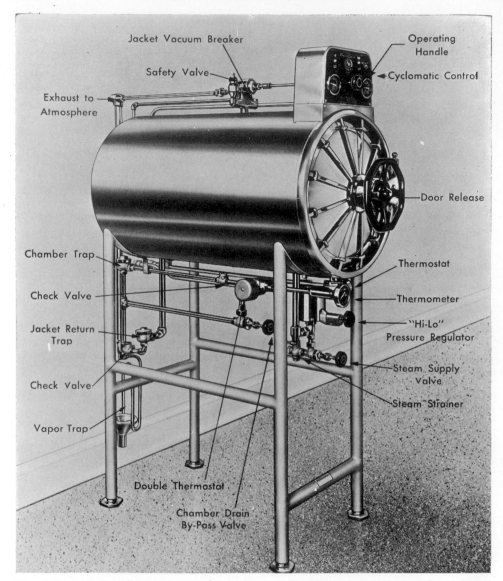

Fig. 168. A modern laboratory sterilizer, steam jacketed type, equipped with automatic controls.

the air has been evacuated from the chamber, then saturated steam follows the air, contacts the thermostatic element of the trap, and it gradually closes off and controls the flow. Thereafter the trap will open slightly and close again to permit the escape of air pockets and condensate as they accumulate in the lower areas of the chamber.

All laboratory sterilizers should have the indicating thermometer located in the chamber discharge line. The purpose is primarily to detect any interruption in the normal flow of air and condensate from the chamber. If the discharge line becomes clogged with sediment or residue from spillage of media in the chamber, there will be no prompt advance in temperature, even though the pressure may rise to the normal operating range. When this occurs, stratification of air and steam in the chamber takes place with the steam concentrated in the upper part of the chamber. A thermometer located at the top of the chamber will then indicate the temperature of relatively pure steam, while the lower or bottom area will be filled with air or an air-steam mixture at much lower temperature. When the thermometer is correctly located in the chamber discharge line, it will promptly indicate faulty operation, the need for cleaning or maintenance, and the quality of the steam in contact with the load. In this connection an added safeguard for the laboratory sterilizer is the automatic time-temperature control. The thermostat which actuates the timer should also be located in the chamber discharge line adjacent to the thermometer. Unless the chamber is filled with saturated steam at the right temperature the control will fail to function.

THE ISOTHERMAL CONTROLLED STERILIZER

The last few years have witnessed an expanding need in laboratories for sterilizers with a much wider range of temperature control than is available in sterilizers of standard design. The requirements cover not only sterilization by steam under pressure, but also fractional sterilization, inspissation and pasteurization. For any one sterilizer to perform all of these functions involves a controlled range of operating temperatures extending from 140° F. (60° C.) to 270° F. (132° C.). To the bacteriologist this broad range of temperature is useful, because it permits him to evaluate the properties of solutions and media sterilized at progressively higher temperatures and shorter periods of time. It also permits fractional sterilization and processing of heat coagulable culture media, egg and blood serum slants, and it provides a convenient means of investigating marginal methods of sterilization of solutions or biologics where a moderate degree of heat plus chemical action produces the required sterilizing effect.

The sterilizer shown in Figure 169 is typical of the latest development in laboratory sterilizer design. The chamber is steam jacketed and constructed for a maximum operating pressure of 30 pounds. The operation is governed by automatic controls which may be set for maintenance of steam temperature anywhere in the range of 221°-270° F. (105° C. to 132° C.) with an accuracy of ± 1.3° F. (± 0.7° C.). The automatic control also permits preselection of exposure periods anywhere in the range of 0 to 90 minutes. For low temperature operation an isothermal control system is employed to prevent air-steam stratification in the chamber. Temperatures may be selected on the thermostat dial anywhere in the range of 140°-219° F. (60° C. to 104° C.) with an average deviation in the chamber of ± 3.3° F.

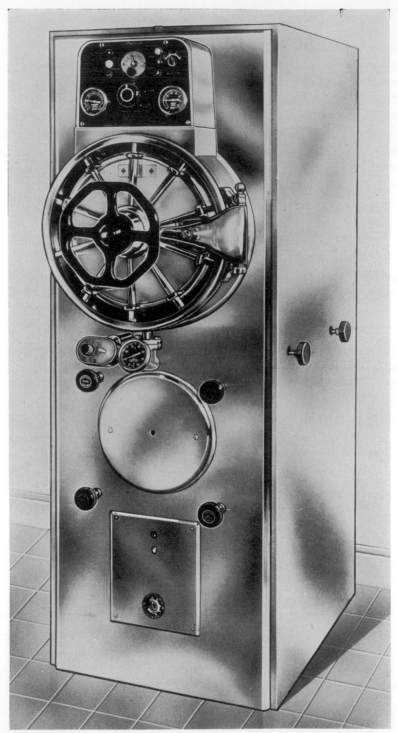

Fig. 169. This unit is typical of one of the latest developments in laboratory sterilizer design. The Isothermal Control provides a range of operating temperatures from 140° F. to 220° F. The automatic pressure control regulator extends the range from 221° F. to 270° F.

(± 1.8° C.). When operating under isothermal control the atmospheric conditions in the chamber approximate saturation with water vapor throughout the cycle.

A diagram of the principle of operation of the isothermal control is given in Figure 170. Steam from the supply line enters the chamber through the steam nozzle or Venturi device. It immediately contacts the cooling coil through which water circulates and the steam is reduced in temperature before it has an opportunity to reach the chamber proper. As steam passes

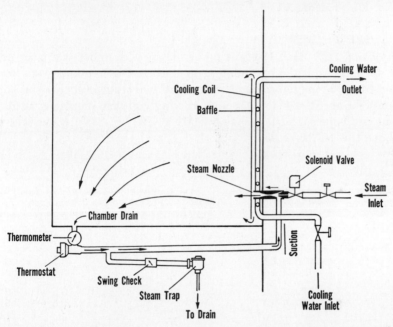

Fig. 170. Diagram of the principle of operation of low temperature Isothermal Control.

through the nozzle and into the chamber, a negative pressure is created at the nozzle which is transmitted to the chamber drain opening through the system of piping. This suction draws incoming steam from the nozzle toward the front end of the chamber and circulates it back to the nozzle via the discharge line and into the chamber again, thereby assuring an isothermal condition throughout the chamber and preventing air-steam stratification. This circulatory process permits the thermometer to function as a true indicator of temperature conditions within the chamber. The supply of steam to the chamber is governed by the solenoid valve which, in turn, is actuated by the thermostat.

Typical of the accuracy of temperature control in processing culture media in the isothermal sterilizer are the following test data:

Sterilizer: 20 x 20 x 36″ Laboratory Sterilizer, steam heat, equipped with Cyclomatic control and Isothermal control.

Load: 235 test tubes (18 x 150 mm.) in baskets, each ⅓ filled with media and stoppered with cotton plugs.

Location of Thermocouples: In tubes located at: 1) front bottom; 2) center, and 3) top rear of chamber. Temperature readings recorded by potentiometer.

Series of Tests

> 5 at 140° F. (60° C.)
> 3 at 160° F. (71° C.)
> 3 at 180° F. (82° C.)
> 3 at 200° F. (93° C.)
> 3 at 210° F. (98.5° C.)

Conditions of Test: Each test was preceded by a chamber warm-up period of 15 minutes at the operating temperature. Observations were continued for a 30-minute period after the load had reached thermostat setting temperature. Water flow through cooling coil was regulated at 20 gallons per hour for all tests below 200° F. (93° C.). No water was used above this temperature.

Results

Thermostat Setting °F. °C.	Thermometer Reading During 30-Min. Period °F. °C.	Time to Heat Load to Processing Temperature Minutes-Average	Deviation of Load Temp. from Thermometer Temp. at Thermocouple Positions °F. °C.
140	141.5 ± 1.5	36	− 5.5 to + 4.5
60	61.0 ± 1.0		− 3.0 to + 2.5
160	163.0 ± 1.0	20	− 6.5 to + 4.0
71	73.0 ± 0.5		− 3.5 to + 2.5
180	181.5 ± 1.0	16	− 3.5 to + 3.5
82	83.0 ± 0.5		− 2.0 to + 2.0
200	200.0 ± 1.0	9	− 1.0 to + 3.0
93	93.0 ± 0.5		− 0.5 to + 1.5
210	210.0 ± 0.5	10	− 1.5 to + 0.
99	99.0 ± 0.3		− 0.8 to + 0.

STERILIZATION OF LIQUIDS

The sterilization of liquids in flasks, bottles or test tubes involves a different use of steam than is required for sterilization of dry goods. In the latter case it is necessary to permeate the porous materials with steam in order that both heat and moisture shall be absorbed by the fibers. In solution sterilization the problem is simply a matter of absorbing heat from the steam. The solution, if aqueous, contains the necessary moisture. When steam contacts the cold flasks or bottles it condenses, and the condensate drains to the bottom of the sterilizer and then out to the waste by means of the chamber discharge line. This process will continue until the solution has been heated to the temperature of the surrounding steam. The time required for heating governs the exposure period. This will vary with the size and shape of the container, the volume of liquid, the thickness of the container walls and the heat conductivity of the container. Measurements to determine the time required for a given container of solution to attain a temperature of 250° F. (121° C.) are usually made by means of a thermo-

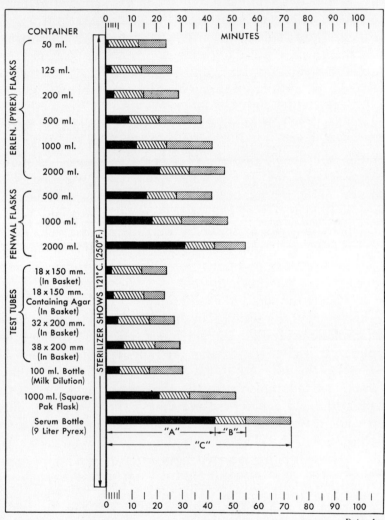

Data from Perkins[3]

Fig. 171. Comparison of the different rates of heating of solutions in commonly used containers. Section "A" of each bar represents the additional time required for the solution in the container to reach 250° F. after the sterilizer thermometer shows this temperature. Section "B" is the holding period (minimum standard) after the solution has reached 250° F. "A" plus "B" equals the required exposure period. The entire bar length designated "C" is the total time that the solution remains above 212° F. during the entire sterilizing cycle, including slow exhaust. (Sterilizer equipped with automatic control.)

couple and potentiometer. The graphic data given in Figure 171 are illustrative of the different rates of heat transfer through commonly used flasks and bottles.

Common errors in solution sterilization can often be avoided through a clear understanding of the operating cycle. During the period of heating the solution and as long as the exposure continues, there will be no visible indication of boiling of the liquid, even though the temperature may be far above the normal boiling point of water at atmospheric pressure. This is due to steam pressure maintained in the sterilizer, at all times equal to or in excess of the pressure possible to develop from the heat in the liquid. Until this condition reverses there can be no ebullition. When the chamber pressure is reduced, after sterilization, the pressure corresponding to the temperature of the liquid will then be greater than the steam pressure and the liquid will begin to boil. If chamber pressure is exhausted rapidly, boiling will be so violent that stoppers will be blown out of the flasks and some of the solution will escape into the chamber. Experience has shown that when pressure is exhausted at a uniform rate through a period of not less than 10 to 15 minutes, the solution will lose its heat at about the same rate as the pressure reduction, and violent boiling will not occur. With heavy loads of solutions in flasks or bottles it may be necessary to extend the exhaust period to 20 or 30 minutes, depending upon the characteristics of the sterilizer exhaust valve and the type of closure on the flasks or bottles.

Even when the cooling down process is conducted with the greatest of care there will be an evaporation loss of fluid of 3 to 5 per cent, unless the containers are hermetically sealed. This has established the general practice in preparing solutions of adding about 5 per cent more distilled water to the container so that after sterilization the product will have the intended concentration. On the other hand, too slow cooling is objectionable. If the period is over-extended, the effect is the same as over-exposure. If the heat is turned off at the end of the exposure time and the sterilizer allowed to cool down without opening the exhaust, one hour or longer may elapse before the pressure in the chamber is reduced to zero gauge. During this period, the liquid will be maintained between the maximum temperature of 250°-254° F. (121°-123° C.) and 212° F. (100° C.). For many solutions this prolonged exposure to temperatures above 212° F. (100° C.) is not harmful, but for bacteriological media containing carbohydrates or agar the destructive influence is marked.

Assuming that a modern sterilizer is in use, destructive effects usually follow the incorrect practice of sterilizing all loads of solutions for the same period, the old "15 pounds for 20 minutes" rule or something equally unscientific. It takes much longer to sterilize a 1000 ml. flask of liquid than a test tube containing 10 ml., yet it is not uncommon to find laboratory sterilizers filled with large flasks and small tubes, all in the same load. The size and type of flask used, not the number of flasks in the sterilizer, establishes the exposure period. If the flasks are all alike, the exposure period will be the same for one or any number placed in the sterilizer. The time required to heat the containers to the sterilizing temperature will, of course, vary with the size of load, but exposure period should not vary. Containers should not be filled to more than 75 per cent of their capacity, to allow for fluid expansion and to prevent overflow.

EXPOSURE PERIODS FOR SOLUTIONS

The following exposure periods for aqueous solutions or liquids in various types of containers will afford a reasonable factor of safety in sterilization:

Container	Capacity	Minutes Exposure 250°-254° F. (121°-123° C.)
Test Tubes	18 x 150 mm.	12 – 14
Test Tubes	32 x 200 mm.	13 – 17
Test Tubes	38 x 200 mm.	15 – 20
Erlenmeyer (Pyrex) Flask	50 ml.	12 – 14
Erlenmeyer (Pyrex) Flask	125 ml.	12 – 14
Erlenmeyer (Pyrex) Flask	200 ml.	12 – 15
Erlenmeyer (Pyrex) Flask	500 ml.	17 – 22
Erlenmeyer (Pyrex) Flask	1000 ml.	20 – 25
Erlenmeyer (Pyrex) Flask	2000 ml.	30 – 35
Fenwal (Pyrex) Flask	500 ml.	24 – 28
Fenwal (Pyrex) Flask	1000 ml.	25 – 30
Fenwal (Pyrex) Flask	2000 ml.	40 – 45
Square-Pak (Pyrex) Flask	500 ml.	24 – 28
Square-Pak (Pyrex) Flask	1000 ml.	25 – 30
Square-Pak (Pyrex) Flask	2000 ml.	40 – 45
Milk Dilution Bottle	100 ml.	13 – 17
Serum Bottle (Pyrex)	9000 ml.	50 – 55

Minimum exposures as given above represent the least periods under which sterilization should be attempted and the maximum periods should not normally be exceeded.

BACTERIOLOGICAL MEDIA

Various kinds of bacteriological media are known to be heat-sensitive. Prolonged sterilization or excessive heating of media containing sugars, such as glucose, lactose and saccharose, frequently undergo hydrolysis with the production of acid. Phenol red lactose broth, for example, sterilized at 250° F. (121° C.) for 15 minutes, or sterilized by filtration, produces no demonstrable amount of acid when inoculated with S. *typhosa,* but when sterilized for 30 to 45 minutes at this temperature an appreciable amount of acid is produced. Excessive heating may also result in the formation of a precipitate in agar media. Over-exposure may cause an increase in acidity, break down the peptones, and diminish the ability of the agar to produce a firm jell. Media, such as wort agar, with a normal pH of 4.8, will upon over-sterilization, cause destruction of the agar. Nutrient agar should be sterilized immediately after it is made and while still fluid because of the destructive influence attendant with each additional heating. Most sugars contained in media can be sterilized by autoclaving if overheating is avoided. In fact, it has been shown[1] that maltose and lactose undergo less destruction by rapid autoclaving than by fractional or intermittent sterilization in the Arnold apparatus. If the medium is contained in test tubes, the tubes placed in wire baskets (not overloaded), so that steam can circulate freely around each tube, an exposure period of 12 minutes at 250° F. (121° C.) will usually be found satisfactory.

FRACTIONAL STERILIZATION

Occasionally it is necessary to sterilize bacteriological media at temperatures no higher than that of atmospheric steam. Also, solutions of certain chemicals, such as cocaine and epinephrine, which are unstable at autoclaving temperatures, can best be sterilized with flowing steam. For this purpose a special type of non-pressure sterilizer (Arnold) is commonly used in which the material is subjected to the free-flowing steam from boiling water for periods of time varying from 20 to 60 minutes on each of three consecutive days. The modern laboratory sterilizer of the type shown in Figure 168 will also permit operation with non-pressure or flowing steam. Between exposures to steam the material is kept at incubation temperature or room temperature. The principle of this method is that the first exposure to flowing steam destroys the vegetative forms of bacteria but not the spores. Then when the material is incubated overnight or for 24 hours, most of the spores will develop into the vegetative stage and they will be killed by the second period of heating. Again the material is incubated, allowing the remainder of the spores to germinate so that they may be killed on the third heating. Although sterilization usually results after the third period of heating, failures may also occur. Optimum conditions must prevail in the media in order for the spores to develop into vegetative forms during the incubation period. The presence of proper nutrients, correct pH, and the absence of bacteriostatic substances influence the effectiveness of the process.

INSPISSATION

The process of inspissation is a combination of pasteurization with intermittent or discontinuous heating for a period of 4 to 7 days. It consists of heating the solution or material in a water bath or an inspissator once daily for 30 to 60 minutes at 140° F. (60° C.) to 176° F. (80° C.), or at the highest temperature below 212° F. (100° C.) which the substance can tolerate without change, for from 4 to 7 days. It is not regarded as a reliable method of sterilization, but frequently must be used for heat-sensitive pharmaceuticals or chemicals which are injured by higher temperatures. A bacteriostatic agent is usually added to the medicinal preparations sterilized by this process.

One of the most useful applications of the inspissation process is the preparation of heat-coagulable media for use in diagnostic bacteriology. Loewenstein's, Jensen's, Petroff's, Locke's, blood serum and other heat-coagulable media call for special treatment in order to prepare culture slants with the proper degree of hardness and to avoid formation of broken bubbles on the surface caused by engendered pressure. Many laboratories process such media in the Arnold sterilizer or in the autoclave with air trapped in the chamber so that the partial pressure of steam in the air-steam mixture produces a temperature of 176° F. (80° C.) to 200° F. (93° C.). Neither of these methods is satisfactory because of the difficulty in maintaining accurate temperature control, the non-uniformity of temperature throughout the chamber and the load, and the long time required for inspissation. Even with a specially designed electrically heated inspissator the time required to produce a satisfactory medium is 2 hours.[2] The isothermal controlled sterilizer (Fig. 170) functions ideally for the processing of heat-coagulable media. Slants coagulate satisfactorily at 176° F. (80° C.) for 30 minutes or 200° F. (93° C.) for 20 minutes. The degree of hardness may be altered as desired by increasing temperature and/or lengthening exposure period.

STERILIZATION OF EMPTY FLASKS OR BOTTLES

Empty flasks or bottles can be sterilized in the autoclave if they are placed on their sides in the chamber so as to provide a horizontal path for the escape of air. If the container has no stopper or cover air will be displaced quickly in this position and sterilization will occur in 15 minutes at 250° F. (121° C.). If the container is tightly sealed or stoppered sterilization will not occur, regardless of the position of the container, because steam will be excluded. Even when flasks are lightly stoppered with cotton, placed bottom side up in the sterilizer, air evacuation will be somewhat retarded and exposure should be not less than 30 minutes. This method of sterilizing lightly stoppered containers can only be recommended with reservation because of the uncertainty of air elimination. It is preferable to sterilize stoppered flasks by the hot air method.

HOT AIR STERILIZATION OF GLASSWARE

Exposure to hot air is the method of choice for the routine sterilization of glassware common to the bacteriological laboratory. This includes such items as Petri dishes and pipettes (wrapped in paper or placed in special metallic holders), empty test tubes (plugged), centrifuge tubes, fermentation tubes, bottles, flasks, and any other empty glass, porcelain or metallic containers required as sterile stock laboratory supplies. Prior to sterilization, all glassware must be thoroughly cleaned and free from traces of organic matter, otherwise during the heating process the residue may char and leave stains on the containers after sterilization. Glassware containing cultures or infectious material should first be sterilized by means of steam under pressure, then emptied, and thoroughly cleaned in hot detergent solution. A temperature of 340° F. (170° C.) for at least one hour is recommended for the hot air sterilization of glassware. Although a prolonged exposure to this temperature is not deleterious to the glassware, excessive heating will definitely char the paper wrappers or cotton plugs.

REFERENCES

1. BENTON, A. AND LEIGHTON, A.: Actual Temperatures Attained by Mediums in Autoclave Sterilization. *J. Infect. Dis.*, 37:353-358, 1925.
2. LEVIN, W., BRANDON, G. R. AND MCMILLEN, S.: The Culture Method of Laboratory Diagnosis of Tuberculosis. *Am. J. Pub. Health*, 40:1305-1310, 1950.
3. PERKINS, J. J.: Bacteriological and Surgical Sterilization by Heat. From REDDISH, G. F., *Antiseptics, Disinfectants, Fungicides and Sterilization*. Philadelphia, Lea & Febiger, p. 697, 1954.

Gaseous Sterilization With Ethylene Oxide

RESEARCH STUDIES in the past decade have yielded important findings in the field of gaseous sterilizing agents. The cause of these investigations is the ever-present need for a reliable "cold" sterilizing process, whereby a variety of materials of low thermostability may be rendered sterile with comparative ease, rapidity and economy. Of chief importance are those studies relating to the microbicidal action of the compound known as ethylene oxide, in both liquid and gaseous states. The methodology of handling ethylene oxide is rapidly expanding and, today, equipment and procedures are being used for sterilization purposes in the pharmaceutical and surgical dressings industry, research institutions and in some hospitals.

The discussion which follows is intentionally restricted to as brief a summary on gaseous sterilization as is deemed advisable at the present time. Any attempt to discuss the subject on the same established basis as that of heat sterilization could hardly be justified. Developments resulting from current studies in this field will undoubtedly have a marked influence on existing methods and applications for gaseous sterilization in the reasonably near future.

PROPERTIES OF ETHYLENE OXIDE

Ethylene oxide is an extremely reactive and useful chemical. It is classified chemically as a cyclic ether, the structure of which may be represented as:

$$\begin{array}{ccc} H & & H \\ HC & \!\!\!\!\!\!\!\rule[0.3em]{3em}{0.4pt}\!\!\!\!\!\! & CH \\ & \diagdown\;\diagup & \\ & O & \end{array}$$

It is manufactured on a large scale in the United States, principally for use as an intermediate in the synthesis of other organic compounds, not the least of which are the synthetic detergents. Ethylene oxide will react with substances such as water, alcohols, ammonia, amines, organic and mineral acids. At ordinary temperatures and pressures it is a colorless gas with an ethereal like odor. Below its boiling point of 51.3° F. (10.7° C.) it is a colorless liquid, miscible with water in all proportions. It is irritating to the skin and mucous membranes in both the liquid and vapor forms. Exposure of the skin to the liquid, concentrated or dilute, can cause severe burns. A maximum allowable concentration of 100 parts per million of ethylene oxide by volume in air has been suggested by several agencies[1] as the safe concentration for an 8-hour working day exposure.

Liquid ethylene oxide is flammable and the vapors form flammable and explosive mixtures with air in all proportions from 3 to 80 per cent by volume.[2] Because of the potential fire and explosive hazard pure ethylene oxide in either the liquid or vapor form cannot be recommended for routine use as a sterilizing agent. Fortunately this hazard can be eliminated when ethylene oxide is mixed or diluted with an inert gas, such as carbon dioxide, in a concentration of not less than 7.5 volumes of carbon dioxide per volume of ethylene oxide. The commercial product known as "Carboxide"[*] is a safe and practical mixture for sterilization purposes. It consists of 10 per cent ethylene oxide and 90 per cent carbon dioxide, supplied in 30 and 60 pound cylinders with specially constructed eductor tubes to insure that the ratio of ethylene oxide to carbon dioxide emerging from the nozzle is within the safe range.

Unlike formaldehyde or other gaseous disinfectants, ethylene oxide and Carboxide possess the ability to diffuse and penetrate through a mass of dry material with ease. Phillips[3] presented data to show that cloth impregnated with bacterial spores and placed inside unsealed paper envelopes could be sterilized by exposure to ethylene oxide vapor at 450 mg. per liter (0.45 ounces per cubic foot) concentration at room temperature in 4 to 6 hours, even though the envelopes were protected by many layers of clothing. According to Lorenz *et al.*,[4] this gas will also penetrate through unbroken egg shells and sterilize the contents within. A good example of the penetrating power of Carboxide in an air evacuated chamber is the sterilization of small surgical dressings, hermetically sealed in cellophane envelopes, packaged in small cartons and the cartons, in turn, placed in large fiberboard sealed shipping containers. Under vacuum treatment the gas readily permeates the containers, diffuses through the cellophane barrier, without rupture, and sterilizes the dressings in 4-6 hours exposure at 110° F. (43° C.) and a concentration of 450 mg. per liter of ethylene oxide. Both ethylene oxide and Carboxide possess the desirable characteristic of being quickly dissipated from materials following sterilization. Thus, a wide variety of materials can be sterilized effectively without undesirable side effects caused by excessive temperatures, or undesirable after effects caused by retention of harmful residues of the sterilizing agent for long periods of time.

MICROBICIDAL ACTION OF ETHYLENE OXIDE

The germicidal properties of ethylene oxide have been noted by a number of investigators, particularly those associated with the food processing

---

[*] A product of Carbide and Carbon Chemicals Corp., New York.

industry, where ethylene oxide and Carboxide have been used for many years as insecticidal and fumigating agents. In 1936, a patent was issued to Schrader and Bossert[5] on a fumigant composition consisting of a mixture of ethylene oxide or alkylene oxides with an inert gas, such as carbon dioxide. Mention is made in this patent of the powerful germicidal and pest exterminating effect as well as the incombustible properties of the mixture. This is probably the earliest reference in the literature to the antibacterial properties of ethylene oxide. It is generally accepted that the sterilizing action of gaseous ethylene oxide was not well known until the appearance of a series of papers by Phillips and Kaye[6, 7, 8, 9] in 1949. These studies demonstrated the sporicidal activity of the gas as well as the effects of concentration, time, temperature and moisture upon sterilization. Other workers[10] have shown that ethylene oxide is capable of destroying the highly resistant thermophilic bacteria frequently encountered in food materials.

Ginsberg and Wilson[11] reported on the inactivation of several viruses by liquid ethylene oxide. Also, Klarenbeek and Tongeren[12] showed that gaseous ethylene oxide in conjunction with carbon dioxide inactivated the vaccinia virus and Columbia-SK-encephalomyelitis virus in 8 hours at room temperature. Mold spores[13] and pathogenic fungi[14] are likewise destroyed by exposure to adequate concentrations of the gas. Wilson and Bruno[15] demonstrated that liquid ethylene oxide will kill *Mycobacterium tuberculosis,* and Carboxide gas under proper conditions is also effective against the BCG strain of this organism.[16] It appears that one of the virtues of ethylene oxide gas as a sterilizing agent is its effectiveness in the presence of large amounts of extraneous materials. Phillips,[3] for example, mentioned that dry bacterial spores mixed with raw eggs, feces, petroleum jelly and motor oil could be sterilized by exposing the mixture to an atmosphere containing ethylene oxide, provided the depth through which the gas had to diffuse was not too great. Caution should be exercised, however, in the treatment of foods or experimental animal diets with ethylene oxide because of the possibility of impairment of nutritional properties.[17, 18]

FACTORS WHICH INFLUENCE THE STERILIZING EFFICIENCY OF ETHYLENE OXIDE

There are several factors which markedly influence the sterilizing efficiency of ethylene oxide and Carboxide. One serious obstacle frequently encountered is the moisture content of the material undergoing sterilization. Dry powdered materials of very low moisture content are considerably more difficult to sterilize than those which are relatively moist. Protein powder, for example, heavily contaminated and with a moisture content of 0.5 per cent, could not be sterilized in 16 hours exposure to ethylene oxide in a concentration of 450 mg. per liter at 115° F. (46° C.). When the powder was equilibrated beforehand against a 60 per cent relative humidity sterilization was accomplished in the same period of exposure, concentration and temperature. The effect of the moisture factor on the sterilizing action of ethylene oxide, as related to various materials, is not well defined. Practical industrial applications in the sterilization of dry materials would seem to indicate that best results are obtained when the materials are in equilibrium with relative humidities ranging from 30 to 60 per cent prior to sterilization. In general, this supports the findings of Kaye and Phillips[9] that when ethylene oxide vapor is applied to highly evacuated systems from which almost all air and moisture have been removed before admission of the vapor, sterilization becomes more difficult.

The concentration of ethylene oxide, the temperature, and the exposure time are other factors which determine the efficiency of the sterilizing process. When using Carboxide in commercial sterilizing chambers, designed for a maximum operating pressure of 20 psig., it is not possible to obtain an ethylene oxide concentration much greater than 400 mg. per liter or 0.4 ounce per cubic foot. At this level and with ambient temperatures ranging from 75° to 100° F. (24° to 38° C.), it is not advisable to attempt sterilization of bulk materials in less than 16 hours' exposure or overnight. A more practical procedure with a much greater factor of safety is to use a sterilizing chamber designed for a maximum operating pressure of 33 psig. This will permit the introduction of sufficient Carboxide so as to obtain an ethylene oxide concentration of 450 to 550 mg. per liter in the temperature range of 75° to 100° F. Under these conditions the exposure period can be safely reduced to 4-8 hours.

CARBOXIDE STERILIZERS FOR BULK MATERIALS

From the standpoint of safety, ethylene oxide should always be used in combination with an inert gas such as carbon dioxide. When this mixture is contained within vacuum-pressure chambers of correct design, under intelligent operation, it provides a reliable means for sterilization of heat-sensitive and moisture-sensitive materials. Articles made of plastic, rubber, leather, delicate instruments, laboratory apparatus, mattresses and bedding, surgical dressings and pharmaceuticals may be sterilized by this process. The sterilizing chamber should be designed and constructed to withstand a working pressure of 33 pounds per square inch. This will permit the admission of a sufficient amount of Carboxide to give a concentration of 450 to 525 mg. per liter of ethylene oxide, with chamber temperature maintained in the range of 100° to 130° F. (38° to 54° C.). An efficient vacuum pump with adequate capacity to remove air and residual gas from the chamber and the load is also essential (see Fig. 172).

The chief difficulty encountered in Carboxide sterilization, to date, has been the lack of a standardized and controlled method of dispensing the gas from the high pressure cylinder into the sterilizing chamber. The standard cylinder of Carboxide is provided with an internal eductor tube of special design, the purpose of which is to insure that the discharged mixture will be in the non-explosive range and yet contain sufficient ethylene oxide to make it an effective sterilizing agent. These two conditions can be met only if the cylinder is discharged under rigidly specified conditions. When the valve on the cylinder is opened, the escaping mixture is both liquid and gas which, under proper conditions of temperature and pressure, will completely vaporize. However, when small portions of the mixture are intermittently withdrawn from the cylinder they are known to be higher in ethylene oxide concentration than 10 per cent, usually in the

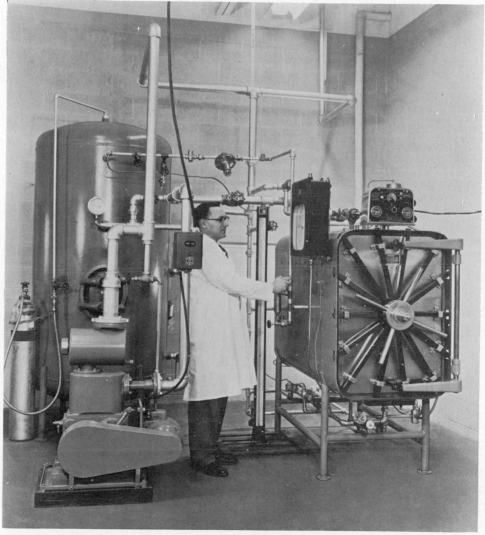

Fig. 172. Carboxide sterilizer for bulk materials. The assembly consists of a 24 cu. ft. chamber with essential controls, expansion tank and vacuum pump.

range of 11 to 12.5 per cent. After approximately 80 per cent of the contents
of the cylinder are withdrawn in this manner the remaining 20 per cent is too
low in ethylene oxide concentration to be of value in sterilization. Figure

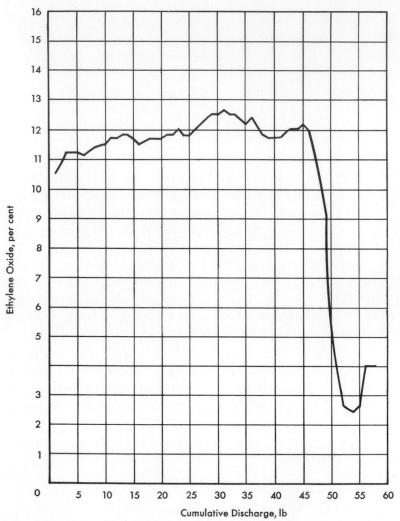

Fig. 173. Composition of the discharged mixture when Carboxide is withdrawn intermittently in 1-pound increments from a standard cylinder.

173 shows the composition of the discharge when the Carboxide is withdrawn intermittently in 1-pound increments from a standard cylinder. It
can be seen that the ethylene oxide concentration is appreciably higher
than 10 per cent in the first 46 pounds discharged, and drops too low in the
final 10 pounds, when mostly vapor is being withdrawn. This means that
when small increments are withdrawn from a Carboxide cylinder to directly
charge sterilizing chambers of less than 50 cubic feet capacity, there is no

alternative other than to discard (not use) the last 20 per cent remaining in the cylinder.

Experimentation has also shown that it is not advisable to directly charge the sterilizer from the Carboxide cylinder for three reasons: First, the incoming mixture of liquid and gas undergoes a marked drop in temperature when permitted to expand in the sterilizer. This cooling effect retards sterilizing action. Secondly, if the incoming ethylene oxide in the liquid phase contacts the materials undergoing sterilization harmful effects may occur. Plastics and certain types of packaging materials are often damaged for this reason. Thirdly, there is no provision for automatic make-up of Carboxide in the sterilizer should leakage occur during the exposure period. To overcome these unfavorable conditions it is desirable to first release the Carboxide from the cylinder into an intermediate chamber or expansion tank. This tank should be uniformly heated to a temperature required to maintain the mixture in the gas phase. The sterilizing chamber may then be charged directly from the expansion tank under ideal conditions. With equipment of the type shown in Figure 172, the following procedure is recommended for the sterilization of bulk materials:

1) Use a jacketed pressure chamber, fabricated of carbon steel or stainless clad steel, designed for a maximum working pressure of 33 pounds per square inch. Low pressure steam thermostatically controlled should be supplied to jacket so as to maintain a chamber temperature in the range of 115°-130° F. (46°-54° C.).

2) Admit the entire contents of two 30-pound Carboxide cylinders into an evacuated, heated expansion tank of about 70 cubic feet capacity, located adjacent to the sterilizer. It is desirable to use a jacketed expansion tank heated with low pressure steam under thermostatic control so as to maintain the Carboxide in the gas phase at all times.

3) Remove the air from the sterilizer chamber and the load by drawing a vacuum of 27-28 inches in no more than 5 minutes. *Avoid holding vacuum for long periods.*

4) Immediately admit the heated gas from the expansion tank to the sterilizing chamber, by means of an automatic pressure regulator, until a chamber pressure of 25-28 pounds is attained.

5) The exposure period is largely dependent upon the type and degree of contamination present on the materials. For heavily contaminated materials containing 1 million or more resistant spores per gram or the equivalent, the exposure period should be not less than 7 hours. For most articles it is rarely necessary to exceed 4 hours' exposure under the above conditions.

6) At the end of the exposure period the gas in the sterilizer is exhausted to the atmosphere outside the building, followed by drawing a vacuum of 28-29 inches to remove residual gas from the load.

7) The final vacuum in the sterilizer is relieved by admission of room air to atmospheric pressure through a bacteria-retentive air filter.

AUTOMATICALLY CONTROLLED CARBOXICLAVE

The full value of Carboxide gas as a sterilizing agent cannot be realized until such time as suitable equipment is commercially available for routine

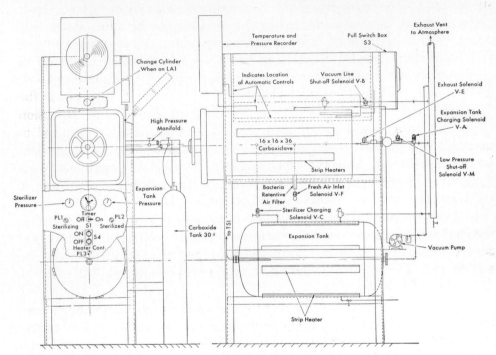

Fig. 174. Schematic diagram of an automatically controlled "Carboxiclave," complete with auxiliary equipment.

and experimental use in hospitals and laboratories. The sterilizing equipment and procedure described above is well suited to the treatment of bulk materials, but it is poorly adapted to the sterilization of the many small articles of a heat-sensitive nature required in hospitals and laboratories. To meet this latter requirement for institutional use, it is necessary that the Carboxide sterilizer be subject to fully automatic control. Typical of one of the latest developments in Carboxide sterilizer design with automatic control is the schematic diagram shown in Figure 174. The sterilizing chamber has dimensions of 16 x 16 x 36 inches with a useful capacity of 5.3 cu. ft. The auxiliary equipment essential to safe operation includes an expansion tank mounted directly under the sterilizer, a small vacuum pump located at the rear of the expansion tank, and a pressure-temperature recorder.

The control mechanism is mounted on a concealed panel located on the upper righthand side of the sterilizer. Both the sterilizing chamber and the expansion tank are maintained at constant temperature by means of external strip (electric) heaters. The instrument panel on the front of the sterilizer contains an adjustable timer with settings from 0 to 18 hours, pressure gauges for expansion tank and chamber, indicator signal lights and manual control switches. Carboxide gas is supplied to the expansion tank from the high pressure cylinder via the manifold connector. The automatic controls prevent charging the sterilizer until the gaseous mixture in the expansion tank is at the correct temperature and pressure. The pressure in the sterilizer is maintained constant during the entire exposure period. A complete cycle of operation comprises the following sequence of events:

After loading the sterilizer, locking door, and setting timer, the main switch "S-1" is turned on. Air is automatically discharged from the chamber by means of the vacuum pump. When a vacuum of 28 inches is reached in the chamber the pump stops and a solenoid valve (VC) opens between expansion tank and chamber. Carboxide gas at the correct temperature is then released into the chamber until a pressure of 27 pounds is attained. The valve (VC) closes and the timer begins to operate. At the end of the exposure period valve (VE) opens and the gas in the chamber is discharged to the atmosphere via the exhaust vent. After pressure in the chamber is reduced to zero gauge, valve (VE) closes, and valve (VB) opens, the vacuum pump starts, and the chamber is evacuated to 28 inches. This step removes residual gas from the load. The pump then stops, valve (VB) closes, and valve (VF) opens. Filtered air is then permitted to enter the chamber to relieve the final vacuum. At this point an alarm rings informing the operator that the cycle of sterilization is complete. The load may then be removed from the sterilizer.

In closing, it may be appropriate to mention that recognition of ethylene oxide as a sterilizing agent has renewed scientific interest in the microbicidal action of other gases as well as the mode of action of gaseous agents upon the bacterial cell. What the future may hold in this field of endeavor is difficult to predict. It is probable that other gases or combinations thereof will eventually be found which are superior to ethylene oxide, both in sterilizing efficiency and economy. Or, perhaps, future investigations in this area will give way to even more challenging methods of "cold" sterilization by means of ionizing radiations. Recent advances in the application of cathode rays and gamma rays for sterilization purposes have been encouraging, particularly in the food processing and pharmaceutical industries. However, much research still remains to be done. How soon or to what extent these newer sterilizing agents will invade and possibly replace the time-honored methods of heat sterilization is a topic for future discussion.

REFERENCES

1. *Operating Procedures for Ethylene Oxide.* Carbide and Carbon Chemicals Corp., New York, 1952, p. 4.

2. JONES, G. W. AND KENNEDY, R. E.: Extinction of Ethylene Oxide Flames with Carbon Dioxide. *Indust. and Engin. Chem.*, 22:146-147, 1930.

3. PHILLIPS, C. R.: *Practical Aspects of Sterilization with Ethylene Oxide Vapor.* Bact. Proc., 50th Meeting, Soc. Am. Bact., 23-24, 1950.

4. LORENZ, F. W., STARR, P. B. AND BOUTHILET, R. J.: Fumigation of Shell Eggs with Ethylene Oxide. *Poultry Sc.*, 29:545-547, 1950.

5. SCHRADER, H. AND BOSSERT, E.: *Fumigant Composition.* U.S. Patent 2,037,439, April 14, 1936.

6. PHILLIPS, C. R. AND KAYE, S.: The Sterilizing Action of Gaseous Ethylene Oxide. I. Review. *Am. J. Hyg.*, 50:270-279, 1949.

7. PHILLIPS, C. R.: II. Sterilization of Contaminated Objects with Ethylene Oxide and Related Compounds: Time, Concentration and Temperature Relationships. *Am. J. Hyg.*, 50:280-288, 1949.

8. KAYE, S.: III. The Effect of Ethylene Oxide and Related Compounds upon Bacterial Aerosols. *Am. J. Hyg.*, 50:289-295, 1949.

9. KAYE, S. AND PHILLIPS, C. R.: IV. The Effect of Moisture. *Am. J. Hyg.*, 50:296-306, 1949.

10. PAPPAS, H. J. AND HALL, L. A.: The Control of Thermophilic Bacteria. *Food Tech.*, 6:456-458, 1952.

11. GINSBERG, H. S. AND WILSON, A. T.: Inactivation of Several Viruses by Liquid Ethylene Oxide. *Proc. Soc. Exper. Biol. & Med.*, 73:614-616, 1950.

12. KLARENBEEK, A. AND TONGEREN VAN, H. A. E.: *On the Virucidal Action of Gaseous Ethylene Oxide in Conjunction with Carbon Dioxide.* From Dept. of Bact. and Exper. Path., Netherlands Institute for Preventive Medicine, Leiden, Holland.

13. KIRBY, G. W., ATKIN, L. AND FREY, C. N.: Recent Progress in "Rope" and Mold Control, *Food Indust.*, 8:450, 1936.

14. FULTON, J. D. AND MITCHELL, R. B.: Sterilization of Footwear. *U.S. Armed Forces Med. J.*, 3:425-439, 1952.

15. WILSON, A. T. AND BRUNO, P.: The Sterilization of Bacteriological Media and Other Fluids with Ethylene Oxide. *J. Exper. Med.*, 91:449-458, 1950.

16. KAYE, S.: The Use of Ethylene Oxide for the Sterilization of Hospital Equipment. *J. Lab. & Clin. Med.*, 35:823-828, 1950.

17. HAWK, E. A. AND MICKELSEN, O.: Nutritional Changes in Diets Exposed to Ethylene Oxide. *Science, 121*:442-444, 1955.

18. BARLOW, J. S. AND HOUSE, H. L.: Ethylene Oxide for Sterilizing Diets. *Science, 123*:229, 1956.

Index

A

Actinomyces, heat resistance of, 37
Air
  adverse effects on sterilization, 59
  air-steam mixtures, 53, 55
  density of, 56
  discharge of, from sterilizers, 28, 54, 61, 62
  filter on water sterilizers, 151, 152
  in instrument boilers, 199
  in utensil boilers, 199
  pressure on earth, 48
  stratification of in sterilizer, 57
Alcohol
  antiseptic, 215
  disinfectant for plastic tubing, 219
  ethyl, 215
  isopropyl, 215
Aluminum
  metal for water still, 269
  tubing for transmission of distilled water, 269
American Sterilizer Company, 21
Amines, anti-corrosive agents, 123
Ampoules
  disinfection of, 221
Antiseptic
  definition, 214
  surgery, 13
Appert, Nicolas, 30
Autoclave
  laboratory, types of, 312
  term defined, 73

B

Bacilli, thermal resistance of, 37, 38
Bacillus stearothermophilus, resistance of spores, 234
Bacillus subtilis, resistance of spores, 234
Bacteria
  death, cause of, 33
  discovery of, 4
  order of death, 33
  pyrogenic in water, 264
  resistance to heat, 11, 37, 40, 160, 162
  thermal death point, 35
  thermal death time, 35
  thermal destruction of, 33, 42, 160, 162
Bacteriological media, 321

Basins
  disinfection by boiling, 199
  incorrect packaging, 99
  sterilization, 143
Bedpans
  disinfection, 204
  handling of, 206
  oil in, removal of, 206
  washer for, 208
Bedpan washer-disinfector, 204, 210
Biosorb, glove powder, 120
Boiling water
  alkali, addition of, 199
  bactericidal efficiency of, 199
  for disinfection of instruments, 197, 200
  for disinfection of utensils, 199, 203
  for sanitization of dishes, 201
  scale formation, 199
  state of, 196
Budenberg steam disinfector, *illus.* 18

C

Carboxide
  composition, 326
  sterilizer, for bulk materials, 328
  sterilizer, automatically controlled, 332
Carboy, for distilled water, *illus.* 266
Catheters
  cleaning of, 123
  packaging of, 123
  sterilization of, 123, 125
  woven, care of, 123
Central (supply) service department
  advantages of, 240
  definition, 239
  equipment for, 250
  location, 246
  planning the department, 241
  purpose of, 239
  space assignment, 244
  staffing, 251
  sterile supplies, storage period, 254
Charcoal, activated, for pyrogen removal, 264
Chamberland, Charles, 9, 30
Chamberland's autoclave, *illus.* 10
Chemical disinfection
  cause of, 214
  definition, 196, 213
  factors which influence, 214

335